A Comprehensive Guide to Non-alcoholic Fatty Liver Disease

Edited by Ju-Seop Kang

Published in London, United Kingdom

A Comprehensive Guide to Non-alcoholic Fatty Liver Disease
http://dx.doi.org/10.5772/intechopen.1001700
Edited by Ju-Seop Kang

Contributors
Alejandra Díaz García, Ana-Marija Liberati Pršo, Auwal A. Bala, Cristian Alexis Oviedo Garza, Daozhen Chen, Eron G. Manusov, Hyun-Jin Kim, Inyoung Hwang, Iris Pinheiro, Jacob A. Galan, John Blangero, Ju-Seop Kang, Leila Ghahremani, Mahin Nazari, Marcio Almeida, Marco A. Arriaga, María del Rosario Herrero Macedo, Narges Mobasheri, Natasha S. Garcia-Rodriguez, Paulin Bilonda Kabeya, Renee Hernandez, Sandica Bucurica, Sang-Won Lee, Sarah Williams-Blangero, Satish Kumar, Scherezada Maria Isabel Mejia Loza, So-Jung Lim, Vincent P. Diego, Xinyi Lu, Yu Chen, Zhengyang Bao, Željko Krznarić

First published in London, United Kingdom, 2025 by IntechOpen
IntechOpen is the global imprint of INTECHOPEN LIMITED, registered in England and Wales, registration number: 11086078, 167-169 Great Portland Street, London, W1W 5PF, United Kingdom

For EU product safety concerns: IN TECH d.o.o., Prolaz Marije Krucifikse Kozulić 3, 51000 Rijeka, Croatia, info@intechopen.com or visit our website at intechopen.com.

British Library Cataloguing-in-Publication Data
A catalogue record for this book is available from the British Library

A Comprehensive Guide to Non-alcoholic Fatty Liver Disease
Edited by Ju-Seop Kang
p. cm.
Print ISBN 978-1-83634-026-3
Online ISBN 978-1-83634-025-6
eBook (PDF) ISBN 978-1-83634-027-0

Meet the editor

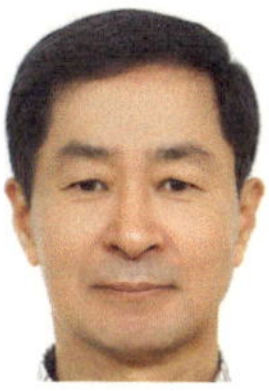

Prof. Ju-Seop Kang received his medical degree from Hanyang University College of Medicine, South Korea. He is currently the director of the Department of Pharmacology and Clinical Pharmacology Lab at the same university. He is also a member of the Research Integrity Committee at Hanyang University and a member of the appraisal committee of the Korea Medical Dispute Mediation and Arbitration Agency under the Ministry of Health and Welfare. He is also the Former President of the Korean Pharmacology Society (2024), Standing Chairman of the Drug Prevention and Rehabilitation Education Committee (2024-2027), and a member of the National Academy of Medicine of Korea (2023-2028). He has published more than 150 papers in peer-reviewed international journals and 20 book chapters. He serves as a reviewer for 10 international journals and is a member of the editorial board of several others. He was selected as a person of scientific merit by the Korean Ministry of Science and Technology in 2025 and received the Minister's Award.

Contents

Preface

Non-alcoholic fatty liver disease (NAFLD), which affects approximately 25% of the global adult population, represents the most common cause of chronic liver disease worldwide. Approximately 20% of individuals with NAFLD progress to non-alcoholic steatohepatitis (NASH), a more severe phenotype associated with an increased risk of cirrhosis and hepatocellular carcinoma (HCC). Notably, liver cancer is the second leading cause of years of life lost among all cancers.

NAFLD imposes a significant economic burden through sustained healthcare costs and productivity losses and is associated with a reduction in health-related quality of life. NAFLD is widely regarded as the hepatic manifestation of metabolic syndrome (MetS) and is increasingly recognized as a multisystem disease.

The prevalence of NAFLD is markedly elevated in individuals with type 2 diabetes mellitus (T2DM) compared to the general population, and conversely, the incidence of T2DM is higher among individuals with NAFLD. Cardiovascular disease (CVD) remains the leading cause of mortality in patients with NAFLD, followed by extrahepatic malignancies and liver-related complications.

NAFLD is strongly correlated with obesity, with prevalence rates rising proportionally with increasing body mass index (BMI); however, lean NAFLD can occur, particularly among Asian populations. The global burden of NAFLD is expected to rise in the coming decades, driven by increasing rates of obesity, T2DM, and an ageing population.

Management of NAFLD is stage-dependent. Lifestyle modification, including dietary changes and physical activity, alongside the management of underlying metabolic risk factors, forms the foundation of therapy. In patients at increased risk of disease progression, pharmacological interventions may be warranted.

This book aims to enhance the general public's comprehensive understanding of non-alcoholic fatty liver disease (NAFLD) by describing its general characteristics and its associations with metabolic disorders, nutrition, diet, gut microbiome, pregnancy, and lifestyle factors. It has been published as a sequel to the previous volume, *Non-alcoholic Fatty Liver Disease – New Insight and Glance Into Disease Pathogenesis*, which focused on the pathophysiology of NAFLD.

This book includes nine chapters as follows:

1. An Overview of Non-alcoholic Fatty Liver Diseases (NAFLD)

2. The Role of Gut Microbiota in Metabolic Dysfunction-Associated Fatty Liver Disease (MASLD)

3. The Role of the Intestinal Microbiota in NAFLD Onset and Progression

4. Principles of Nutrition in Patients with Non-alcoholic Fatty Liver Disease

5. Role of Micronutrients in MAFLD

6. Lifestyle Intervention of Metabolic Dysfunction-Associated Steatotic Liver Disease

7. Pregnancy and Metabolic Dysfunction-Associated Steatotic Liver Disease (MASLD): Relationship with Obesity, Clinical Outcomes, and Diagnosis

8. Gene-Environment Interactions in Non-alcoholic Fatty Liver Disease: Insights from Mexican American Populations

9. Non-alcoholic-Related Fatty Liver Disease (NAFLD) as a Risk Factor for Atherosclerotic Cardiovascular Disease: The Hidden Link – ASCVD Risk Factors from NAFLD

Ju-Seop Kang MD, Ph.D.
Professor of Department of Pharmacology and
Clinical Pharmacology Laboratory,
College of Medicine,
Hanyang University,
Seoul, South Korea

Chapter 1

An Overview of Non-alcoholic Fatty Liver Diseases (NAFLD)

Ju-Seop Kang, Hyun-Jin Kim, So-Jung Lim, Sang-Won Lee and Inyoung Hwang

Abstract

Non-alcoholic fatty liver disease (NAFLD) is an umbrella term that encompasses a diverse range of clinicopathological findings of largely unknown etiology. It refers to conditions characterized by steatosis in more than 5% of hepatocytes, often associated with metabolic risk factors such as obesity and type 2 diabetes. Non-alcoholic fatty liver disease (NAFLD) encompasses a range of liver conditions characterized by fat accumulation in liver cells, including simple steatosis (non-alcoholic fatty liver, NAFL), non-alcoholic steatohepatitis (NASH), NASH-associated fibrosis, cirrhosis, and hepatocellular carcinoma (HCC), all of which occur without significant alcohol intake or other chronic liver disorders. Pathohistologically, NAFLD is defined by steatosis with or without mild inflammation (NAFL) and a necroinflammatory subtype (NASH), which is characterized by hepatocellular injury, including hepatocyte ballooning. Affecting approximately one-quarter of the global adult population, NAFLD poses a significant health and economic burden on societies, yet no definitive or approved pharmacotherapies currently exist. Often asymptomatic, NAFLD is frequently identified incidentally during investigations for other health issues. A hallmark of this condition is the accumulation of lipid droplets in hepatocytes, which contain triglycerides, cholesterol esters, and other lipid species. To better reflect its metabolism-related etiology, a recent consensus has proposed renaming the condition to metabolic dysfunction-associated fatty liver disease (MAFLD). This chapter aims to educate the general public about NAFLD, providing an overview that establishes a foundation for understanding the subsequent chapters of this book.

Keywords: non-alcoholic fatty liver disease (NAFLD), metabolic dysfunction-associated fatty liver disease (MAFLD), fibrosis, cirrhosis, hepatocellular carcinoma

1. Introduction

Non-alcoholic fatty liver disease (NAFLD) represents the most prevalent form of liver disease globally, characterized by the excessive accumulation of hepatic fat in the absence of secondary etiologies or underlying hepatic disorders [1]. The NAFLD is on the rise, driven by the rising prevalence of physical inactivity and nutritionally inadequate dietary patterns [1]. NAFLD constitutes a substantial global public health challenge, with an estimated 882 million cases reported in 2017. This figure is likely an underestimation, attributable to incomplete screening of high-risk, asymptomatic populations [2]. Furthermore, the reliance on inaccurate biomarkers for predicting disease progression and the lack of approved therapeutic interventions hinder the effective management of NAFLD. Treatment primarily focuses on lifestyle and dietary modifications, although numerous novel therapeutics are currently undergoing evaluation. NAFLD represents a continuum of hepatic conditions, spanning from isolated hepatic steatosis (non-alcoholic fatty liver, NAFL) to the more advanced stage of non-alcoholic steatohepatitis (NASH), NASH-related fibrosis, cirrhosis, and, in many instances, hepatocellular carcinoma (HCC) (**Figure 1**) [1, 6]. Histologically, NAFLD shares characteristics with alcoholic liver disease (ALD); however, it is distinguished by the level of alcohol intake. The precise threshold for defining 'non-alcoholic' remains an area of active research and debate [7]. Alcohol consumption is conventionally classified based on daily intake levels: mild (≤20 g/day for women and ≤ 30 g/day for men), moderate (21–39 g/day for women and 31–59 g/day for men), and heavy (≥40 g/day for women and ≥ 60 g/day for men) [8]. However, the threshold for harmful alcohol intake remains poorly defined in the publications. The National Institute on Alcohol Abuse and Alcoholism (NIAAA) defines heavy drinking as exceeding 4 alcoholic drink equivalents (ADEs, standard drinks, approximately 40–60 g of alcohol) on a single day or more than 14 ADEs per week (approximately 196 g) for men, and exceeding 3 ADEs (approximately 30–40 g) on any day or more than 7 ADEs per week (approximately 98 g) for women [9]. Additionally, binge drinking is defined as the consumption of more than 5 ADEs (50–70 g) for men and more than 4 ADEs (40–50 g) for women within 2 hours [10]. Importantly, although certain studies indicate that the style or manner in which alcohol consumed and drinking behaviors may affect the progression and severity of ALD, further research is needed to clarify these associations. Hepatic steatosis (HS) is frequently identified in the initial stages of ALD, facilitating earlier diagnosis when detected, whether through targeted screening or incidental findings. It is estimated that steatosis occurs

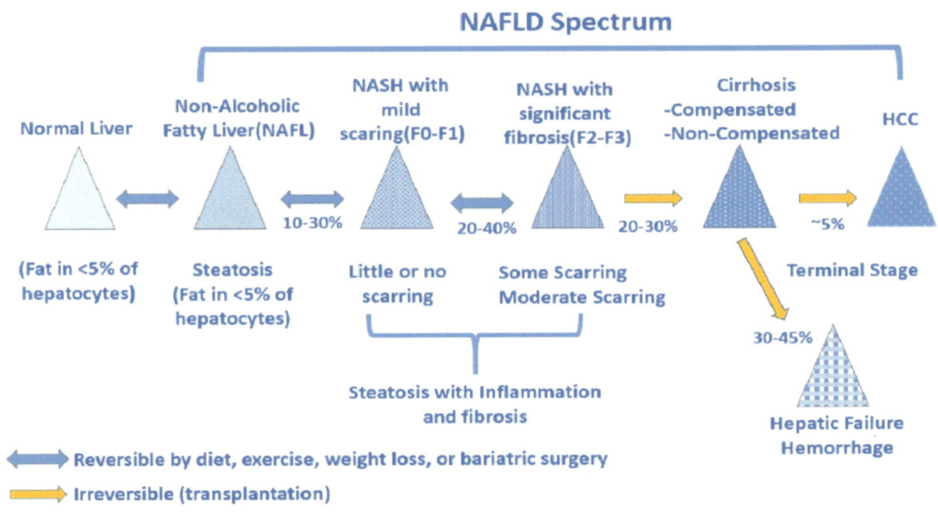

Figure 1.
Spectrum, pathogenesis, stages, and natural course of NAFLD [3–5].

in over 90% of individuals consuming 4–5 ADEs per day [11]. The current nomenclature characterizes NAFLD as primarily a diagnosis of exclusion, and ongoing debate persists regarding the limitations inherent in the existing terminology and diagnostic criteria [12, 13]. In 2020, an international panel of clinical experts introduced the concept of metabolic dysfunction-associated fatty liver disease (MAFLD), highlighting the significance of cardiometabolic risk factors in the pathogenesis and deterioration of hepatic disease, even in patients with coexisting hepatic pathology [14]. However, the term 'MAFLD' has not yet achieved widespread endorsement by the American Association for the Study of Liver Diseases or the European Association for the Study of the Liver. In contrast, NAFLD remains an umbrella designation encompassing a broad spectrum of clinicopathological features. Histologically, NAFLD comprises a spectrum of pathologies, as depicted in **Figure 1**, extending from simple steatosis, with or without mild inflammatory changes (non-alcoholic fatty liver, NAFL), to a necroinflammatory subtype (non-alcoholic steatohepatitis, NASH), which is further distinguished by hepatocellular injury, including hepatocyte ballooning [15]. The primary determinants of disease can vary significantly among patients with NAFLD, and both disease progression and treatment responses exhibit heterogeneity across different populations. Understanding disease activity, particularly the extent of liver fibrosis, is critical for assessing disease severity and informing treatment strategies. The integration of insights from metabolomics, genomics, and related fields will enhance our capacity to characterize disease phenotypes and facilitate future disease categorization [15].

2. Epidemiology and pathology of NAFLD

NAFLD requires the fulfillment of two criteria: (1) the presence of HS, confirmed through imaging techniques or histological evaluation, and (2) the exclusion of secondary causes of hepatic fat accumulation, including excessive alcohol consumption, extended use of steatogenic medications, or monogenic hereditary conditions. NAFLD is commonly associated with concurrent metabolic abnormalities such as obesity, diabetes mellitus (DM), and dyslipidemia. Histologically, NAFLD can be classified into two distinct categories such as NAFL and NASH (**Table 1**) [16]. NAFL is characterized by the presence of at least 5% HS without evidence of hepatocellular injury, such as hepatocyte ballooning. In contrast, NASH is defined by the presence of at least 5% HS accompanied by inflammation and hepatocellular injury (e.g., ballooning), with or without fibrosis. When referring to 'advanced' fibrosis, this document specifically highlights stages 3 and 4, known as bridging fibrosis and cirrhosis (**Figure 1**) [17].

NAFLD affects approximately one-quarter of the adult population worldwide, constituting a significant health and economic burden for many societies [14, 18, 19], yet it currently lacks definitive or approved pharmacotherapy. NAFLD has evolved from a relatively obscure condition to the leading cause of chronic liver disease globally. Presently, consensus defines NAFLD as an umbrella term that encompasses a variety of conditions characterized by hepatic steatosis in more than 5% of hepatocytes, in conjunction with metabolic risk factors such as obesity and T2DM, without significant alcohol consumption or other chronic liver diseases [17, 20]. Globally, the predominant phenotype of patients with NAFLD consists of men with an average age of 51.7 years, who frequently present with obesity and/or type 2 diabetes mellitus (T2DM) [21]. A linear increase in the prevalence of NAFLD, T2DM, and metabolic

Item/score or code	0	1	2	3	4
1. Steatosis (Grade)*					
Parenchymal involvement (%)	5%↓	5–33%	33–66%	66%↑	
Microvesicular (contiguous patches)	Zone 3	Zone 1	Azonal	Peracinar	
	No	Present			
2. Fibrosis (Stage)	No	Presinosoidal or periportal	Presinosoidal and periportal	Bridging fibrosis	Cirrhosis
		1A (mild, Zone3)			
		1B (moderate, Zone3)			
		1C (portal/periprotal			
3. Inflammation**					
Lobular inflammatory foci(x200)	No	2 foci↓	2–4 foci	4 foci↑	
Microglonulomas (macrophage aggregate)	No	Present			
Large lipogranulamas (portal triad area)	None-minimal	Minimal↑			
4. Liver cell injury Ballooning***	None	Few	Many/prominent		
5. Diagnostic steatohepatitis	None	Possible/borderline	Definite		

**Percent of hepatocytes with fat droplets identified at low- to medium-power evaluation of hepatic involvement.*
***Overall assessment of all inflammatory foci per one x 200 field.*
****Few indicates rare and definite ballooned hepatocytes or borderline ballooning.*

Table 1.
NASH Clinical Research Network Scoring System definitions and scores [16].

disorders has been observed and documented [22, 23], particularly among individuals with central obesity, T2DM, and metabolic syndrome [24, 25]. Additional concurrent metabolic disorders include hypertension (37%) and metabolic syndrome (40%) among affected individuals [21]. The prevalence of NAFLD in individuals with T2DM can be as high as 70% [26], and these patients experience a twofold increased risk of all-cause mortality [27, 28]. In patients with severe obesity, the prevalence of NAFLD may rise to 90% [28]. Consequently, the prevalence of NAFLD represents a significant global health burden that requires urgent clinical attention and management. NAFLD is explicitly defined by the presence of excessive hepatic fat accumulation in the absence of other causative factors that include, but are not limited to, significant alcohol consumption, viral hepatitis, the use of steatogenic medications such as amiodarone or tamoxifen, and concurrent liver diseases [29]. In contrast, when excessive alcohol consumption leads to fat deposition and tissue damage within the liver, the condition is referred to as ALD. In cases where a patient has a history of heavy alcohol use along with hepatic fat accumulation, the diagnosis may favor ALD over NAFLD. It is important to note that individuals with risk factors for NAFLD who also engage in excessive alcohol intake may concurrently present with both NAFLD and ALD. Currently, no specific diagnostic tests exist that can accurately determine the extent to which each condition contributes to hepatic pathology [30]. NAFLD is defined as the excessive accumulation of hepatic fat in the absence of other identifiable etiological factors, such as significant alcohol consumption, viral hepatitis, the administration of steatogenic medications (e.g., amiodarone, tamoxifen), or coexisting liver diseases (e.g., autoimmune hepatitis, Wilson's disease) [29]. Conversely, when excessive alcohol intake induces fat deposition and resultant tissue damage in the liver, the condition is classified as ALD. In cases where a patient exhibits both a history of heavy alcohol consumption and hepatic fat accumulation, a diagnosis of ALD may take precedence over NAFLD. Importantly, individuals with risk factors for NAFLD who consume excessive alcohol may present with features of both conditions. Currently, there are no standardized diagnostic tests available that can accurately delineate the contributions of each condition to the overall hepatic pathology [30].

NAFLD is categorized into two subtypes: NAFL and NASH, with the latter indicating the presence of significant hepatic inflammation [17, 30]. While NAFL is generally regarded as less harmful than NASH and has a lower likelihood of progression to the latter [30], progression can occur, potentially resulting in severe complications such as cirrhosis, hepatocellular carcinoma, liver failure, or cardiovascular disorders [30]. The NAFLD spectrum includes a range of abnormalities, from simple increases in intrahepatic lipid content (termed simple steatosis or NAFL) to NASH, which is characterized by varying degrees of necroinflammatory activity, fibrosis, and, ultimately, cirrhosis (**Figure 1**) [31]. NAFL and NASH are differentiated by examining liver histology for key pathological characteristics, particularly steatosis, lobular inflammation, and hepatocyte ballooning, typically found in zone 3, with or without peri-sinusoidal fibrosis (**Table 1**) [16].

Furthermore, the progression of liver fibrosis is strongly linked to increased morbidity and mortality rates [32]. Importantly, advanced fibrosis, defined as stage 2 or higher, is associated with a significantly heightened risk of liver-specific as well as all-cause mortality [33]. Consequently, the population most urgently requiring therapeutic intervention comprises individuals diagnosed with NASH and significant fibrosis. The global prevalence of NAFLD continues to rise, paralleling the increasing incidence of obesity-related metabolic syndrome [13, 34]. Definitions of conditions associated with NAFLD are detailed in **Table 2**. NAFLD is linked not only to an elevated risk of

NAFLD	Refers to all stages of FLD in those who consume minimal or no alcohol, starting with simple steatosis and advancing to HS and cirrhosis.
NAFL	Hepatic steatosis (HS) is characterized by fat accumulation in at least 5% of hepatocytes without accompanying hepatocellular injury, such as hepatocyte ballooning or fibrosis. In such cases, the risk of progression to cirrhosis or liver failure is considered minimal.
NASH	The presence of HS involving at least 5% of hepatocytes, accompanied by inflammation and hepatocellular injury, including ballooning, with or without associated fibrosis. This condition has the potential to progress to cirrhosis, liver failure, and, in rare instances, hepatocellular carcinoma. • *Type 1*: A zone 3-centered or confluent injury pattern characterized by hepatocyte ballooning. • *Type 2*: A zone 1 (portal area)-centered injury pattern with periportal to panacinar steatosis, accompanied by portal inflammation, with or without hepatocyte ballooning. • *Pediatric*: An umbrella term encompassing zone 3 NASH, zone 1 NASH, and borderline NASH in children (age ≤ 17 years).
NAFLD fibrosis	NAFL or NASH with periportal, portal, or sinosoidal fibrosis.
NAFLD cirrhosis	NAFL or NASH with bridging fibrosis, architectural distortion, or nodule formation, accompanied by current or previous histological evidence of steatosis or HS.
Cryptogenic cirrhosis	Bridging fibrosis with architectural distortion without overt liver disease. These patients often exhibit a high prevalence of metabolic risk factors, including obesity, T2DM, and other MetS.
NAS	A non-weighted aggregate score combining steatosis, lobular inflammation, and hepatocyte ballooning is commonly utilized to evaluate histological changes in patients with non-alcoholic fatty liver disease (NAFLD), while fibrosis is assessed independently [35].
SAF score	A semi-quantitative scoring system that evaluates the extent of steatosis, the activity (combining lobular inflammation and hepatocyte ballooning), and the degree of fibrosis [36].
ALD	Liver damage caused by drinking too much alcohol for a long time.
SH	An advanced stage of MASLD

Abbreviations: FLD, fatty liver disease; HS, hepatic steatosis; NAFL, non-alcoholic fatty liver; NAFLD, non-alcoholic fatty liver disease; NASH, non-alcoholic steatohepatitis; NAS, NAFLD Activity Score; ALD, alcoholic liver disease; SH, steatohepatitis; metabolic dysfunction-associated steatotic liver disease, MASLD; MetS, metabolic syndrome.

Table 2.
NAFLD and related definitions [17].

hepatocellular carcinoma but also to cardiovascular diseases and complications of T2DM, including diabetic nephropathy and neuropathy [37, 38]. Therefore, elucidating the mechanisms driving NAFLD pathogenesis is critical for the effective management of both NAFLD and its associated comorbidities [39]. Hepatic steatosis (fatty liver) has long been recognized as prevalent among individuals with excessive alcohol consumption and obesity [40, 41]. Additionally, it may result from the use of various therapeutic agents [42]. Regardless of etiology, steatosis can progress to necroinflammation and fibrosis, culminating in the development of steatohepatitis, which may further advance to cirrhosis [43]. Notably, steatohepatitis induced by alcohol, drugs, or NASH shares many histopathological features [44]. This raises the question of whether these distinct etiologies of steatohepatitis and its complications, such as cirrhosis or liver failure, are driven by one or more common molecular mechanisms. A comprehensive unifying model must explain why, in certain individuals, hepatic steatosis—irrespective of its cause—fails to progress to steatohepatitis [45], as well as account for the variable incidence and severity of steatohepatitis (SH) and fibrosis observed across different etiologies of fatty liver. A hallmark of NAFLD is the expansion of hepatocyte lipid droplets, containing triglycerides, cholesterol esters, and other lipid species [46–49]. Reflecting its metabolic-related pathogenesis, a recent consensus proposed renaming this condition to MAFLD, following endorsement by 70% of a panel of experts [12]. This nomenclature change was formally adopted in 2023 [50, 51].

The diagnosis of MAFLD should be based on the presence of at least one cardiometabolic risk factor in individuals with evident hepatic steatosis. MAFLD can coexist with other conditions [52], and patients with both MAFLD and ALD form a significant group that warrants further investigation, particularly regarding etiology and hepatic histopathology. This raises concerns about the applicability of evidence derived from NAFLD definitions to individuals with MASLD. However, a re-evaluation of existing cohort studies suggests that findings from NAFLD research are largely applicable to MASLD. For example, analyses of a large tertiary care NAFLD cohort and the population-based NHANES III survey showed a nearly complete overlap between NAFLD and MASLD populations, with a 99.8% concordance rate in the NAFLD cohort. Conversely, only 5.3% of individuals classified as NAFLD in NHANES III did not meet MASLD criteria [53]. Furthermore, clinical characteristics were nearly indistinguishable between the two groups, and non-invasive diagnostic tests demonstrated equivalent accuracy and cutoff values for both NAFLD and MASLD definitions [53]. Long-term follow-up data indicated comparable mortality rates, though mortality was marginally elevated in the MASLD cohort compared to NAFLD [53]. Consequently, we consider NAFLD research evidence applicable to MASLD and use both terms as equivalents. However, it is crucial to acknowledge that MASLD with moderate alcohol consumption (MetALD) constitutes a distinct entity, and recommendations based on the 'pure' NAFLD criteria may not be directly applicable to this subgroup (**Figure 2**).

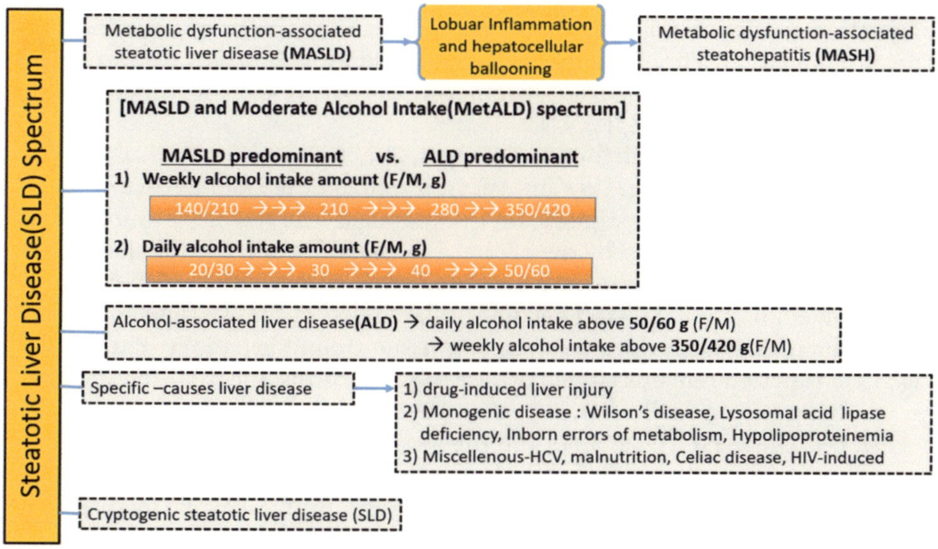

Figure 2.
Spectrum of SLD and definition of MASLD. Abbreviations: ALD, alcohol-related liver disease; MASH, metabolic dysfunction-associated steatohepatitis; MASLD, metabolic dysfunction-associated steatotic liver disease; MetSLD, MASLD with moderate alcohol consumption; SLD, steatotic liver disease; HCV, hepatitis C virus.

At the histological level, lipid accumulation within hepatocytes can occur in the absence of inflammation, a condition termed metabolic dysfunction-associated fatty liver (MAFL). However, this may progress to chronic inflammation and tissue damage, known as SH, often accompanied by varying degrees of fibrosis. The hallmark of fibrosis is collagen deposition, which occurs due to the activation and transformation of hepatic stellate cells into fibroblast-like forms. While SH itself is not acutely critical and dangerous, it significantly increases the potential for advanced liver diseases, including fibrosis, cirrhosis, and hepatocellular carcinoma, as well as cardiovascular disease, which is the leading cause of mortality in individuals with MAFLD [49, 54, 55].

Current literature proposes two models for the pathogenesis of NAFLD: the 'double-hit' [56] and 'multiple-hit' [57] hypotheses. The double-hit model posits that the initial hit involves intrahepatic FA accumulation, which sensitizes hepatocytes to subsequent insults, leading to inflammation and fibrosis [58]. However, this model has been challenged by evidence indicating that inflammation can precede hepatic TAG accumulation and that steatosis may serve a protective role against liver injury. This suggests that NAFLD progression is driven by multiple concurrent factors rather than a sequential process [59]. According to the 'multiple-hit' hypothesis, primary factors such as insulin resistance, obesity, T2DM, and metabolic syndrome promote hepatic accumulation of free fatty acids, resulting in simple steatosis [59]. Disease progression occurs when additional 'hits'—including oxidative stress, inflammatory mediators, apoptosis, immune cell activation, gut-derived endotoxins, and mitochondrial dysfunction—contribute to liver injury and the advancement of NAFLD [57]. In the 'three-hit' model of NAFLD progression, the increasing prevalence of obesity and metabolic syndrome has led to the widespread development of NAFL in individuals without significant alcohol intake. In many cases, simple steatosis progresses to NASH, with a subset of patients subsequently developing fibrosis, which can advance to cirrhosis. This model suggests that the 'first hit' involves an imbalance between hepatic lipid uptake and either lipid oxidation or secretion. The 'second hit' entails dysregulation of pro-inflammatory and anti-inflammatory pathways, leading to hepatic inflammation. The 'third hit' is characterized by an imbalance between pro-fibrotic and antifibrotic mechanisms, promoting the progression of hepatic fibrosis and, in some cases, cirrhosis [3].

NAFLD progresses through four main stages, although most individuals remain asymptomatic in the first stage. In some cases, if undiagnosed and untreated, the disease can advance and cause significant liver damage. The stages are as follows: ① simple steatosis, characterized by the benign accumulation of fat within hepatocytes, typically detected incidentally during unrelated medical evaluations; ② NASH, marked by liver inflammation and hepatocellular injury; ③ fibrosis, where chronic inflammation promotes the formation of scar tissue around hepatic structures, though liver function remains largely preserved; ④ cirrhosis, the final and most severe stage, involving extensive fibrosis, liver shrinkage, and architectural distortion. At this stage, the damage is irreversible, and the liver is at risk of failure or hepatocellular carcinoma. The progression from fibrosis to cirrhosis typically occurs over years, underscoring the importance of early intervention and lifestyle modification to prevent further disease advancement (**Figure 3**) [60]. NAFLD is closely linked to metabolic risk factors, leading a panel of experts to advocate for its reclassification as MAFLD in order to emphasize the role of metabolic dysregulation and recognize its co-occurrence with other liver diseases. However, this revised nomenclature has not yet been universally accepted (**Table 3**) [14].

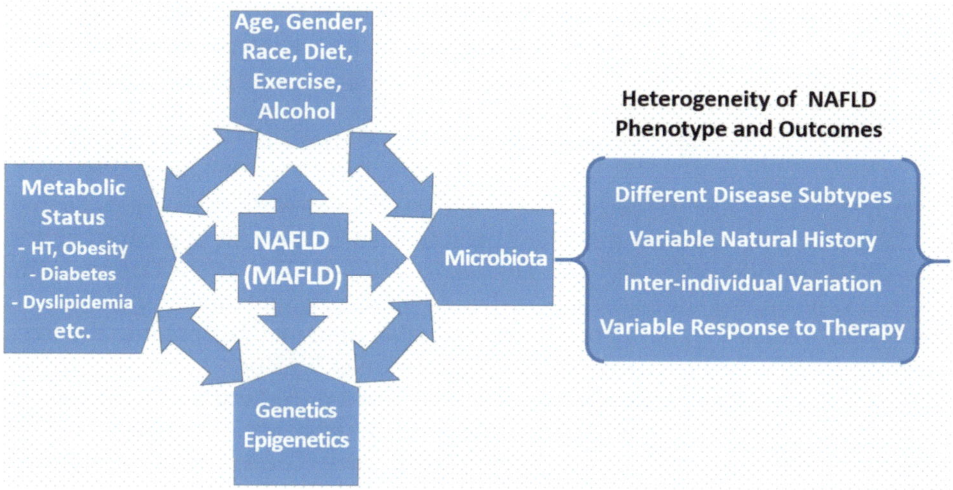

Figure 3.
Heterogeneity of course, clinical features, and outcomes of NAFLD (MAFLD).

Metabolic risk factor	Adult criteria	Contents
Overweight or obesity	BMI	• ≥25 kg/m2(≥23 kg/m^2 in Asian ethnicity)
	Waist circumference	• ≥94 cm(M)/≥80 cm(F) in Europeans
		• ≥90 cm(M)/≥80 cm(F) in South Asians and Chinese
		• ≥85 cm(M)/≥80 cm(F) in Japanese
Dysglycemia or T2DM	Prediabetes	• HbA1c (5.7–6.4%) or fasting plasma glucose (100–125 mg/dl) or
		• 2-hr plasma glucose during OGTT (140–199 mg/dl)
	T2DM	• HbA1c (≥6.5%) of fasting plasma glucose (≥126 mg/dl) or
		• 2-hr plasma glucose during OGTT (≥200 mg/dl) or
	Tx for T2DM	• During treatment
Plasma TG	• ≥1.7 mmol/L(≥150 mg/dl) or	
	• lipid-lowering drug	
HDL-cholesterol	• ≤1.0 mmol/L(≤39 mg/dl, M) and ≤ 1.3 mmol/L(≤50 mg/dl, F) or	
	• lipid-lowering drug	
Blood pressure	• ≥130/85 mmHg or	
	• antihypertensive treatment	

BMI, body mass index; M/F, male/female; HbA1c, glycated hemoglobin; HDL, high-density lipoprotein; OGTT, oral glucose tolerance test.

Table 3.
Cardiometabolic risk factors in the definition of MASLD (modified Rinella et al. [8]).

NAFLD is a heterogeneous disorder, with cardiovascular disease being the predominant cause of mortality in affected individuals. Notably, certain genetic polymorphisms that heighten susceptibility to liver disease may paradoxically offer protection against cardiovascular disease [61]. This heterogeneity—characterized by diverse primary drivers and co-occurring disease modifiers—poses a significant challenge to the development of effective pharmacotherapies. The phenotypic expression of fatty liver disease likely emerges from complex, system-wide interactions among these factors, highlighting the need for a personalized therapeutic approach tailored to an individual's phenotype and genetic background [47, 62]. Various factors, including age, sex, hormonal status, ethnicity, dietary habits, alcohol intake, smoking, genetic predispositions, gut microbiota composition, and metabolic status, are likely to modulate the clinical presentation and progression of NAFLD.

NAFLD reflects a complex phenotype arising from the interaction between genetic susceptibility, environmental influences, components of metabolic syndrome, and demographic characteristics such as sex. The impact of genetic variants and primary drivers varies considerably among individuals, underscoring the importance of identifying key factors in each NAFLD patient to inform personalized treatment strategies. The clinical outcomes of NAFLD arise from a complex interplay of multiple factors, each influencing the disease's manifestations and progression. In the United States, NAFLD is the second leading cause of liver transplantation [63] and a growing contributor to the incidence of hepatocellular carcinoma [64–66]. While the global prevalence of NAFLD is estimated at 25%, only a subset of individuals is at risk of progression. In the United States, NAFLD ranks as the second leading cause of liver transplantation [63] and represents an increasingly significant contributor to the incidence of HCC [64–66]. Although the global prevalence of NAFLD is estimated to be approximately 25%, only a specific subset of individuals exhibits a risk of disease progression. Although liver biopsy remains the gold standard for differentiating NAFL from NASH, it is invasive, expensive, and impractical for broad application, with substantial intra- and inter-observer variability, even among experts [67, 68].

3. Origin of nomenclature of NAFLD

Is NAFLD still an appropriate term for metabolic liver disease? Emerging insights into its pathophysiology suggest otherwise. Several key considerations highlight the need to redefine and rename NAFLD, with this consensus focusing on four primary aspects [14].

Initially, NAFLD was considered a diagnosis of exclusion, identified only after ruling out other conditions such as viral hepatitis, autoimmune diseases, or significant alcohol consumption [69–71]. However, recent findings suggest that NAFLD should be characterized by inclusion, as it frequently coexists with these conditions and can exacerbate their progression [72, 73]. Given its high prevalence in populations with Westernized diets, there is a need for the nomenclature and diagnostic criteria to evolve to reflect this broader understanding.

Second, the safe threshold for alcohol intake remains a subject of debate. Revising NAFLD diagnostic criteria to mandate zero or near-zero alcohol consumption, as some have suggested, is impractical [62]. Moreover, assessing alcohol intake *via* questionnaires presents significant methodological challenges, including the difficulty of accurately documenting lifetime consumption, accounting for low-level intake, patient underreporting, recall bias, and the inconsistent definitions of terms such as 'social drinking' and 'binge drinking' in NAFLD patients. Thus, associating metabolic fatty liver disease—a distinct condition—with alcohol in its nomenclature is problematic. The inclusion of the term 'nonalcoholic' can be discouraging for patients who abstain from alcohol and perpetuates the stigma of alcohol consumption. Misleading terminology should be revised, as evidenced by the renaming of primary biliary cirrhosis to primary biliary cholangitis, where more accurate, albeit sometimes redundant, terms have provided clarity [74] . Additionally, it is essential to recognize patients with overlapping metabolic and ALD to ensure they receive appropriate treatment, as they constitute a distinct group from those with predominantly alcohol-induced cirrhosis. Currently, these patients are excluded from NASH trials, underscoring the need for clearer diagnostic criteria.

Third, while current clinical practice differentiates patients into those with NASH and those without, this classification remains controversial. Given the significant plasticity in metabolic liver disease over the lifespan, and the well-established role of fibrosis as the primary determinant of adverse outcomes [75], this dichotomous approach may be misleading. It may be more appropriate to consider MAFLD in a manner akin to other chronic liver diseases, characterized by varying degrees of activity and stages of fibrosis, rather than stratifying patients strictly into NASH and non-NASH categories. From a pathological standpoint, this would improve disease classification, particularly in the context of liver biopsy [76].

Fourth, the diverse and multifaceted nature of fatty liver diseases highlights the necessity of recognizing them as distinct conditions rather than a singular entity and of employing tailored management strategies. Overlooking this variability compromises our capacity to accurately delineate the natural history of the various fatty liver phenotypes, identify suitable participants for clinical trials with meaningful endpoints, and perform reliable comparisons or meta-analyses of clinical trial data. Therefore, revising the disease nomenclature is crucial for addressing its complexity and advancing our understanding of its varied manifestations (**Figure 3**) [77].

4. The overlap between ALD and NAFLD

The intersection between ALD and NAFLD underscores shared pathophysiological mechanisms and risk factors, complicating their differentiation and highlighting the need for refined diagnostic criteria to better classify and manage patients with overlapping or coexisting liver disease phenotypes [78]. While NAFLD and ALD are traditionally considered distinct entities in academic medicine and are often studied independently, clinical practice frequently reveals their coexistence, with alcohol consumption and metabolic dysfunction jointly contributing to hepatic steatosis [79]. This intersection is highlighted by shared pathophysiological mechanisms, common genetic and epigenetic susceptibilities, a similar histopathological progression from steatosis to SH and cirrhosis, and overlapping clinical characteristics, excluding alcohol-related hepatitis. An unhealthy lifestyle characterized by poor dietary patterns, physical inactivity, and excessive alcohol consumption supports similar pathogenic pathways [66, 80]. In NAFLD, obesity-induced adipose tissue hypertrophy triggers localized inflammation and metabolic dysregulation, fostering the development of insulin resistance, adipokine imbalance, and augmented lipolysis. This heightened lipolysis leads to an increased influx of free fatty acids (FFA) into the liver, thereby facilitating hepatic lipid accumulation. The accumulation of excess lipid, particularly in the form of toxic species such as ceramides and sphingolipids, instigates lipotoxicity, resulting in mitochondrial dysfunction, ROS production, ER stress, impaired autophagic activity, apoptosis, inflammasome activation, and the secretion of extracellular vesicles. Extracellular vesicles mediate hepatic inflammation, while platelet-derived growth factor (PDGF) stimulates hepatic stellate cell activation, driving fibrogenesis. Similarly, ethanol intake disrupts adipose tissue function, increases fatty acid uptake of hepatocyte, and promotes hepatic *de novo* lipogenesis *via* sterol regulatory element-binding protein 1c (SREBP1c) activation. Alcohol metabolites, particularly acetaldehyde, exacerbate cellular stress pathways implicated in NAFLD, leading to hepatocellular injury and apoptosis—critical factors driving progression toward advanced fibrosis and cirrhosis. In cases of SH, inflammation, hepatocellular proliferation, and immune dysregulation further increase the risk of hepatocellular carcinoma. Additionally, dysbiosis and heightened intestinal permeability substantially worsen liver injury in both NAFLD and ALD. NAFLD is characterized by hepatic steatosis without significant alcohol consumption or other underlying factors contributing to liver fat buildup, with ethanol intake thresholds defined as less than 20 g per day for women and less than 30 g per day for men [50]. Insulin resistance is prevalent among NAFLD patients, and both obesity and T2DM are major risk factors that influence the severity and progression of the disease [81]. The pathogenesis of hepatic steatosis in both NAFLD and ALD involves intricate mechanisms, and notably the initiation of inflammatory and fibrogenic pathways in the liver leads to hepatocyte damage, disease advancement, and compromised liver function (**Figure 1**). An early pathological hallmark of both NAFLD and ALD is impaired lipid processing within hepatocytes, leading to macrovesicular steatosis, characterized by the displacement of the nucleus to the peripheral cytoplasm by a single lipid macrovacuole [36, 82]. Lipid droplets—intracellular organelles composed of a neutral lipid core, primarily triacylglycerols and sterol esters, encased by a phospholipid monolayer with associated proteins—are synthesized in the endoplasmic reticulum (ER) and function as essential fat storage reservoirs [83]. Dysregulation of hepatic lipid homeostasis, due to disruptions in the processes of lipid uptake, synthesis, breakdown, and FFA export contribute to the formation of lipid droplets [84]. In NAFLD, hepatic lipid accumulation results from systemic metabolic disturbances characterized by elevated fat accumulation and reduced insulin sensitivity [85]. Insulin resistance in adipose tissue promotes lipolysis, raising circulating FFA levels and enhancing hepatic FFA influx [86]. This influx facilitates lipid accumulation in hepatocytes, supported by fatty acid transporters such as CD36, FATP2, and FATP5, as well as fatty acid-binding proteins (FABPs), particularly FABP1, which mediates accumulation of lipids within cells by targeting fatty acids to organelles. A major contributor to hepatic lipid accumulation is the upregulation of *de novo* lipogenesis, driven by sterol regulatory element-binding protein 1c (SREBP1c), which induces enzymes such as acetyl-CoA carboxylase (ACC), stearoyl-CoA desaturase 1 (SCD1), and fatty acid synthase (FAS) [87, 88]. While decreased FAO, reduced lipid droplet catabolism, and impaired VLDL secretion may contribute to hepatic steatosis, they are not considered predominant mechanisms in NAFLD [87].

5. Molecular mechanisms underlying hepatocyte injury in fatty liver diseases, including NAFLD and ALD

This section outlines the molecular mechanisms underlying the pathogenesis of fatty liver disease. In a subset of individuals with hepatic steatosis, progression to hepatocellular injury and inflammation occurs, a condition termed SH [89]. Understanding the molecular mechanisms that trigger inflammation and drive the progression from simple steatosis to SH in both NAFLD and ALD is crucial for developing targeted treatments [90]. Cellular stress responses induced by both metabolic dysfunction and chronic alcohol consumption contribute to hepatocyte damage and death, thus advancing disease progression [91]. Sublethal hepatocyte injury, predominantly triggered by lipotoxicity—the toxic accumulation of lipid species—constitutes a critical event in the progression of NAFLD [92]. Toxic lipid species, such as saturated fatty acids, ceramides, free cholesterol, sphingolipids, and glycerophospholipids [93, 94], induce cellular impairment and dysfunction *via* mechanisms such as ER stress, mitochondrial dysfunction, impaired autophagy, and lysosomal membrane permeabilization [89]. This cellular damage leads to the release of pro-inflammatory cytokines and damage-associated molecular patterns (DAMPs) into the extracellular matrix, which are pivotal in initiating inflammation and fibrosis [95]. Notable DAMPs in NAFLD include HMGB1, DNA, RNA, S100 proteins, heat shock proteins, hyaluronan, and sonic hedgehog ligands [81]. The activation of resident macrophages and the recruitment of various myeloid cells amplify the inflammatory cascade, ultimately resulting in cell death [96]. In NAFLD, hepatocyte death mainly occurs *via* apoptosis, involving both extrinsic (death receptor) and intrinsic (mitochondrial) pathways [97]. Research suggests that tumor necrosis factor (TNF)-related apoptosis-inducing ligand receptor 2 (TRAILR2) activation is involved in caspase-dependent hepatocyte death, which plays a central role in NASH progression [98]. TRAILR2 activation can occur without ligand binding, driven by the rearrangement of plasma membrane domains, which leads to receptor clustering and subsequent activation [99]. This process, induced by saturated fatty acids such as palmitate or endoplasmic reticulum stress [94], initiates hepatocyte death through caspase-8, a critical player in linking both apoptotic pathways [100]. Multiple cell death mechanisms, including necroptosis, pyroptosis, and ferroptosis, have been implicated in the pathogenesis of NAFLD and are considered key drivers of inflammation in this disease [91]. These processes are characterized by rapid membrane disruption, leading to the release of cytoplasmic contents, which then trigger sterile inflammation [101]. The simultaneous activation of pyroptosis, apoptosis, and necroptosis has introduced the concept of 'PANoptosis,' a newly recognized pathway of cell death [102]. However, the exact role of PANoptosis in non-alcoholic steatohepatitis (NASH) remains to be fully explored. Similarly, chronic alcohol consumption leads to various forms of cell death, with apoptosis being well-characterized in both animal models of ALD and *in vitro* systems [93, 103]. Alcohol-induced increases in ROS and ER stress activate both extrinsic and intrinsic apoptotic pathways. The extrinsic pathway is triggered by ligands such as TNF, FAS ligand, and TRAIL, while the intrinsic pathway involves BCL-2 family proteins that regulate mitochondrial membrane permeability and promote the release of cytochrome c, leading to caspase activation [80]. Additionally, other cell death modalities like PANoptosis have been observed in chronic ethanol-fed animal models, though their clinical relevance remains unclear. Dysregulated autophagy also plays a significant role in both NAFLD and ALD [104]. Autophagy, a process responsible for the removal of damaged proteins and organelles, when disrupted, can contribute to cell death, inflammation, and fibrosis. Both experimental and clinical studies have shown impaired autophagic flux in NAFLD patients, with chronic ethanol intake exacerbating this dysfunction, contributing to steatosis, cell death, and the development of HCC in both NAFLD and ALD [105, 106].

6. Concise overview: The gut-liver axis and its relationship with microbiota in NAFLD and ALD

The gut-liver axis plays a pivotal role in the pathophysiology of both NAFLD and ALD, with dysregulation of the intestinal microbiome implicated in the etiology of both conditions, though the exact mechanisms remain incompletely understood [107, 108]. Alterations in the gut microbiome, noted in both animal studies and individuals with NAFLD, contribute to disease progression by enhancing intestinal permeability, impairing energy balance, modifying choline and bile acid metabolism, and triggering hepatic immune responses through metabolites and molecular signals derived from the microbiome [51, 109, 110]. Recent studies indicate that distinct microbial patterns could function as diagnostic biomarkers for NAFLD and help predict the progression of the disease [111]. Similarly, the intestinal microbiota composition in ALD has been shown to correlate with fibrosis stage [112]. Alcohol consumption disrupts tight junction proteins, leading to increased intestinal permeability [113, 114] and facilitating the translocation of lipopolysaccharides and bacterial DNA into the portal circulation. This translocation activates Kupffer cells through Toll-like receptors 4 (TLR4) and 9 (TLR9), contributing to steatosis and fibrosis in murine models [115]. Furthermore, alcohol impairs gut adaptive immunity, particularly in the early stages of ALD [116]. Endogenous ethanol production by the gut microbiota has also been implicated in the pathogenesis of NAFLD, potentially revealing shared pathophysiological mechanisms between NAFLD and ALD [117, 118].

7. Conclusion

This chapter outlines the definition and core pathophysiology of fatty liver disease (FLD), encompassing both NAFLD and ALD. NAFLD represents a spectrum of liver conditions, ranging from simple steatosis (non-alcoholic fatty liver, NAFL) to more severe forms such as NASH, which can progress to fibrosis, cirrhosis, and HCC, all in the absence of significant alcohol intake or other chronic liver disorders. Pathologically, NAFLD is defined by hepatic steatosis, with NAFL exhibiting minimal inflammation, while NASH is characterized by marked hepatocellular injury. Affecting nearly 25% of the global population, NAFLD imposes a substantial health and economic burden, yet there are currently no approved pharmacological therapies available. This chapter provides a foundational understanding of NAFLD, setting the stage for more detailed exploration in subsequent sections.

Author details

Ju-Seop Kang[1*], Hyun-Jin Kim[1], So-Jung Lim[1], Sang-Won Lee[1,2] and Inyoung Hwang[2]

1 Department of Pharmacology and Clinical Lab, Hanyang University College of Medicine, Seoul, South Korea

2 Department of Clinical Pharmacology, Hanyang Medical Center, Seoul, South Korea

*Address all correspondence to: jskang@hanyang.ac.kr

References

[1] Sayiner M, Koenig A, Henry L, Younossi ZM. Epidemiology of nonalcoholic fatty liver disease and nonalcoholic steatohepatitis in the United States and the rest of the world. Clinics in Liver Disease. 2016;**20**(2):205-214

[2] Ge X, Zheng L, Wang M, Du Y, Jiang J. Prevalence trends in non-alcoholic fatty liver disease at the global, regional and national levels, 1990-2017: A population-based observational study. BMJ Open. 2020;**10**(8):e036663

[3] Bosserhoff A, Hellerbrand C. Obesity and fatty liver are 'grease' for the machinery of hepatic fibrosis. Digestive Diseases. 2011;**29**(4):377-383

[4] Guo X, Yin X, Liu Z, Wang J. Non-alcoholic fatty liver disease (NAFLD) pathogenesis and natural products for prevention and treatment. International Journal of Molecular Sciences. 2022;**23**(24):15489

[5] Sebastiani G, Patel K, Ratziu V, Feld JJ, Neuschwander-Tetri BA, Pinzani M, et al. Current considerations for clinical management and care of non-alcoholic fatty liver disease: Insights From the 1st International Workshop of the Canadian NASH Network (CanNASH). Canadian Liver Journal. 2022;**5**(1):61-90

[6] Metrakos P, Nilsson T. Non-alcoholic fatty liver disease–A chronic disease of the 21st century. Journal of Biomedical Research. 2018;**32**(5):327

[7] Wandji LCN, Gnemmi V, Mathurin P, Louvet A. Combined alcoholic and non-alcoholic steatohepatitis. JHEP Reports. 2020;**2**(3):100101

[8] Rinella ME, Lazarus JV, Ratziu V, Francque SM, Sanyal AJ, Kanwal F, et al. A multisociety Delphi consensus statement on new fatty liver disease nomenclature. Hepatology. 2023;**78**(6):1966-1986

[9] NIAAA. Drinking Levels Defined: NIH; Rockville, MD. 2023. Available from: https://www.niaaa.nih.gov/alcohol-health/overview-alcohol-consumption/moderate-binge-drinking

[10] Arab JP, Roblero JP, Altamirano J, Bessone F, Araujo RC, Higuera-De la Tijera F, et al. Alcohol-related liver disease: Clinical practice guidelines by the Latin American Association for the Study of the liver (ALEH). Annals of Hepatology. 2019;**18**(3):518-535

[11] Osna NA, Donohue TM Jr, Kharbanda KK. Alcoholic liver disease: Pathogenesis and current management. Alcohol Research: Current Reviews. 2017;**38**(2):147

[12] Eslam M, Newsome PN, Sarin SK, Anstee QM, Targher G, Romero-Gomez M, et al. A new definition for metabolic dysfunction-associated fatty liver disease: An international expert consensus statement. Journal of Hepatology. 2020;**73**(1):202-209

[13] Younossi ZM, Stepanova M, Younossi Y, Golabi P, Mishra A, Rafiq N, et al. Epidemiology of chronic liver diseases in the USA in the past three decades. Gut. 2020;**69**(3):564-568

[14] Eslam M, Sanyal AJ, George J, Sanyal A, Neuschwander-Tetri B, Tiribelli C, et al. MAFLD: A consensus-driven proposed nomenclature for

metabolic associated fatty liver disease. Gastroenterology. 2020;**158**(7):1999-2014 e1

[15] Powell EE, Wong VW-S, Rinella M. Non-alcoholic fatty liver disease. The Lancet. 2021;**397**(10290):2212-2224

[16] Kleiner DE, Brunt EM, Van Natta M, Behling C, Contos MJ, Cummings OW, et al. Design and validation of a histological scoring system for nonalcoholic fatty liver disease. Hepatology. 2005;**41**(6):1313-1321

[17] Chalasani N, Younossi Z, Lavine JE, Charlton M, Cusi K, Rinella M, et al. The diagnosis and management of nonalcoholic fatty liver disease: Practice guidance from the American Association for the Study of Liver Diseases. Hepatology. 2018;**67**(1):328-357

[18] Younossi Z, Anstee QM, Marietti M, Hardy T, Henry L, Eslam M, et al. Global burden of NAFLD and NASH: Trends, predictions, risk factors and prevention. Nature Reviews Gastroenterology & Hepatology. 2018;**15**(1):11-20

[19] Sarin SK, Kumar M, Eslam M, George J, Al Mahtab M, Akbar SMF, et al. Liver diseases in the Asia-Pacific region: A lancet gastroenterology & hepatology commission. The Lancet Gastroenterology & Hepatology. 2020;**5**(2):167-228

[20] Milić S, Lulić D, Štimac D. Non-alcoholic fatty liver disease and obesity: Biochemical, metabolic and clinical presentations. World Journal of Gastroenterology: WJG. 2014;**20**(28):9330

[21] Le MH, Yeo YH, Li X, Li J, Zou B, Wu Y, et al. 2019 Global NAFLD prevalence: A systematic review and meta-analysis. Clinical Gastroenterology and Hepatology. 2022;**20**(12):2809-17. e28

[22] Calzadilla Bertot L, Adams LA. The natural course of non-alcoholic fatty liver disease. International Journal of Molecular Sciences. 2016;**17**(5):774

[23] Kanwar P, Kowdley KV. The metabolic syndrome and its influence on nonalcoholic steatohepatitis. Clinics in Liver Disease. 2016;**20**(2):225-243

[24] Browning JD, Szczepaniak LS, Dobbins R, Nuremberg P, Horton JD, Cohen JC, et al. Prevalence of hepatic steatosis in an urban population in the United States: Impact of ethnicity. Hepatology. 2004;**40**(6):1387-1395

[25] Pouwels S, Sakran N, Graham Y, Leal A, Pintar T, Yang W, et al. Non-alcoholic fatty liver disease (NAFLD): A review of pathophysiology, clinical management and effects of weight loss. BMC Endocrine Disorders. 2022;**22**(1):63

[26] Ali A, Amin MJ, Ahmed MU, Taj A, Aasim M, Tabrez E. Frequency of non-alcoholic fatty liver disease (NAFLD) and its associated risk factors among Type-2 diabetics. Pakistan Journal of Medical Sciences. 2022;**38**(1):28

[27] Allen AM, Therneau TM, Larson JJ, Coward A, Somers VK, Kamath PS. Nonalcoholic fatty liver disease incidence and impact on metabolic burden and death: A 20 year-community study. Hepatology. 2018;**67**(5):1726-1736

[28] Alexander M, Loomis AK, Fairburn-Beech J, van der Lei J, Duarte-Salles T, Prieto-Alhambra D, et al. Real-world data reveal a diagnostic gap in non-alcoholic fatty liver disease. BMC Medicine. 2018;**16**:1-11

[29] Dash S, Xiao C, Morgantini C, Lewis GF. New insights into the regulation of chylomicron production. Annual Review of Nutrition. 2015;**35**(1):265-294

[30] NIH(NIDDK). Nonalcoholic Fatty Liver Disease & NASH: NIH. Rockville, MD; 2023. Available from: https://www.niddk.nih.gov/health-information/liver-disease/nafld-nash

[31] Pafili K, Maltezos E, Papanas N. Ipragliflozin and sodium glucose transporter 2 inhibitors to reduce liver fat: Will the prize we sought be won? Expert Opinion on Pharmacotherapy. 2018;**19**(3):185-187

[32] Younossi ZM, Koenig AB, Abdelatif D, Fazel Y, Henry L, Wymer M. Global epidemiology of nonalcoholic fatty liver disease—Meta-analytic assessment of prevalence, incidence, and outcomes. Hepatology. 2016;**64**(1):73-84

[33] Dulai PS, Singh S, Patel J, Soni M, Prokop LJ, Younossi Z, et al. Increased risk of mortality by fibrosis stage in nonalcoholic fatty liver disease: Systematic review and meta-analysis. Hepatology. 2017;**65**(5):1557-1565

[34] Younossi ZM, Golabi P, de Avila L, Paik JM, Srishord M, Fukui N, et al. The global epidemiology of NAFLD and NASH in patients with type 2 diabetes: A systematic review and meta-analysis. Journal of Hepatology. 2019;**71**(4):793-801

[35] Kleiner DE, Brunt EM. Nonalcoholic fatty liver disease: Pathologic patterns and biopsy evaluation in clinical research. Seminar Liver Disease. 2012;**32**:3-13

[36] Bedossa P. Pathology of non-alcoholic fatty liver disease. Liver International. 2017;**37**:85-89

[37] Targher G, Lonardo A, Byrne CD. Nonalcoholic fatty liver disease and chronic vascular complications of diabetes mellitus. Nature Reviews Endocrinology. 2018;**14**(2):99-114

[38] Anstee QM, Targher G, Day CP. Progression of NAFLD to diabetes mellitus, cardiovascular disease or cirrhosis. Nature Reviews Gastroenterology & hepatology. 2013;**10**(6):330-344

[39] Pafili K, Roden M. Nonalcoholic fatty liver disease (NAFLD) from pathogenesis to treatment concepts in humans. Molecular Metabolism. 2021;**50**:101122

[40] Day CP, Yeaman SJ. The biochemistry of alcohol-induced fatty liver. Biochimica et Biophysica Acta (BBA)-lipids and lipid. Metabolism. 1994;**1215**(1-2):33-48

[41] Braillon A, Capron J, Herve M, Degott C, Quenum C. Liver in obesity. Gut. 1985;**26**(2):133-139

[42] Fromenty B, Pessayre D. Inhibition of mitochondrial beta-oxidation as a mechanism of hepatotoxicity. Pharmacology & Therapeutics. 1995;**67**(1):101-154

[43] Bacon BR. Nonalcoholic steatohepatitis : An expanded clinical entity. Gastroenterology. 1994;**107**:1103-1109

[44] Diehl A, Goodman Z, Ishak K. Alcohollike liver disease in nonalcoholics: A clinical and histologic comparison with alcohol-induced liver injury. Gastroenterology. 1988;**95**(4):1056-1062

[45] Teli MR, James OF, Burt AD, Bennett MK, Day CP. The natural history of nonalcoholic fatty liver: A follow-up study. Hepatology. 1995;**22**(6):1714-1719

[46] Haas JT, Francque S, Staels B. Pathophysiology and mechanisms of nonalcoholic fatty liver disease. Annual Review of Physiology. 2016;**78**(1):181-205

[47] Friedman SL, Neuschwander-Tetri BA, Rinella M, Sanyal AJ.

Mechanisms of NAFLD development and therapeutic strategies. Nature Medicine. 2018;**24**(7):908-922

[48] Samuel VT, Shulman GI. Nonalcoholic fatty liver disease as a nexus of metabolic and hepatic diseases. Cell Metabolism. 2018;**27**(1):22-41

[49] Deprince A, Haas JT, Staels B. Dysregulated lipid metabolism links NAFLD to cardiovascular disease. Molecular Metabolism. 2020;**42**:101092

[50] Rinella ME, Neuschwander-Tetri BA, Siddiqui MS, Abdelmalek MF, Caldwell S, Barb D, et al. AASLD practice guidance on the clinical assessment and management of nonalcoholic fatty liver disease. Hepatology. 2023;**77**(5):1797-1835

[51] Jennison E, Byrne CD. The role of the gut microbiome and diet in the pathogenesis of non-alcoholic fatty liver disease. Clinical and Molecular Hepatology. 2021;**27**(1):22

[52] Tacke F, Horn P, Wong VW-S, Ratziu V, Bugianesi E, Francque S, et al. EASL–EASD–EASO clinical practice guidelines on the management of metabolic dysfunction-associated steatotic liver disease (MASLD). Journal of Hepatology. 2024;**81**:492-542

[53] Younossi ZM, Paik JM, Stepanova M, Ong J, Alqahtani S, Henry L. Clinical profiles and mortality rates are similar for metabolic dysfunction-associated steatotic liver disease and non-alcoholic fatty liver disease. Journal of Hepatology. 2024;**80**(5):694-701

[54] Targher G, Day CP, Bonora E. Risk of cardiovascular disease in patients with nonalcoholic fatty liver disease. New England Journal of Medicine. 2010;**363**(14):1341-1350

[55] Schwabe RF, Tabas I, Pajvani UB. Mechanisms of fibrosis development in nonalcoholic steatohepatitis. Gastroenterology. 2020;**158**(7):1913-1928

[56] Day CP, James OF. Steatohepatitis: A tale of two "hits"? Gasteroenterology. 1998;**114**(4):842-845

[57] Petagine L, Zariwala MG, Patel VB. Non-alcoholic fatty liver disease: Immunological mechanisms and current treatments. World Journal of Gastroenterology. 2023;**29**(32):4831

[58] Imajo K, Yoneda M, Kessoku T, Ogawa Y, Maeda S, Sumida Y, et al. Rodent models of nonalcoholic fatty liver disease/nonalcoholic steatohepatitis. International Journal of Molecular Sciences. 2013;**14**(11):21833-21857

[59] Tilg H, Moschen AR. Evolution of inflammation in nonalcoholic fatty liver disease: The multiple parallel hits hypothesis. Hepatology. 2010;**52**(5):1836-1846

[60] Website N. Non-alcoholic Fatty Liver Disease (NAFLD): NHS for England. Unites Kingdom; 2023. Available from: https://www.nhs.uk/conditions/non-alcoholic-fatty-liver-disease/

[61] Stefan N, Häring H-U, Cusi K. Non-alcoholic fatty liver disease: Causes, diagnosis, cardiometabolic consequences, and treatment strategies. The Lancet Diabetes & Endocrinology. 2019;**7**(4):313-324

[62] Eslam M, George J. Genetic insights for drug development in NAFLD. Trends in Pharmacological Sciences. 2019;**40**(7):506-516

[63] Kwong A, Kim W, Lake J, Smith J, Schladt D, Skeans M, et al. OPTN/SRTR 2018 annual data report: Liver.

American Journal of Transplantation. 2020;**20**:193-299

[64] Younossi Z, Stepanova M, Ong JP, Jacobson IM, Bugianesi E, Duseja A, et al. Nonalcoholic steatohepatitis is the fastest growing cause of hepatocellular carcinoma in liver transplant candidates. Clinical Gastroenterology and Hepatology. 2019;**17**(4):748-755 e3

[65] Haldar D, Kern B, Hodson J, Armstrong MJ, Adam R, Berlakovich G, et al. Outcomes of liver transplantation for non-alcoholic steatohepatitis: A European liver transplant registry study. Journal of Hepatology. 2019;**71**(2):313-322

[66] Loomba R, Wong R, Fraysse J, Shreay S, Li S, Harrison S, et al. Nonalcoholic fatty liver disease progression rates to cirrhosis and progression of cirrhosis to decompensation and mortality: A real world analysis of Medicare data. Alimentary Pharmacology & Therapeutics. 2020;**51**(11):1149-1159

[67] Ratziu V, Charlotte F, Heurtier A, Gombert S, Giral P, Bruckert E, et al. Sampling variability of liver biopsy in nonalcoholic fatty liver disease. Gastroenterology. 2005;**128**(7):1898-1906

[68] Merriman RB, Ferrell LD, Patti MG, Weston SR, Pabst MS, Aouizerat BE, et al. Correlation of paired liver biopsies in morbidly obese patients with suspected nonalcoholic fatty liver disease. Hepatology. 2006;**44**(4):874-880

[69] Brunt EM, Ramrakhiani S, Cordes BG, Neuschwander-Tetri BA, Janney CG, Bacon BR, et al. Concurrence of histologic features of steatohepatitis with other forms of chronic liver disease. Modern Pathology. 2003;**16**(1):49-56

[70] Sánchez-Muñoz D, Castellano-Megías VM, Romero-Gómez M. Case report: Histologic features of Steatohepatitis in patients with a clinical diagnosis of autoimmune cholestasis. Digestive Diseases and Sciences. 2004;**49**(11-12):1957

[71] Cotrim HP, Andrade ZA, Parana R, Portugal M, Lyra LG, Freitas LA. Nonalcoholic steatohepatitis: A toxic liver disease in industrial workers. Liver. 1999;**19**(4):299-304

[72] Choi HS, Brouwer WP, Zanjir WM, de Man RA, Feld JJ, Hansen BE, et al. Nonalcoholic steatohepatitis is associated with liver-related outcomes and all-cause mortality in chronic hepatitis B. Hepatology. 2020;**71**(2):539-548

[73] Chiang DJ, McCullough AJ. The impact of obesity and metabolic syndrome on alcoholic liver disease. Clinics in Liver Disease. 2014;**18**(1):157-163

[74] Beuers U, Gershwin EM, Gish RG, Invernizzi P, Jones DE, Lindor K, et al. Changing nomenclature for PBC: From 'cirrhosis' to 'cholangitis'. Official Journal of the American College of Gastroenterology – ACG. 2015;**110**(11):1536-1538

[75] Vilar-Gomez E, Calzadilla-Bertot L, Wong VW-S, Castellanos M, Aller-de la Fuente R, Metwally M, et al. Fibrosis severity as a determinant of cause-specific mortality in patients with advanced nonalcoholic fatty liver disease: A multi-national cohort study. Gastroenterology. 2018;**155**(2):443-457 e17

[76] Pelusi S, Cespiati A, Rametta R, Pennisi G, Mannisto V, Rosso C, et al. Prevalence and risk factors of significant fibrosis in patients with nonalcoholic

fatty liver without steatohepatitis. Clinical Gastroenterology and Hepatology. 2019;**17**(11):2310-2319 e6

[77] Eslam M, Sanyal AJ, George J. Toward more accurate nomenclature for fatty liver diseases. Gastroenterology. 2019;**157**(3):590-593

[78] Díaz LA, Arab JP, Louvet A, Bataller R, Arrese M. The intersection between alcohol-related liver disease and nonalcoholic fatty liver disease. Nature Reviews Gastroenterology & Hepatology. 2023;**20**(12):764-783

[79] Idalsoaga F, Kulkarni AV, Mousa OY, Arrese M, Arab JP. Non-alcoholic fatty liver disease and alcohol-related liver disease: Two intertwined entities. Frontiers in Medicine. 2020;**7**:448, 1-17

[80] Wu X, Fan X, Miyata T, Kim A, Cajigas-Du Ross CK, Ray S, et al. Recent advances in understanding of pathogenesis of alcohol-associated liver disease. Annual Review of Pathology: Mechanisms of Disease. 2023;**18**(1):411-438

[81] Arrese M, Cabrera D, Kalergis AM, Feldstein AE. Innate immunity and inflammation in NAFLD/NASH. Digestive Diseases and Sciences. 2016;**61**:1294-1303

[82] Greuter T, Malhi H, Gores GJ, Shah VH. Therapeutic opportunities for alcoholic steatohepatitis and nonalcoholic steatohepatitis: Exploiting similarities and differences in pathogenesis. JCI Insight. 2017;**2**(17):e95354, 1-18

[83] Mashek DG, Khan SA, Sathyanarayan A, Ploeger JM, Franklin MP. Hepatic lipid droplet biology: Getting to the root of fatty liver. Hepatology. 2015;**62**(3):964-967

[84] Gluchowski NL, Becuwe M, Walther TC, Farese RV. Lipid droplets and liver disease: From basic biology to clinical implications. Nature Reviews Gastroenterology & Hepatology. 2017;**14**(6):343-355

[85] Arab JP, Arrese M, Trauner M. Recent insights into the pathogenesis of nonalcoholic fatty liver disease. Annual Review of Pathology: Mechanisms of Disease. 2018;**13**(1):321-350

[86] Lee E, Korf H, Vidal-Puig A. An adipocentric perspective on the development and progression of non-alcoholic fatty liver disease. Journal of Hepatology. 2023;**78**(5):1048-1062

[87] Ipsen DH, Lykkesfeldt J, Tveden-Nyborg P. Molecular mechanisms of hepatic lipid accumulation in non-alcoholic fatty liver disease. Cellular and Molecular Life Sciences. 2018;**75**:3313-3327

[88] Lambert JE, Ramos-Roman MA, Browning JD, Parks EJ. Increased de novo lipogenesis is a distinct characteristic of individuals with nonalcoholic fatty liver disease. Gastroenterology. 2014;**146**(3):726-735

[89] Musso G, Cassader M, Paschetta E, Gambino R. Bioactive lipid species and metabolic pathways in progression and resolution of nonalcoholic steatohepatitis. Gastroenterology. 2018;**155**(2):282-302 e8

[90] Singal AK, Shah VH, Malhi H. Emerging targets for therapy in ALD: Lessons from NASH. Hepatology. 2024;**80**(1):223-237

[91] Gautheron J, Gores GJ, Rodrigues CM. Lytic cell death in metabolic liver disease. Journal of Hepatology. 2020;**73**(2):394-408

[92] Ibrahim SH, Hirsova P, Gores GJ. Non-alcoholic steatohepatitis

pathogenesis: Sublethal hepatocyte injury as a driver of liver inflammation. Gut. 2018;**67**(5):963-972

[93] Schwabe RF, Luedde T. Apoptosis and necroptosis in the liver: A matter of life and death. Nature Reviews Gastroenterology & Hepatology. 2018;**15**(12):738-752

[94] Hatting M, Zhao G, Schumacher F, Sellge G, Al Masaoudi M, Gaβler N, et al. Hepatocyte caspase-8 is an essential modulator of steatohepatitis in rodents. Hepatology. 2013;**57**(6):2189-2201

[95] Geng Y, Faber KN, de Meijer VE, Blokzijl H, Moshage H. How does hepatic lipid accumulation lead to lipotoxicity in non-alcoholic fatty liver disease? Hepatology International. 2021;**15**:21-35

[96] Peiseler M, Schwabe R, Hampe J, Kubes P, Heikenwälder M, Tacke F. Immune mechanisms linking metabolic injury to inflammation and fibrosis in fatty liver disease–novel insights into cellular communication circuits. Journal of Hepatology. 2022;**77**(4):1136-1160

[97] Hirsova P, Gores GJ. Death receptor-mediated cell death and proinflammatory signaling in nonalcoholic steatohepatitis. Cellular and Molecular Gastroenterology and Hepatology. 2015;**1**(1):17-27

[98] Feldstein AE, Gores GJ. Apoptosis in alcoholic and nonalcoholic steatohepatitis. Frontiers in Bioscience. 2005;**10**(3):3093-3099

[99] Idrissova L, Malhi H, Werneburg NW, LeBrasseur NK, Bronk SF, Fingas C, et al. TRAIL receptor deletion in mice suppresses the inflammation of nutrient excess. Journal of Hepatology. 2015;**62**(5):1156-1163

[100] Eguchi A, Du Jeu XDM, Johnson CD, Nektaria A, Feldstein AE. Liver bid suppression for treatment of fibrosis associated with non-alcoholic steatohepatitis. Journal of Hepatology. 2016;**64**(3):699-707

[101] Wiering L, Tacke F. Treating inflammation to combat non-alcoholic fatty liver disease. Journal of Endocrinology. 2022;**256**:e220194, 1-20

[102] Vitale I, Pietrocola F, Guilbaud E, Aaronson SA, Abrams JM, Adam D, et al. Apoptotic cell death in disease—Current understanding of the NCCD 2023. Cell Death & Differentiation. 2023;**30**(5):1097-1154

[103] Shojaie L, Iorga A, Dara L. Cell death in liver diseases: A review. International Journal of Molecular Sciences. 2020;**21**(24):9682

[104] Wu Y, Tan HWS, Lin J-Y, Shen H-M, Wang H, Lu G. Molecular mechanisms of autophagy and implications in liver diseases. Liver Research. 2023;**7**(1):56-70

[105] Chao X, Wang S, Zhao K, Li Y, Williams JA, Li T, et al. Impaired TFEB-mediated lysosome biogenesis and autophagy promote chronic ethanol-induced liver injury and steatosis in mice. Gastroenterology. 2018;**155**(3):865-879 e12

[106] Las G, Serada SB, Wikstrom JD, Twig G, Shirihai OS. Fatty acids suppress autophagic turnover in β-cells. Journal of Biological Chemistry. 2011;**286**(49):42534-42544

[107] Betrapally NS, Gillevet PM, Bajaj JS. Changes in the intestinal microbiome and alcoholic and nonalcoholic liver diseases: Causes or effects? Gastroenterology. 2016;**150**(8):1745-1755 e3

[108] Sharpton SR, Ajmera V, Loomba R. Emerging role of the gut microbiome in nonalcoholic fatty liver disease:

From composition to function. Clinical Gastroenterology and Hepatology. 2019;**17**(2):296-306

[109] Leung H, Long X, Ni Y, Qian L, Nychas E, Siliceo SL, et al. Risk assessment with gut microbiome and metabolite markers in NAFLD development. Science translational Medicine. 2022;**14**(648):eabk0855

[110] Liu Y, Meric G, Havulinna AS, Teo SM, Åberg F, Ruuskanen M, et al. Early prediction of incident liver disease using conventional risk factors and gut-microbiome-augmented gradient boosting. Cell Metabolism. 2022;**34**(5):719-30. e4

[111] Oh TG, Kim SM, Caussy C, Fu T, Guo J, Bassirian S, et al. A universal gut-microbiome-derived signature predicts cirrhosis. Cell Metabolism. 2020;**32**(5):878-888 e6

[112] Fairfield B, Schnabl B. Gut dysbiosis as a driver in alcohol-induced liver injury. JHEP Reports. 2021;**3**(2):100220

[113] Jew MH, Hsu CL. Alcohol, the gut microbiome, and liver disease. Journal of Gastroenterology and Hepatology. 2023;**38**(8):1205-1210

[114] Leclercq S, Matamoros S, Cani PD, Neyrinck AM, Jamar F, Stärkel P, et al. Intestinal permeability, gut-bacterial dysbiosis, and behavioral markers of alcohol-dependence severity. National Academy of Sciences of the United States of America. 2014;**111**(42):E4485-E4E93

[115] Mutlu EA, Gillevet PM, Rangwala H, Sikaroodi M, Naqvi A, Engen PA, et al. Colonic microbiome is altered in alcoholism. American Journal of Physiology-Gastrointestinal and Liver Physiology. 2012;**302**(9):G966-GG78

[116] Maccioni L, Loriot A, Dewulf J, Bommer G, Horsmans Y, Lanthier N, et al. Duodenal CD8+ T resident memory cell apoptosis contributes to gut barrier dysfunction and microbial translocation in early alcohol-associated liver disease in humans. Alimentary Pharmacology & Therapeutics. 2022;**56**(6):1055-1070

[117] Zhu L, Baker SS, Gill C, Liu W, Alkhouri R, Baker RD, et al. Characterization of gut microbiomes in nonalcoholic steatohepatitis (NASH) patients: A connection between endogenous alcohol and NASH. Hepatology. 2013;**57**(2):601-609

[118] Meijnikman AS, Davids M, Herrema H, Aydin O, Tremaroli V, Rios-Morales M, et al. Microbiome-derived ethanol in nonalcoholic fatty liver disease. Nature Medicine. 2022;**28**(10):2100-2106

Chapter 2

The Role of Gut Microbiota in Metabolic Dysfunction-Associated Fatty Liver Disease (MASLD)

Sandica Bucurica

Abstract

Gut microbiota plays a critical role in developing and progressing metabolic dysfunction-associated steatotic liver disease (MASLD). Studies show reduced microbial diversity and specific shifts in bacterial populations in MASLD patients, with harmful species increasing and beneficial ones decreasing. These changes contribute to liver fat accumulation by impairing fiber fermentation, disrupting bile acid metabolism, increasing intestinal permeability, and promoting inflammation. The progression of MASLD is linked to evolving microbiota changes, and probiotics like *Lactobacillus plantarum* show potential in mitigating disease by restoring gut balance. Thus, gut microbiota serves as both a key factor and therapeutic target in MASLD. Interventions on microbiota are possible targets in treating MASLD or preventing progression toward advanced stages. At the same time, prebiotics and probiotics have shown results in ameliorating MASLD, post-biotic therapy, immuno-nutrition, bacteria engineering, or phages, which have been applied only in experimental studies.

Keywords: MASLD, NAFLD, gut microbiota, gut-liver axis, liver steatosis

1. Introduction

Following the multi-society Delphi consensus, the former nonalcoholic fatty liver disease was renamed metabolic dysfunction-associated steatotic liver disease (MASLD) in 2023. The complex pathogenesis of MASLD remains open to research since not all pathways are elucidated. Current knowledge comprises many aspects, such as metabolic disturbances of lipids and glucose, oxidative stress and pro-inflammatory response, altered functionality of intracellular organelles, inherited predisposition and epigenomic influences, imbalanced gut microbiota, and gut-liver axis engagement. Gut microbiota represents an enormous biosystem. So far, more than 3500 microbial species have been described, most belonging to six main phyla that populate the gut; there are also fungi, viruses, and phages. The phyla found in the gut microbiota are *Bacteroidetes, Firmicutes, Proteobacteria, Actinobacteria, Fusobacteria, and Verrucomicrobia*. Studies have shown a decreased variety in gut microbiota species in MASLD, alongside anomalies of the bacterial populations in contrast with the gut microbiota of healthy individuals.

Former nonalcoholic fatty liver disease was renamed following the multi-society Delphi consensus as Metabolic dysfunction-associated steatotic liver disease (MASLD) in 2023 [1]. This new nomenclature is meant to encompass the various factors accompanying the metabolic links of fatty liver with overweight or obesity, lipid metabolism disturbances, impaired glucose tolerance/diabetes mellitus, or cardiovascular dysfunction [2].

The most recent collaborative guideline for the management of MASLD was released in September 2024, and three European societies contributed: the European Association for the Study of Diabetes (EASD), the European Association for the Study of Obesity (EASO), and the European Association for the Study of the Liver (EASL) [3].

According to the latest data, the general prevalence of MASLD globally has increased by 5% in the last 8 years, with an ascending incidence trend [4–6].

It is essential to highlight that the EASL-EASD-EASO guideline states that NAFLD-related research may be applied to MASLD, supported by a concordance of NAFLD studied population for more than 99% of the MASLD patients. Moreover, the clinical characteristics and paraclinical tests overlap for NAFLD and MASLD. Consequently, this guideline considers that the new MASLD and former NAFLD share the same evidence [3].

This chapter will also use the term NAFLD to highlight all the previous background and scientific results published regarding the progression of hepatic steatosis. The evolution of sequence analysis technologies and metabolite profiling led to a better description of the specific gut microbiome and microbiota features, their interaction through the gut-liver axis, and their involvement in developing liver steatosis [7].

The complex pathogenesis of MASLD remains open to research since not all pathways are elucidated. Current knowledge comprises many aspects, such as metabolic disturbances of lipids and glucose, oxidative stress and pro-inflammatory response, altered functionality of intracellular organelles, inherited predisposition and epigenomic influences, imbalanced gut microbiota, and gut-liver axis engagement [8].

The gut microbiota has excellent plasticity, and intercurrent diseases, infections, antibiotics, and environmental factors might influence its dynamics. Still, chronic long-term exposure to stressful factors could induce irremediable changes in gut microbiota composition and variety, leading to sub-clinically chronic inflammation and reduced ability to maintain homeostasis [9].

2. Molecular mechanisms of fatty liver transformation

The mechanisms involved in hepatic steatosis comprise various pathways of the inflammatory cascade. Dietary lipids and carbohydrates in excess are the initiators of inflammation cycle activation through the purinergic receptor P2X7 receptor and NOD-, LRR-, and pyrin domain-containing protein 3 (NLRP3) [10]. The shifting process from normal to liver steatosis occurs in multiple steps. The progression toward the fatty transformation of the liver starts through overexpression of mRNA and protein of chemokine monocyte chemoattractant protein 1 (MCP-1) [10]. Consequently, the sequence of inflammation markers exhibits tumor necrosis factor-α (TNF-α) and interleukin-1β (IL-1β) at the hepatic level in the first instance and following that in the serum [10]. The inflammasome pathway is involved in most metabolic disorders, such as obesity, diabetes mellitus, and MASLD [11]. Experimental studies have shown that the NLRP3 inflammasome is involved in the liver's steatosis, inflammation, and fibrotic processes [12]. The most studied NLRP3 is a cellular sensing element that responds to various exogenous and endogenous hostile or threatening elements, such as microbial particles [13].

Steatotic changes in the liver occur through the progressive assimilation of fatty acids, enabled by fatty transport protein (FATP)-2 and 5 carriers alongside the cluster of differentiation-36 (CD-36) [14]. When their activity is high, the hepatic intracellular transport of fatty acids is increased, and the lipids depositing into the hepatocyte are also increased. Moreover, the intervention of CD-36 through hepatic receptors – liver X, pregnane X, and peroxisome proliferator-activated receptor-ϒ (PPAR-ϒ) facilitates the accumulation of long-chain fatty acids [14]. In the hepatocyte, fatty acids binding proteins-1 (FABP-1) carry the long-chain fatty acids toward specialized intracellular organelle where the process of lipids oxidation, lipogenesis, and very low-density lipoproteins (VLDL) are synthesized [14].

The main organelle involved in lipid synthesis is the mitochondria, which have structural and functional alterations in the steatotic liver. The mitochondria exert an essential role in modulating oxidative stress, and the hepatic cell mitochondrial apparatus participates in altered lipid oxidation [15]. Thus, a low level of oxidative phosphorylation proteins (OXPHOS) indicates fibrosis progression. Excessive lipid accumulation impedes their oxidation or export and release as very low-density lipoproteins (VLDL) [16]. Acetyl-coenzyme A is involved in endogenous lipid synthesis by conversion into palmitate, which has a pro-inflammatory action and contributes to the progression of steatohepatitis [17]. The mitochondrial sirtuin-3 proteins (SIRT3) are predominant in situations of increased metabolic activity and influence the response to oxidative stress. In progression to MASLD, disturbed oxidative stress results in a high production of reactive oxygen species, and SIRT-3 regulates fatty acid oxidation (**Figure 1**) [18].

The circulating lipids transport to hepatocytes is facilitated by fatty acids transporters (FATP) and cluster differentiation-36 (CD-36), which are regulated by

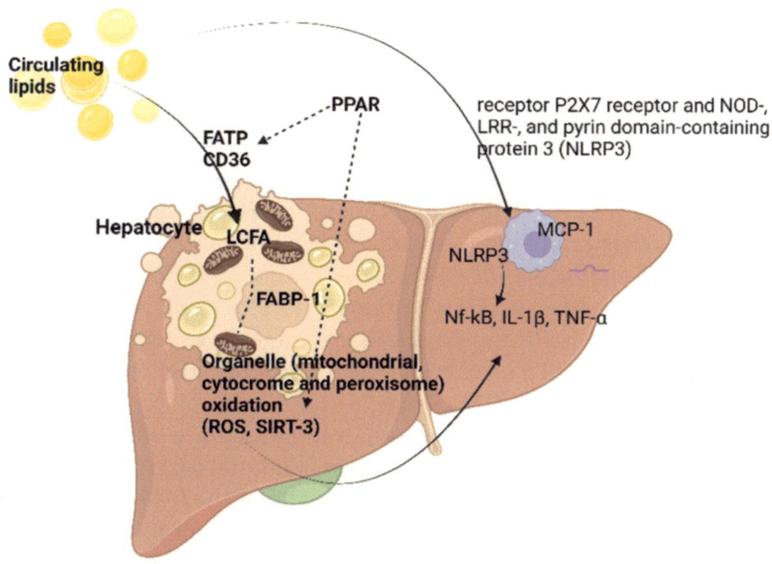

Figure 1.
Gut microbiota-derived metabolites and Metabolic-Associated Fatty Liver Disease (MAFLD).

peroxisome proliferator-activated receptor (PPAR). Intra-hepatocytes, the transportation to cellular organelle is enabled by fatty acid binding protein-1 (FABP-1). At the mitochondrial level, the oxidation process takes place (which is also controlled by PPAR by stimulating the utilization of fats as an energetic substrate). The lipids overload and mitochondrial dysfunctions generate reactive oxygen species (ROS), which favor inflammation. Simultaneously, high-level circulating lipids induce the inflammasome pathways through the purinergic receptor P2X7 receptor, NOD-, LRR-, and pyrin domain-containing protein 3 (NLRP3). As a result, the NF-kB, IL-1β, and TNF-α are released, starting the inflammation cycle [14, 18].

Another important protein in MASLD development is Fibroblast growth factor 19 (FGF-19), a hormone that regulates the diurnal secretion of biliary acids related to food ingestion. FGF-19 is regulated in the ileum under the farnesoid X receptor (FXR) response to fluctuation of bile acid concentrations. The hepatic response is the stimulation of the membranous FGFR4-KLB complex [19, 20]. The duality of FGF-19 action is exerted by lowering the bile acids at the hepatocyte level through Cyp7A1 influence and decreased production of lipids through FGFR 1c and FGFR4 [19, 21].

Different from FGF-19, FGF-21 has a broader metabolic effect. High serum glucose levels stimulate hepatic expression of FGF-21, influencing the metabolism of free fatty acids, energetic balance, and the metabolic pathways of glucose, fats, and adipose tissue [22].

At the nuclear level, Peroxisome proliferator-activated receptor-ϒ (PPAR-ϒ) is a receptor that modulates inflammation pathways. It is linked to lipid processing by favoring fatty acid production and lipid deposits (it is highly expressed in adipose tissue). The activated PPAR promotes hepatic fat accumulation and progression to MASLD, while inhibition has the opposite effect [23].

The AMP-activated protein kinase pathway (AMP), which participates in energetic metabolism and cellular expansion modulation, is the intracellular mechanism involved in progressing to hepatic steatosis [24].

3. The role of gut microbiota in gut-liver axis

Gut microbiota represents an enormous biosystem. So far, more than 3500 microbial species have been described, most belonging to bacteria except 17 that belong to the Archaea domain (mainly represented by *Methanobrevibacter smithii*) [25]. Alongside the six main phyla that populate the gut, there are also fungi, viruses, and phages. The phyla found in the gut microbiota are *Bacteroidetes*, *Firmicutes*, *Proteobacteria*, *Actinobacteria*, *Fusobacteria*, and *Verrucomicrobia*, while the most described fungi are *Candida*, *Saccharomyces*, *Malassezia*, and *Cladosporium* [26]. The dominant phyla are Firmicutes and Bacteroidetes, and the remaining phyla represent the rest of 10% [9]. It is also suggested that changes in the ratio of Firmicutes/Bacteroidetes might represent a marker of dysbiosis; some studies described it as an increase in metabolic diseases [9, 27].

Since the gastrointestinal tract has a broad luminal surface interaction, the intestinal barrier represents the first defense between alimentary particles and the human organism [28]. Essential elements define the integrity of the intestinal barrier (such as the mucus layer, commensal microbial organisms, antimicrobial proteins, secretory immunoglobulin A, mono-layered cells with specialized epithelial cells and lamina propria, which contain immune cells), and all these should function as a well-coordinated team to maintain a normal barrier [28]. The integrity of the intestinal barrier is essential for preventing endotoxemia in MASLD. Disruption of the intestinal barrier could appear at the physical or molecular level of defense [29]. A lack of intestinal barrier integrity appears early in the development of MASLD and enables bacterial translocation through gut vascular barrier impairment [30].

Tight intercellular connections characterize the normal mucosal layer of the intestinal lumen, and underneath the vascular barrier, the blood flow supports nutritive and functional circulation [29]. Loosening the tight junctions leads to increased permeability or "leaky gut," which facilitates the passage of pathogen-associated molecular patterns [31].

One of the proteins involved in regulating intestinal barrier permeability is Zonulin, which acts as a modulator of the epithelial and vascular barrier. A high release of Zonulin characterizes imbalanced gut microbiota, consequently allowing microbial microparticles to enter the bloodstream and favoring endotoxemia [32].

The relationship between gut microbiota and the intestinal barrier starts at birth and continuously changes throughout one's life [33, 34].

The gut microbiota microorganisms could presumably influence mucus secretion and quality by stimulating the enteric and colonic cells [33]. Another significant influence of gut microbiota on the intestinal barrier is regulating intestinal barrier immunity. Moreover, it is involved in the development of enteric nervous system.

The gut microbiota supports the intestinal barrier by promoting mucus production, strengthening tight junctions, and regulating immune responses. Disruption of the microbiota can weaken the barrier, leading to increased permeability ("leaky gut") and inflammation [33].

Besides those above, a chemical barrier encompasses defense substances such as antimicrobial-effect proteins that prevent intestinal barrier erosion. These bile acids modulate gut epithelium growth and regeneration, mucus and mucin, and enzymes. The microbial protection of the small bowel is done by gastric low pH, which inhibits the colonization of the intestine [29].

The interaction of gut microbiota with the host is a complex symbiotic relationship since the state of eubiosis (that represents a balanced microbial population) influences the host's overall health through immune regulation, protection against pathogens, and metabolic and enzymatic processing of nutrients. Nevertheless, gut microbiota synthesizes bioactive peptides containing neurotransmitters, secondary bile acid conversion, short-chain fatty acids, branched-chain amino acids, intestinal hormones, and vitamins [26]. All bioactive peptides described are part of a complex of gut-brain and gut-liver axes signals [35]. The short-chain fatty acids enter the bloodstream and send signals to the brain, being part of this gut-brain axis, concomitantly stimulating the hypothalamus-pituitary-adrenal axis or influencing the mucosal immune system. As a result, it indirectly deteriorates the central nervous system (CNS) transmission. The gut-brain axis is between the GI tract and the central nervous system (CNS), and the gut GI plays an important role. In this process, neural, endocrine, and immune systems are involved, running in an almost perfectly more extensive bidirectional information interaction system that influences the regulation of each participant (up-down regulation, down-up regulation) [36]. Furthermore, the gut and liver are interconnected through anatomical and functional portal and systemic circulation [35, 37]. The gut-liver axis is a bidirectional system representing the interplay between the gut microbial population and the liver. An imbalanced and inappropriate microbiota population characterizes the state of gut dysbiosis, and it is linked to various diseases, including hepatic disorders [38]. The liver reacts to gut microbiota dysbiosis by an abnormal immune response, biliary duct and hepatocyte inflammation, fibrogenesis, or inhibited regeneration [39].

Concurrently, dysregulated microbial development is controlled by the hepatic excretion of bile salts and antimicrobial peptides [35]. Thus, the impaired hepatic functionality influences the extent of gut dysbiosis [35, 37].

Hepatic immune function is innate, and defense against pathogens is assured mainly by tissue-resident immune cells—the Kupfer cells—and around 10% by monocyte-derived macrophages [40]. These are sensitive to bacterial endotoxins, which modulate their activity and memory [40].

NLRP3 is mainly involved in launching the inflammatory reaction when an imbalanced microbiota triggers it *via* the gut-liver axis [11].

The host's response materializes by releasing the interleukin-1β (IL-1β) precursor (pro-IL1β) through Kupfer cells and macrophage activation, and NLRP3 favors the Caspase-1 proteolytic cleavage of pro-IL-1β form to IL-1β. These are implicated in the process of fatty liver transformation, promoting the evolution toward steatosis and fibrosis [11].

Microparticles or bacterial components from the gut microbial population trigger inflammation, such as lipopolysaccharides from Gram-negative bacterial walls, peptidoglycans from the rigid layer of Gram-positive bacteria, and lipoteichoic acids (LTA). This initiates the inflammation process by stimulating immune Kupffer cells in the liver. The mechanism is endotoxemia, which triggers the hepatic immune system through the gut-liver axis [9, 41, 42]. In metabolic disturbances, the LPSs from the Bacteroidetes envelope have lower endotoxic effects than those from Proteobacteria [9].

In the liver, Kupffer cells respond by mediating and maintaining inflammation by overexpressing the cluster of differentiation (CD) 11b, CD 68, and CD 163 in the fatty liver transformation process. Initially, M2 macrophages are involved, and later, M1 macrophages are involved as the disease progresses toward advanced liver stages [10].

Microbe-associated molecular patterns (MAMPs) are detected by Toll-like receptors (TLRs) and nucleotide-binding oligomerization domain-like receptors (NLRs). Lipids are ligands for TLR 1, 2, 4, and 6 subfamilies, and nucleic acids are ligands for TLR 3, 7, 8 and 9 [43].

The liver participates in microbial defense and gut microbiota modulation by bile acid secretion. Bile acids suffer a deconjugating process into the gut lumen and influence the microbiota by damaging the bacterial envelope. In MASLD (former NAFLD), when the integrity of the intestinal barrier is damaged, and the secretion of bile acids is impaired, the MAMPs access the liver *via* the gut-liver axis [29].

The progression of MASLD to advanced stages was correlated with increased serum bile acid levels. The nuclear receptor FXR intervenes as a modulator of bile acids, and it is expressed in hepatic, fatty, intestine, renal, and adrenal tissue. Medication targeting the FXR (FXR agonists) reduced endotoxemia through the gut-liver axis [29].

Moreover, the intestines function as an immune organ because the epithelium releases T lymphocytes and goblet cells, which are actually antigen-presenting cells. The antigens are directed toward lamina propria dendritic cells, which promote the immune response [29].

4. Gut microbiota roles in MASLD

A large amount of literature sustains the involvement of gut microbiota in the etiopathogenic pathways of fatty liver. Studies have shown a decreased variety in gut microbiota species in MASLD, alongside anomalies of the bacterial populations in contrast with the gut microbiota of healthy individuals [44, 45].

The metabolic interplay between gut microbiota and MASLD has features similar to obesity and type 2 diabetes mellitus. Some microbiota changes, such as for *Clostridium* and *Lactobacillus* species, overlap with obesity, type 2 diabetes mellitus, and MASLD [46].

The influence is attributable to the bacterial inability to ferment non-digestible fiber from the diet since a healthy microbiota produces succinate and short-chain fatty acids through fiber fermentation. These exert preventive roles in lipids accumulation, and disturbances in these pathways result in the production of harmful metabolites such as ammonia and phenols (through protein distal intestinal catabolism and branched-chain fatty acids) [47].

The link between gut microbiota and hepatic steatosis is bidirectional. Experimental studies have shown that changes in microbiota influence hepatic metabolism, similar to a high-fat diet. Besides a neuroendocrine lipids modulation capability, gut microbiota affects intestinal permeability, might maintain chronic subtle inflammation, interferes with bile acids and choline metabolic pathways, and is a source of endogenous ethanol production [48, 49]. Microbiota changes in MASLD varied in clinical and preclinical studies. In the study of Boursier et al., an inverse proportionality between Bacteroides and Prevotella was found in favor of *Bacteroides* in patients with nonalcoholic liver steatosis [48]. Moreover, in patients with MASLD-progression toward fibrosis, *Rumminococcus* genus was predominant [48]. Alcohol-producing species such as *Klebsiella pneumoniae* also participate in the development of steatotic transformation of the liver since it was reported in preclinical studies that it was associated twice more with MASLD (former NAFLD) [50].

Meanwhile, *Coprococcus* and *Faecalibacterium* were deficient in patients with MASLD; other studies found that Escherichia, Streptococcus, and Prevotella were predominant [51].

Regarding the strains of Gram-positive acid-lactic producing Lactobacilli, *Lactobacillus plantarum* proved to reduce at half the levels of cholesterol and the accumulation of triglycerides in hepatocytes, with an inhibition of the molecules that promote the fatty liver progression. Thus, the PPAR-ϒ and SREBP were inhibited, CYP7A1 was upregulated in HepG2 nonalcoholic steatohepatitis experimental model substrates, and *L. platarum* was proposed as a probiotic with action on the nonalcoholic steatohepatitis [52].

A recent comparative study using 16S rRNA gene sequencing and metagenomic sequencing showed that the microbiota of patients with MASLD differed significantly from that of healthy individuals [53]. This study confirmed that healthy individuals' gut microbiota diversity was higher. In MASLD, the variety of the population decreased, with no differences between the patients with MASLD (no regard for the biochemical changes in hepatic enzymes in the MASLD group) [53]. Moreover, the study showed that *Dorea*, *Megaspheraea*, and *Lactobacillus* were more predominant in MASLD patients, and *Ruminococus obeum* and *Allistipes* were deficient compared to non-MASLD subjects. The *Alistipes* favored a better glucose and liver enzymes biochemical profile (**Table 1**) [53].

The changes in gut microbiota composition vary through different phases of the progression of MASLD. The changes appear relatively early and are characterized by decreased *Bifidobacterium* and *Lactobacillus genus* in favor *of Lactoccocus and Akkermansia.* The changes are more profound as the disease progresses to fibrotic stages (**Table 1**) [55].

Decreased species	Increased species	Variates in different stages of liver damage
Flavonifaractor [54]	*Clostridium* [54]	*Bifidobacterium* [55, 56]
Odoribacter [54]	*Anaerobacter* [54]	*Bacteroides* [48]
Alistipes [53, 54]	*Streptococcus* [54]	*Ruminococcus obeum* [53, 57]
Coprococcus [56]	*Escherichia coli* [46]	*Lactobacillus* [55]
Fecalibacterium [56]	*Proteobacteria* [46]	*Prevotella* [48, 57]
Coprococcus [51]	*Firmicutes* [58]	*Akkermansia muciniphila* [55, 59]
Eubacterium [46, 56]	*Lactococcus* [55]	
Oscillospira [57]	*Klebsiella pneumoniae* [50]	
Fecalibacterium [51]	*Dorea* [57]	
	Megaspheraea [53]	

Table 1.
The MASLD-associated gut microbiota changes.

Most gut microbiota changes are represented by a change in *Firmicutes* and *Bacteroidetes* ratio in MASLD [58].

Other studies reported a predominance of *the Clostridium, Anaerobacter, and Streptococcus* genera in MASLD-associated gut microbiota signatures and a decreased content of *Favonifaractor, Odoribacter,* and *Alistipes* species [54]. Another overgrowth gut-populating microorganism found in patients with fatty liver transformation was *Proteobacteria* [46].

The pathogen bacterial population was found to be increased in MASLD-associated gut microbiota, with representatives from *Proteobacteria*, *Enterobacteriaceae*, and *Escherichia* species. The microorganisms responsible for producing beneficial short-chain fatty acids and butyrate were found in deficit in MASLD cases, especially with a relative scarcity of *Faecalibacterium prausnitzii*, *Eubacterium rectale*, and *Eubacterium haldi.* Moreover, *Fecalibacterium prausnitzii* was reported as decreased in cirrhosis patients' microbiota [46]. Antibiotic administration could counteract the overgrowth of likely pathogenic bacteria. Still, this therapy affects the helpful commensal bacteria. Specific strains such as *Lactobacillus rhamnosus GG, Lactobacillus reuteri, Lactobacillus plantarum*, or *Bifidobacterium lactis* might rebalance it [60].

Another beneficial bacteria, *Akkermansia muciniphila*, responsible for mucin production in the gut, was found in reduced amounts in Satapathy et al.'s study; the butyrate-producing bacteria enhances its beneficial activity and exerts protective mucosal effects by itself [59]. The microbiota evolves from birth in the first years of childhood, but it is influenced through all phases of life, although it prefigures adult microbiota features from earlier years [61]. In pediatric patients with MASLD, a deficient amount of *Oscillospira* species and higher populations of *Dorea*, *Prevotella*, and *Ruminoccoccus* species were found, in contrast with normal pediatric gut microbiota populations (**Table 2**) [57].

It is important to emphasize that gut bacterial populations influence the occurrence or progression of MASLD or the progression of MASLD to fibrosis stages not only by their physical presence but also by acting as pro-inflammatory triggers and various serum metabolites [77]. In this regard, Caussy et al. reported that MASLD (former NAFLD) was associated with increased growth of Gram-negative microorganisms, especially Escherichia coli, which relates to high serum levels of 3-(4-hydroxyphenyl)-lactate and phenyl-lactate. This study also suggested that this metabolite plays a role in the genetics of MASLD [77].

Species	Effect	Mechanisms
Lactobacillus rhamnosus	Beneficial	Lowering adiponectin levels Increasing FGF-21 [52, 62] inflammation, increasing SCFA, lower body weight and intrahepatic fat, evaluated through magnetic resonance imaging (MRI) and the proton density fat fraction (PDFF) [52, 63, 64]
Lactobacillus plantarum	Beneficial	decreasing serum triglyceride levels, gamma-glutamyl-transferase and C-reactive protein, Improved liver steatosis index [65–68]
Bifidobacterium	Beneficial	Increased activation of liver FXR Decreased expression of intestinal FXR Strengthening of intestinal tight junctions [64, 69] Producing high levels of acetate [33]
Felicalibacterium prausnitzii	Beneficial	producing SCFAs in the gut and butyrate inhibiting NF-*k*B and pro-inflammatory cytokines IL-6 and TNF-α increasing anti-inflammatory cytokines IL-10 [70, 71]
Akkermansia muciniphila	Beneficial	stimulating the SCFAs, preventing leaky gut, stimulating GLP-1 [72, 73]
Pseudomonas	Harmful	Outer membrane vesicles induce glucose and insulin impairment in adipose tissue, and exacerbate liver inflammation by Toll-like receptor 4 (TLR4) activation [74]
Klebsiella pneumoniae	Harmful	Toxic effect of endogenous alcohol-producing [75]
Clostridioides Escherichia coli Enterococcus	Harmful	Microbial particles promote acute inflammation *via* TLR2- and TLR4-signaling and potentially trigger TLR-dependent accumulation of neutrophils and T-cells toxin production [76]

SCFA – short-chain fatty acids, NF-kB (nuclear factor kappa-light-chain-enhancer of activated B cells), short-chain fatty acids (SCFAs), glucagon-like peptide-1 (GLP-1).
FXR-farnesoid X receptor, FGF-21-fibroblast growth factor-21.

Table 2.
Gut-populating microorganisms beneficial and harmful effects in MASLD.

Other metabolites incriminated as an interplay between imbalanced microbiota and the onset of steatotic alterations in the liver are bile acidic compounds, short-chain fatty acids, trimethylamine N-oxide, and tryptophan metabolites (**Figure 2**) [7].

5. Gut microbiota as an interventional therapeutic target in MASLD

Interventions on microbiota are possible targets in treating MASLD or preventing progression toward advanced stages. Diet and lifestyle interventions should be beneficial by creating an environment for beneficial microbiota changes. The Mediterranean diet significantly influences the quality of gut microbiota in terms of variety and composition based on the content of fibers, monosaturated fatty acids, and polyphenols [80]. A healthy diet will also be advantageous for the gut-liver axis by improving the intestinal barrier and regulating the bile acid circuit. Rich-fiber foods will decrease the Firmicutes—Bacteroides ratio, and polyphenol compounds will stimulate Bifidobacteria [80].

Probiotics used as natural or supplement agents may influence the composition of one's gut microbiota. The supplementation of *Lactobacillus rhamnosus GG* favors the growth of helpful microbiota in the ileum, strengthens the intestinal barrier, and promotes anti-inflammatory and anti-steatosis effects [52, 62, 64].

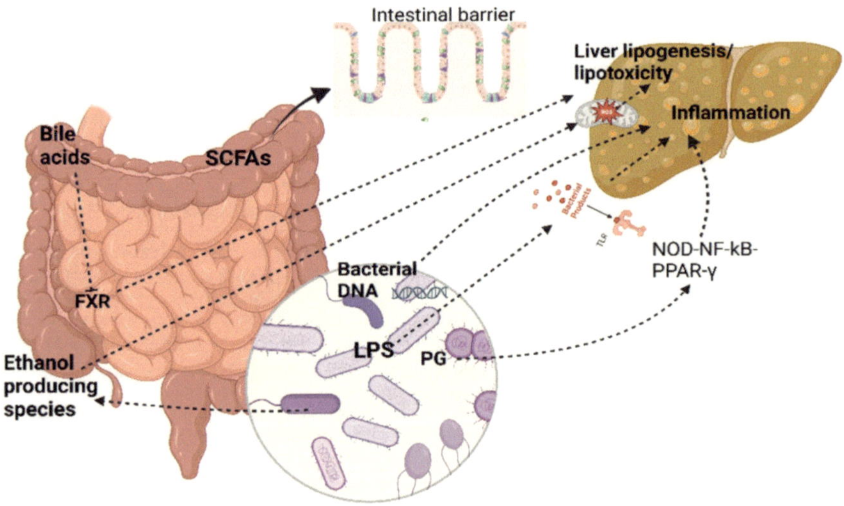

Figure 2.
Microbiota-derived metabolites and MASLD. FXR-farnesoid X factor, LPS-lipopolysaccharides, DNA – deoxyribonucleic acid, PG-peptidoglycans, TLR-Toll-like receptor, SCFAs – short-chain fatty acids (created with Biorender). In the process of fatty liver transformation, the gut microbiota metabolites influence the permeability of the intestinal barrier. The SCFAs are acetate, propionate, and butyrate, resulting from dietary fibers' bacterial fermentation. They exert a protective role on the colonocytes, strengthening the intestinal barrier, besides an immunological role through free fatty acid receptor 2 (FFAR2) and FFAR3. The bacterial cellular components promote liver lipotoxicity by LPS (ligands for TLR4 that promote inflammation); PG favors liver inflammation by the NOD-NF-kB-PPAR-Υ pathway, and microbial DNA maintains chronic inflammation. The microbiota species' endogenous alcohol-producing stimulates lipogenesis by mitochondrial oxidative stress. The bile acids inhibit the FXR and favor endotoxemia and hepatic lipogenesis [56, 78, 79].

VSL#3 is one of the most studied probiotics for metabolic-dysfunction-associated fatty liver disease. After 16 weeks of administration, the hepatic fat burden in both adult and pediatric patients was ameliorated [66–68, 81, 82].

VSL#3 modulated microbiota and was linked to the capacity of *Bifidobacterium longum*, which stimulates the production of conjugated linoleic acid by bacterial microorganisms and could increase glucagon-like peptide 1 (GLP-1) [9]. Regarding gut microbiota-modifying agents used as specific treatments for MASLD, the latest Guideline for MASLD management, released in 2024 by the joint of EASL-EASDO-EASO, recommends caution due to the necessity of large and rigorous RCTs [3]. Published data proved that nutraceutical intervention ameliorated the abnormal liver enzyme profile in patients with MASLD and reduced the steatosis grade [83]. Still, the overall impact of nutraceutical intervention in MASLD was not accurately assessed in terms of severity outcomes of MASLD – such as the necessity for liver transplantation, mortality from MASLD complications, or the occurrence of hepatocarcinoma. Post-biotic therapy intervenes by using components of bacterial cellular walls, inactive specific microbiota cells, or cellular metabolites to enhance the immune response alongside immuno-nutrition, bacteria engineering, or phages, which has been applied only in experimental studies [3, 84].

6. Conclusion

The involvement of gut microbiota in developing and progressing metabolic dysfunction-associated steatotic liver disease (MASLD) is increasingly recognized.

Studies consistently demonstrate reduced microbial diversity and significant shifts in bacterial populations among MASLD patients compared to healthy individuals. Specific bacterial changes, such as decreased beneficial species (e.g., *Bifidobacterium* and *Faecalibacterium*) and increased harmful bacteria (e.g., *Escherichia*, *Streptococcus*, and *Klebsiella*), are associated with disease onset and progression. These microbiota alterations mirror those seen in obesity and type 2 diabetes, with overlapping features in bacterial species such as *Clostridium* and *Lactobacillus*.

Gut microbiota influences MASLD *via* several mechanisms: impaired fiber fermentation, reduced production of protective short-chain fatty acids and accumulation of harmful metabolites like ammonia, disruption of bile acid metabolism, and increased intestinal permeability, inflammation, and endogenous ethanol production. These disturbances collectively contribute to lipid accumulation in the liver, exacerbating the disease.

Changes in microbial composition evolve with disease severity, with species such as *Akkermansia muciniphila* showing protective effects, while others, including *Ruminococcus* and *Proteobacteria*, are linked to advanced fibrosis. Emerging evidence supports the therapeutic potential of probiotics (such as VSL#3) to rebalance the gut microbiota and mitigate MASLD progression by modulating key metabolic pathways. Thus, gut microbiota plays a crucial role in MASLD pathogenesis, serving as both a trigger and a modifiable target for intervention.

Author details

Sandica Bucurica
Carol Davila University of Medicine and Pharmacy, Bucharest, Romania

*Address all correspondence to: sandica.bucurica@umfcd.ro

References

[1] Rinella M et al. A multi society Delphi consensus statement on new fatty liver disease nomenclature. Hepatology. 1 Dec 2023;**78**(6):1966-1986. DOI: 10.1097/HEP.0000000000000520

[2] Hsu CL, Loomba R. From NAFLD to MASLD: Implications of the new nomenclature for preclinical and clinical research. Nature Metabolism. 2024;**6**(4):600-602. DOI: 10.1038/s42255-024-00985-1

[3] Tacke F et al. EASL–EASD–EASO clinical practice guidelines on the management of metabolic dysfunction-associated steatotic liver disease (MASLD). Journal of Hepatology. 2024;**81**(3):492-542. DOI: 10.1016/j.jhep.2024.04.031

[4] Younossi ZM, Golabi P, Paik JM, Henry A, Van Dongen C, Henry L. The global epidemiology of nonalcoholic fatty liver disease (NAFLD) and nonalcoholic steatohepatitis (NASH): A systematic review. Hepatology. 2023;77(4):1335-1347. DOI: 10.1097/HEP.0000000000000004

[5] Quek J et al. Global prevalence of non-alcoholic fatty liver disease and non-alcoholic steatohepatitis in the overweight and obese population: A systematic review and meta-analysis. The Lancet Gastroenterology & Hepatology. 2023;**8**(1):20-30. DOI: 10.1016/S2468-1253(22)00317-X

[6] Le MH et al. Global incidence of non-alcoholic fatty liver disease: A systematic review and meta-analysis of 63 studies and 1,201,807 persons. Journal of Hepatology. 2023;**79**(2):287-295. DOI: 10.1016/j.jhep.2023.03.040

[7] Long Q et al. Gut microbiota and metabolic biomarkers in metabolic dysfunction–associated steatotic liver disease. Hepatology Communications. 2024;**8**(3). DOI: 10.1097/HC9.0000000000000310

[8] Yang K, Song M. New insights into the pathogenesis of metabolic-associated fatty liver disease (MAFLD): Gut–liver–heart crosstalk. Nutrients. 2023;**15**(18):3970. DOI: 10.3390/nu15183970

[9] Magne F et al. The Firmicutes/Bacteroidetes ratio: A relevant marker of gut Dysbiosis in obese patients? Nutrients. 2020;**12**(5):1474. DOI: 10.3390/nu12051474

[10] Ganz M et al. Progression of non-alcoholic steatosis to steatohepatitis and fibrosis parallels cumulative accumulation of danger signals that promote inflammation and liver tumors in a high fat–cholesterol–sugar diet model in mice. Journal of Translational Medicine. 2015;**13**(1):193. DOI: 10.1186/s12967-015-0552-7

[11] Osman HA et al. NLRP3 inflammasome pathway involved in the pathogenesis of metabolic associated fatty liver disease. Scientific Reports. 2024;**14**(1):19648. DOI: 10.1038/s41598-024-69764-y

[12] Colak Y et al. Pathogenetic mechanisms of nonalcoholic fatty liver disease and inhibition of the inflammasome as a new therapeutic target. Clinics and Research in Hepatology and Gastroenterology. 2021;**45**(4):101710. DOI: 10.1016/j.clinre.2021.101710

[13] Swanson KV, Deng M, Ting JP-Y. The NLRP3 inflammasome: Molecular activation and regulation to therapeutics. Nature Reviews. Immunology.

2019;**19**(8):477-489. DOI: 10.1038/s41577-019-0165-0

[14] Ipsen DH, Lykkesfeldt J, Tveden-Nyborg P. Molecular mechanisms of hepatic lipid accumulation in non-alcoholic fatty liver disease. Cellular and Molecular Life Sciences. 2018;**75**(18):3313-3327. DOI: 10.1007/s00018-018-2860-6

[15] Moore MP et al. Compromised hepatic mitochondrial fatty acid oxidation and reduced markers of mitochondrial turnover in human NAFLD. Hepatology. 2022;**76**(5):1452-1465. DOI: 10.1002/hep.32324

[16] Metz M et al. Leptin increases hepatic triglyceride export via a vagal mechanism in humans. Cell Metabolism. 2022;**34**(11):1719-1731.e5. DOI: 10.1016/j.cmet.2022.09.020

[17] Dao AD, Nguyen VH, Ito T, Cheung R, Nguyen MH. Prevalence, characteristics, and mortality outcomes of obese and nonobese MAFLD in the United States. Hepatology International. 2023;**17**(1):225-236. DOI: 10.1007/s12072-022-10436-2

[18] Nassir F. Role of acetylation in nonalcoholic fatty liver disease: A focus on SIRT1 and SIRT3. Exploration of Medicine. 2020;**1**(4):248-258. DOI: 10.37349/emed.2020.00017

[19] Xiaokun Li. FGFR and inhibitors. In: Fibroblast Growth Factors (Second Edition), Academic Press; 2024. pp. 787-908. Available from: https://www.sciencedirect.com/science/ article/pii/B9780443157936000081. DOI: 10.1016/B978-0- 443-15793- 6.00008-1

[20] Henriksson E, Andersen B. FGF19 and FGF21 for the treatment of NASH—Two sides of the same coin? Differential and overlapping effects of FGF19 and FGF21 from mice to human. Frontiers in Endocrinology. 2020;**11**:601349. DOI: 10.3389/fendo.2020.601349

[21] Tian H, Zhang S, Liu Y, Wu Y, Zhang D. Fibroblast growth factors for nonalcoholic fatty liver disease: Opportunities and challenges. International Journal of Molecular Sciences. 2023;**24**(5):4583. DOI: 10.3390/ijms24054583

[22] Tezze C, Romanello V, Sandri M. FGF21 as modulator of metabolism in health and disease. Frontiers in Physiology. 2019;**10**:419. DOI: 10.3389/fphys.2019.00419

[23] Liss KHH, Finck BN. PPARs and nonalcoholic fatty liver disease. Biochimie. 2017;**136**:65-74. DOI: 10.1016/j.biochi.2016.11.009

[24] Fang J et al. Gut dysbiosis in nonalcoholic fatty liver disease: Pathogenesis, diagnosis, and therapeutic implications. Frontiers in Cellular and Infection Microbiology. 2022;**12**:997018. DOI: 10.3389/fcimb.2022.997018

[25] Leviatan S, Shoer S, Rothschild D, Gorodetski M, Segal E. An expanded reference map of the human gut microbiome reveals hundreds of previously unknown species. Nature Communications. 2022;**13**(1):3863. DOI: 10.1038/s41467-022-31502-1

[26] Hou K et al. Microbiota in health and diseases. Signal Transduction and Targeted Therapy. 2022;**7**(1):135. DOI: 10.1038/s41392-022-00974-4

[27] De Filippo C et al. Impact of diet in shaping gut microbiota revealed by a comparative study in children from Europe and rural Africa. Proceedings. National Academy of Sciences. United States of America. 2010;**107**(33):14691-14696. DOI: 10.1073/pnas.1005963107

[28] Vancamelbeke M, Vermeire S. The intestinal barrier: A fundamental role in health and disease. Expert Review of Gastroenterology & Hepatology. 2017;**11**(9):821-834. DOI: 10.1080/17474124.2017.1343143

[29] Liu L et al. Intestinal barrier function in the pathogenesis of nonalcoholic fatty liver disease. Journal of Clinical and Translational Hepatology. 2022;**11**(2):458-452. DOI: 10.14218/JCTH.2022.00089

[30] Mouries J et al. Microbiota-driven gut vascular barrier disruption is a prerequisite for non-alcoholic steatohepatitis development. Journal of Hepatology. 2019;**71**(6):1216-1228. DOI: 10.1016/j.jhep.2019.08.005

[31] Vallianou NG et al. NAFLD/MASLD and the gut–liver Axis: From pathogenesis to treatment options. Metabolites. 2024;**14**(7):366. DOI: 10.3390/metabo14070366

[32] Fasano A. All disease begins in the (leaky) gut: Role of zonulin-mediated gut permeability in the pathogenesis of some chronic inflammatory diseases. F1000Res. 2020;**9**:69. DOI: 10.12688/f1000research.20510.1

[33] Takiishi T, Fenero CIM, Câmara NOS. Intestinal barrier and gut microbiota: Shaping our immune responses throughout life. Tissue Barriers. 2017;**5**(4):e1373208. DOI: 10.1080/21688370.2017.1373208

[34] Bucurica S et al. Estrobolome and hepatocellular adenomas—Connecting the dots of the gut microbial β-Glucuronidase pathway as a metabolic link. International Journal of Molecular Sciences. 2023;**24**(22):16034. DOI: 10.3390/ijms242216034

[35] Ding J-H et al. Role of gut microbiota via the gut-liver-brain axis in digestive diseases. World Journal of Gastroenterology. 2020;**26**(40):40. DOI: 10.3748/wjg.v26.i40.6141

[36] Butler MI, Cryan JF, Dinan TG. Man and the microbiome: A new theory of everything? Annual Review of Clinical Psychology. 2019;**15**(1):1. DOI: 10.1146/annurev-clinpsy-050718-095432

[37] Tripathi A et al. The gut-liver axis and the intersection with the microbiome. Nature Reviews. Gastroenterology & Hepatology. 2018;**15**(7):7. DOI: 10.1038/s41575-018-0011-z

[38] Thursby E, Juge N. Introduction to the human gut microbiota. Biochemical Journal. 2017;**474**(11):1823-1836. DOI: 10.1042/BCJ20160510

[39] Zheng Z, Wang B. The gut-liver Axis in health and disease: The role of gut microbiota-derived signals in liver injury and regeneration. Frontiers in Immunology. 2021;**12**:775526. DOI: 10.3389/fimmu.2021.775526

[40] Wang R, Tang R, Li B, Ma X, Schnabl B, Tilg H. Gut microbiome, liver immunology, and liver diseases. Cellular & Molecular Immunology. 2021;**18**(1):1. DOI: 10.1038/s41423-020-00592-6

[41] Ionita-Radu F et al. Berberine effects in pre-fibrotic stages of non-alcoholic fatty liver disease—Clinical and pre-clinical overview and systematic review of the literature. International Journal of Molecular Sciences. 2024;**25**(8):4201. DOI: 10.3390/ijms25084201

[42] Pouwels S et al. Non-alcoholic fatty liver disease (NAFLD): A review of pathophysiology, clinical management and effects of weight loss. BMC Endocrine Disorders. 2022;**22**(1):63. DOI: 10.1186/s12902-022-00980-1

[43] El-Zayat SR, Sibaii H, Mannaa FA. Toll-like receptors activation, signaling, and targeting: An overview. Bulletin of the National Research Centre. 2019;**43**(1):187. DOI: 10.1186/s42269-019-0227-2

[44] Shen F, Zheng R-D, Sun X-Q, Ding W-J, Wang X-Y, Fan J-G. Gut microbiota dysbiosis in patients with non-alcoholic fatty liver disease. Hepatobiliary & Pancreatic Diseases International. 2017;**16**(4):375-381. DOI: 10.1016/S1499-3872(17)60019-5

[45] Wang B et al. Altered Fecal microbiota correlates with liver biochemistry in nonobese patients with non-alcoholic fatty liver disease. Scientific Reports. 2016;**6**(1):32002. DOI: 10.1038/srep32002

[46] Aron-Wisnewsky J et al. Gut microbiota and human NAFLD: Disentangling microbial signatures from metabolic disorders. Nature Reviews. Gastroenterology & Hepatology. 2020;**17**(5):279-297. DOI: 10.1038/s41575-020-0269-9

[47] Canfora EE, Meex RCR, Venema K, Blaak EE. Gut microbial metabolites in obesity, NAFLD and T2DM. Nature Reviews. Endocrinology. 2019;**15**(5):261-273. DOI: 10.1038/s41574-019-0156-z

[48] Boursier J et al. The severity of nonalcoholic fatty liver disease is associated with gut dysbiosis and shift in the metabolic function of the gut microbiota. Hepatology. 2016;**63**(3):764-775. DOI: 10.1002/hep.28356

[49] Arslan N. Obesity, fatty liver disease and intestinal microbiota. World Journal of Gastroenterology. 2014;**20**(44):16452. DOI: 10.3748/wjg.v20.i44.16452

[50] Yuan J et al. Fatty liver disease caused by high-alcohol-producing Klebsiella pneumoniae. Cell Metabolism. 2019;**30**(4):675-688. DOI: 10.1016/j.cmet.2019.08.018

[51] Li F, Ye J, Shao C, Zhong B. Compositional alterations of gut microbiota in nonalcoholic fatty liver disease patients: A systematic review and meta-analysis. Lipids in Health and Disease. 2021;**20**(1):22. DOI: 10.1186/s12944-021-01440-w

[52] Yang B et al. Screening of the lipid-lowering probiotic Lactiplantibacillus Plantarum SDJ09 and its anti-obesity mechanism. Applied Biochemistry and Biotechnology. 2024. DOI: 10.1007/s12010-024-05034-x

[53] Yang C et al. Characteristics of gut microbiota in patients with metabolic associated fatty liver disease. Scientific Reports. 2023;**13**(1):9988. DOI: 10.1038/s41598-023-37163-4

[54] Jiang W et al. Dysbiosis gut microbiota associated with inflammation and impaired mucosal immune function in intestine of humans with non-alcoholic fatty liver disease. Scientific Reports. 2015;**5**(1):8096. DOI: 10.1038/srep08096

[55] Wang Y et al. Dynamic changes of gut microbiota in mouse models of metabolic dysfunction-associated steatohepatitis and its transition to hepatocellular carcinoma. The FASEB Journal. 2024;**38**(13):e23766. DOI: 10.1096/fj.202400573RR

[56] Ha S, Wong VW-S, Zhang X, Yu J. Interplay between gut microbiome, host genetic and epigenetic modifications in MASLD and MASLD-related hepatocellular carcinoma. Gut. 2024:gutjnl-2024-332398. DOI: 10.1136/gutjnl-2024-332398

[57] Del Chierico F et al. Gut microbiota profiling of pediatric nonalcoholic fatty

liver disease and obese patients unveiled by an integrated meta-omics-based approach. Hepatology. 2017;**65**(2):451-464. DOI: 10.1002/hep.28572

[58] Jadhav K, Cohen TS. Can you trust your gut? Implicating a disrupted intestinal microbiome in the progression of NAFLD/NASH. Frontiers in Endocrinology. 2020;**11**:592157. DOI: 10.3389/fendo.2020.592157

[59] Satapathy SK et al. Characterization of gut microbiome in liver transplant recipients with nonalcoholic Steatohepatitis. Transplantation Direct. 2020;**6**(e612):e625. DOI: 10.1097/TXD.0000000000001033

[60] Mantegazza C, Molinari P, D'Auria E, Sonnino M, Morelli L, Zuccotti GV. Probiotics and antibiotic-associated diarrhea in children: A review and new evidence on lactobacillus rhamnosus GG during and after antibiotic treatment. Pharmacological Research. 2018;**128**:63-72. DOI: 10.1016/j.phrs.2017.08.001

[61] Derrien M, Alvarez A-S, De Vos WM. The gut microbiota in the first decade of life. Trends in Microbiology. 2019;**27**(12):997-1010. DOI: 10.1016/j.tim.2019.08.001

[62] Ritze Y et al. Lactobacillus rhamnosus GG protects against non-alcoholic fatty liver disease in mice. PLoS One. 2014;**9**(1):e80169. DOI: 10.1371/journal.pone.0080169

[63] Ahn SB, Jun DW, Kang B-K, Lim JH, Lim S, Chung M-J. Randomized, double-blind, placebo-controlled study of a multispecies probiotic mixture in nonalcoholic fatty liver disease. Scientific Reports. 2019;**9**(1):5688. DOI: 10.1038/s41598-019-42059-3

[64] Wang G et al. *Bifidobacterium adolescentis* and *lactobacillus rhamnosus* alleviate non-alcoholic fatty liver disease induced by a high-fat, high-cholesterol diet through modulation of different gut microbiota-dependent pathways. Food & Function. 2020;**11**(7):6115-6127. DOI: 10.1039/C9FO02905B

[65] Sun C et al. Lactiplantibacillus plantarum NKK20 alleviates high-fat-diet-induced nonalcoholic fatty liver disease in mice through regulating bile acid anabolism. Molecules. 2023;**28**(10):4042. DOI: 10.3390/molecules28104042

[66] Derosa G et al. Probiotic therapy with VSL#3® in patients with NAFLD: A randomized clinical trial. Frontiers in Nutrition. 2022;**9**:846873. DOI: 10.3389/fnut.2022.846873

[67] Chong PL, Laight D, Aspinall RJ, Higginson A, Cummings MH. A randomised placebo controlled trial of VSL#3® probiotic on biomarkers of cardiovascular risk and liver injury in non-alcoholic fatty liver disease. BMC Gastroenterology. 2021;**21**(1):144. DOI: 10.1186/s12876-021-01660-5

[68] Meroni M, Longo M, Dongiovanni P. The role of probiotics in nonalcoholic fatty liver disease: A new insight into therapeutic strategies. Nutrients. 2019;**11**(11):2642. DOI: 10.3390/nu11112642

[69] Do MH, Oh M-J, Lee H-B, Kang C-H, Yoo G, Park H-Y. Bifidobacterium animalis ssp. lactis MG741 reduces body weight and ameliorates nonalcoholic fatty liver disease via improving the gut permeability and amelioration of inflammatory cytokines. Nutrients. 2022;**14**(9):1965. DOI: 10.3390/nu14091965

[70] Vallianou N, Stratigou T, Christodoulatos GS, Tsigalou C, Dalamaga M. Probiotics, prebiotics,

Synbiotics, Postbiotics, and obesity: Current evidence, controversies, and perspectives. Current Obesity Reports. 2020;**9**(3):179-192. DOI: 10.1007/s13679-020-00379-w

[71] Galeeva JS et al. Microbial signatures in COVID-19: Distinguishing mild and severe disease via gut microbiota. Biomedicine. 2024;**12**(5):996. DOI: 10.3390/biomedicines12050996

[72] Niu H et al. Akkermansia muciniphila: A potential candidate for ameliorating metabolic diseases. Frontiers in Immunology. 2024;**15**:1370658. DOI: 10.3389/fimmu.2024.1370658

[73] Jian H, Liu Y, Wang X, Dong X, Zou X. Akkermansia muciniphila as a next-generation probiotic in modulating human metabolic homeostasis and disease progression: A role mediated by gut–liver–brain axes? International Journal of Molecular Sciences. 2023;**24**(4):3900. DOI: 10.3390/ijms24043900

[74] Villard A, Boursier J, Andriantsitohaina R. Bacterial and eukaryotic extracellular vesicles and nonalcoholic fatty liver disease: New players in the gut-liver axis? American Journal of Physiology-Gastrointestinal and Liver Physiology. 2021;**320**(4):G485-G495. DOI: 10.1152/ajpgi.00362.2020

[75] Gan L et al. Bacteriophage targeting microbiota alleviates non-alcoholic fatty liver disease induced by high alcohol-producing Klebsiella pneumoniae. Nature Communications. 2023;**14**(1):3215. DOI: 10.1038/s41467-023-39028-w

[76] Zhang Y-J, Li S, Gan R-Y, Zhou T, Xu D-P, Li H-B. Impacts of gut bacteria on human health and diseases. International Journal of Molecular Sciences. 2015;**16**(4):7493-7519. DOI: 10.3390/ijms16047493

[77] Caussy C et al. Link between gut-microbiome derived metabolite and shared gene-effects with hepatic steatosis and fibrosis in NAFLD. Hepatology. 2018;**68**(3):918-932. DOI: 10.1002/hep.29892

[78] Dalile B, Van Oudenhove L, Vervliet B, Verbeke K. The role of short-chain fatty acids in microbiota–gut–brain communication. Nature Reviews. Gastroenterology & Hepatology. 2019;**16**(8):461-478. DOI: 10.1038/s41575-019-0157-3

[79] Vallianou N et al. Understanding the role of the gut microbiome and microbial metabolites in non-alcoholic fatty liver disease: Current evidence and perspectives. Biomolecules. 2021;**12**(1):56. DOI: 10.3390/biom12010056

[80] Anania C, Perla FM, Olivero F, Pacifico L, Chiesa C. Mediterranean diet and nonalcoholic fatty liver disease. World Journal of Gastroenterology. 2018;**24**(19):2083-2094. DOI: 10.3748/wjg.v24.i19.2083

[81] Song Y, Guo W, Wang J, Liu S, Li Z, Li Y. Probiotic consumption and hepatic steatosis: Results from the NHANES 2011-2016 and Mendelian randomization study. Frontiers in Nutrition. 2024;**11**:1334935. DOI: 10.3389/fnut.2024.1334935

[82] Alisi A et al. Randomised clinical trial: The beneficial effects of VSL #3 in obese children with non-alcoholic steatohepatitis. Alimentary Pharmacology & Therapeutics. 2014;**39**(11):1276-1285. DOI: 10.1111/apt.12758

[83] Tang Y et al. Effects of probiotics on nonalcoholic fatty

liver disease: A systematic review and meta-analysis. Therapeutic Advances in Gastroenterology. 2019;**12**:1756284819878046. DOI: 10.1177/1756284819878046

[84] Spacova I, Patusco R, Lebeer S, Jensen MG. Influence of biotic interventions on the immune response to vaccines in young and older adults. Clinical Nutrition. 2023;**42**(2):216-226. DOI: 10.1016/j.clnu.2023.01.001

Chapter 3

The Role of the Intestinal Microbiota in NAFLD Onset and Progression

Iris Pinheiro

Abstract

Perturbations in the composition and function of the gut microbiota, termed dysbiosis, are likely to have an impact on nonalcoholic fatty liver disease (NAFLD) onset and progression, and interventions aimed to improve dysbiosis may be of benefit. The existence of a gut-liver axis has long been appreciated. Reports from the 1950s showed that antibiotic treatment delayed cirrhosis in rats fed a choline-deficient diet. More recently, germ-free mice have been shown to be unresponsive to high-fat diet-induced obesity and unable to develop hepatic steatosis. Later, ground-breaking studies demonstrated that obesity is transmissible, that is, germ-free mice that received cecal microbiota collected from obese donors accumulated more fat than those colonized with microbiota from lean donors. An impaired gut microbiota may trigger intestinal inflammation and, consequently, disrupt gut barrier integrity. Following increased intestinal permeability, microbial products can reach the liver to induce hepatic inflammation and liver damage. Presently, numerous luminal metabolites produced or catabolized by intestinal bacteria have been recognized to play key protective or detrimental roles in NAFLD. These include short-chain fatty acids, secondary bile acids, endogenously produced ethanol, and amino acids. In this context, probiotics have been shown to improve liver parameters and other disease outcomes in NAFLD patients and, thus, may offer a promising strategy for the management of the disease.

Keywords: dysbiosis, gut microbiota, gut metabolites, gut-liver axis, NAFLD, NASH

1. Introduction

With the global increase in obesity and related metabolic syndrome, there has been an equally alarming rise in the incidence of nonalcoholic fatty liver disease (NAFLD), the hepatic manifestation of metabolic syndrome, which often co-occurs with obesity, type 2 diabetes mellitus (T2DM), and dyslipidemia (**Figure 1**) [1–3]. NAFLD is the most prevalent chronic liver disease in Western countries, affecting 25% of the population [4]. In the absence of inflammation or fibrosis, it is referred to as isolated steatosis or nonalcoholic fatty liver (NAFL). However, about 20% of NAFL patients will develop nonalcoholic steatohepatitis (NASH) [5], and, as the

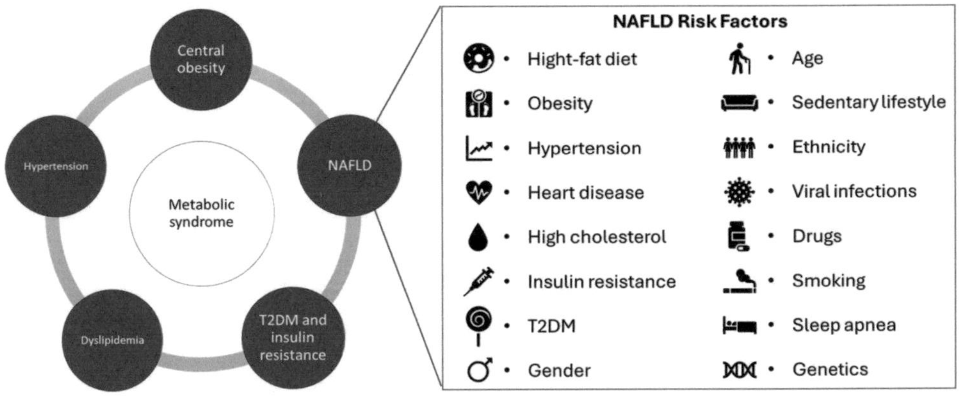

Figure 1.
Metabolic syndrome, NAFLD, and associated risk factors. Metabolic syndrome is a cluster of conditions that co-occur, and which increase the risk of coronary heart disease and stroke. NAFLD is the hepatic manifestation of the metabolic syndrome. NAFLD pathophysiology is multifactorial, involving ecological, genetic, metabolic, and social factors, including a Western diet, a sedentary lifestyle, and smoking.

name indicates, this stage is characterized by the presence of liver steatosis (abnormal accumulation of lipids within the liver), hepatocyte injury (ballooning) [6], and inflammatory alterations, namely, infiltration of immune cells, and production of inflammatory cytokines and reactive oxygen species (ROS) [7]. Ultimately, within a fraction of NASH patients, the disease will progress toward liver cirrhosis and hepatocellular carcinoma (HCC) [1].

Although the pathogenesis of NAFLD is not completely understood, it was first described as a "two-hit" disease. The first "hit" relates to lipid accumulation with ensuing dyslipidemia, obesity, insulin resistance, and dysfunction in adipokine secretion. The second "hit" relates to the subsequent inflammatory alterations, and these are a combination of oxidative stress, lipid peroxidation, mitochondrial dysfunction, bile acid toxicity, chemokine-mediated cell recruitment, and retention of inflammatory cells [8]. However, this model has generated criticism over the years. In the first instance, it is too simplistic to fully describe the pathogenesis of this disease [9]. NAFL and NASH pathophysiology is multifactorial, involving ecological, genetic, metabolic, and social factors, including a Western diet, a sedentary lifestyle, and smoking (**Figure 1**) [10]. Secondly, the idea that steatosis always precedes NASH may be questioned as animal studies have found that inflammation can aggravate hepatic lipid accumulation, suggesting that steatosis may succeed inflammation [11, 12]. Hence, recent hypotheses describe NAFLD pathogenesis as a "multi-hit" model [13], which combines nutritional and environmental factors that together participate in disease onset and progression in genetically predisposed individuals. One of these "multiple hits" comprises the intestinal microbiota.

2. NAFLD: a progressive disease

NAFLD is a chronic liver disease characterized by hepatic fat accumulation in the absence of alcohol abuse (<20 g/day) and other identifiable causes, and it is tightly associated with insulin resistance. It is the most common liver disorder worldwide, particularly in developed countries. The highest rates are described in South America and the Middle East, and then in Asia, the USA, and Europe [14]. NAFLD is prevalent in >90% of obese people, 60% of diabetics, and up to 20% of normal-weight subjects, and it is the leading cause of chronic liver disease and the second most common reason for liver transplant in the USA and Europe. However, NAFLD is an umbrella term used to describe a range of related disorders that represent a continuum spectrum of pathologies that culminate in HCC and liver failure [15, 16]. Generally, the first stage of disease is hepatic steatosis, which is typified by the deposition of triglycerides (TG) as droplets within hepatocytes. Steatosis is described as the presence of hepatic TG levels above 55 mg/g of liver, or the presence of cytoplasmic TG droplets in >5% of hepatocytes. Hepatic steatosis is a self-limiting disorder, but it can evolve into NASH, which distinguishes itself from isolated steatosis by the presence of hepatocyte injury (ballooning and cell death), and by the presence of inflammatory infiltrates and/or collagen deposition (fibrosis). In addition, NASH can progress to cirrhosis, which can occur within 10 years in 10–29% of individuals with NASH [15]. In cirrhosis, hepatocytes are replaced by fibrotic tissue composed mainly of type I collagen. This is produced by stellate cells, which are activated upon liver injury. These cells are fundamental for liver regeneration but are also responsible for liver fibrosis. Ultimately, cirrhosis may, in time, advance to liver cancer.

3. The pathogenesis of steatosis

Hepatic steatosis arises from an imbalance between fat (i.e., triglycerides) acquisition and removal (**Figures 2** and **3**). TGs are the stored form of fatty acids and are assembled by coupling three fatty acids to a glycerol backbone *via* ester bonds. The fatty acids used for hepatic TG assembly originate from three sources: (i) diet, (ii) adipose tissue, and (iii) hepatic *de novo* synthesis (**Figure 3**). Dietary fats taken up in the intestine are packaged into TG-rich chylomicrons and delivered systemically. These TG are then hydrolyzed by the enzyme lipoprotein lipase (LPL), thereby releasing free-fatty acids (FFA) for uptake by peripheral tissues, among which the liver. FFA is also stored in the white adipose tissue (WAT) in the form of TG, that is, bound to glycerol. During fasting or exercise, lipolysis (i.e., the hydrolysis of TG

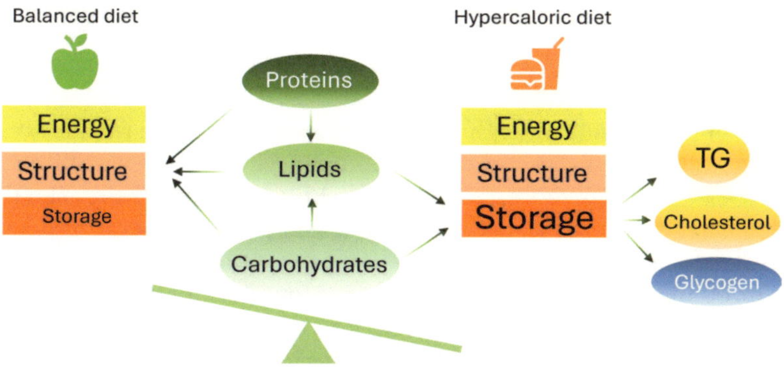

Figure 2.
Progression of liver steatosis. Liver steatosis occurs when there is an excessive caloric intake. In a balanced diet, nutrients (proteins, lipids, carbohydrates) are mostly used for energy production and for the synthesis of cellular structures. Only a small quantity of these nutrients is stored during the fed state to be used during fasted periods. In contrast, a continuous hypercaloric diet is associated with the storage of excess calories. Because cells have a limited capacity to store carbohydrates in the form of glycogen, proteins, and carbohydrates are converted into fatty acids, which are then stored in the form of triglycerides and cholesterol. Figure adapted with permission from Ref. [17].

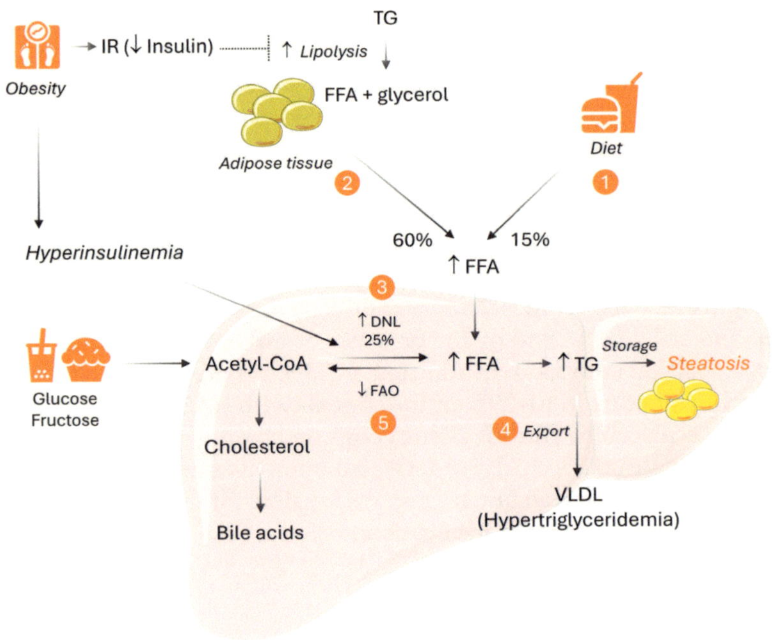

Figure 3.
Sources of increased triglycerides in the liver. Sources of liver fat include: (1) excessive dietary fat intake and delivery of FFA to the liver; (2) excessive FFA influx to the liver from adipose tissue lipolysis; (3) enhanced intrahepatic TG synthesis from de novo *lipogenesis (DNL); (4) diminished export of lipids from the liver; and (5) reduced fatty acid oxidation (FAO). DNL is the metabolic process by which acetyl-CoA is converted to TG for storage in fat. DNL facilitates the synthesis of saturated fatty acids that are esterified to TG to be stored within hepatocytes or, alternatively, packaged into VLDL to be secreted into circulation (and subsequently used in peripheral organs or stored within adipocytes). Thus, the fate of newly formed lipids is to be oxidized, or to be esterified to TG (by incorporation with glycerol), incorporated into VLDL, secreted into systemic circulation, and delivered to peripheral tissues. Insulin secreted by the pancreas regulates these processes: on the one hand, insulin inhibits lipolysis in the adipose tissue leading to a decrease in the delivery of FFA and glycerol to the liver; on the other hand, it promotes DNL. When insulin resistance is installed, lipolysis cannot be inhibited, and the delivery of FFA to the liver increases. CoA: coenzyme A; DNL:* de novo *lipogenesis; FAO: fatty acid oxidation; FFA: free-fatty acids; IR: insulin resistance; TG: triglycerides; VLDL: very-low-density lipoprotein. Figure adapted with permission from Refs. [15, 18].*

into glycerol and FFA) within the WAT is used to mobilize stored energy, thereby releasing FFA into circulation, which will also reach the liver. Finally, carbohydrate feeding promotes *de novo* synthesis of FFA from acetyl-coenzyme A (CoA), a process which is facilitated by insulin and glucose *via* activation of sterol regulatory element-binding protein-1c (SREBP-1c) and carbohydrate responsive element-binding protein (ChREBP), respectively (reviewed in Ref. [15]). FFA in the liver have then three major fates: (i) they can be oxidized in the mitochondria to produce energy and ketone bodies, (ii) they can be re-esterified into TG to be stored in the liver, or (iii) be integrated into apolipoproteins and exported as part of very-low-density lipoproteins (VLDL) (**Figure 3**). Therefore, mutations or malfunctions that impede/prevent removal of TG from the liver, mobilization of FFA from lipid droplets, mitochondrial fatty acid oxidation (FAO), or assembly of TG into functional VLDL particles, do lead to an increase in hepatic steatosis. Thus, in summary, processes that increase hepatic FFA and TG input or reduce FFA and TG output result in hepatic steatosis [15]. Diet composition also impacts hepatic fat deposition. Not only carbohydrates, but particularly fructose, are critical. Fructose consumption conveys dietary carbons directly to the liver to prime *de novo* lipogenesis (DNL) (**Figure 3**). Unlike glucose, circulating fructose is taken up almost entirely by the liver, and cannot be stored in the form of glycogen. Therefore, fructose consumption provides a direct substrate for DNL. The yearly average consumption of fructose has progressively increased in Western countries, thereby most likely contributing to the increased prevalence of NAFLD [15].

4. From NAFL to NASH

Among NAFL patients some will progress to NASH, but the reason why only a fraction of steatotic patients progress to a more severe form of the disease is not totally understood. As outlined above, the excessive accumulation of fat in the liver in the form of TG leads to steatosis. However, in the liver, FFA can also be incorporated into phospholipids and other lipid forms, and these moieties of intracellular fat can have distinct toxic effects. Although arguable, hepatic accumulation of neutral cholesterol esters and TG can be relatively neutral [19–21], but some intermediate products may have more deleterious effects on liver cells. Intermediate lipid products such as diacylglycerol and phospholipids (ceramides and sphingolipids) account for the fatty-acid-induced toxicity and hepatic insulin resistance. This accumulation of

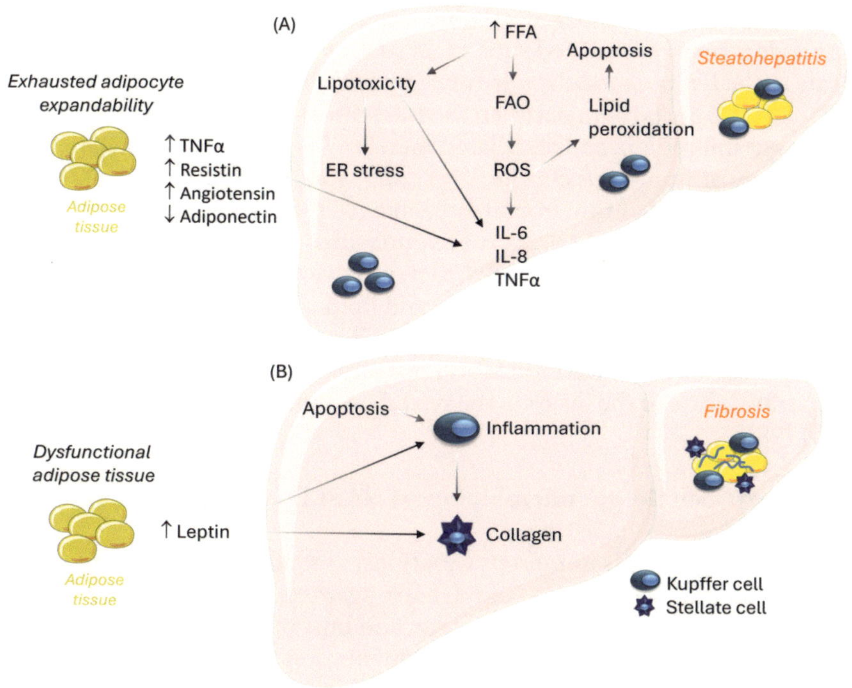

Figure 4.
Hallmarks of steatohepatitis (A) and progression to fibrosis (B). (A) The adipose tissue protects the body from excessive exposure to fatty acids by storing them. When adipocyte expandability is exhausted, allied to peripheral insulin resistance, the adipose tissue acquires a pro-inflammatory profile (i.e., suppression of adiponectin, promotion of adipokines) and once in the liver, these will lead to the activation of Kupffer cells and to the production of inflammatory mediators, such as IL-6, IL-8, and TNFα. (B) This increase in hepatic inflammation, together with the accumulation of lipid toxic species, ROS, and ER stress, will ultimately lead to the activation of stellate cells, and to the progression of liver damage. ER: endoplasmic reticulum; FAO: fatty acid oxidation; FFA: free-fatty acids; IL: interleukin; ROS: reactive oxygen species; TNFα: tumor necrosis factor-alpha. Figure adapted with permission from Ref. [18].

lipid toxic species associated with an altered adipokine profile are suggested to play a pivotal role in the initiation and perpetuation of NASH pathology [22]. The adipose tissue contributes to the systemic production of inflammatory mediators such as interleukin (IL)-6 and tumor necrosis factor (TNF)α, which will alter the inflammatory tone in the liver. In addition, the steady increase in FFA β-oxidation as the result of installed hepatic insulin resistance generates ROS that will activate inflammation and initiate lipid peroxidation. Consequently, necrosis and apoptosis of hepatocytes activate Kupffer cells, thereby perpetuating inflammation and stimulating stellate cells. Stellate cells, in turn, will produce excess amounts of collagen, leading to fibrosis (**Figures 3** and **4**) [15, 18].

5. Microbiota and the gut-liver axis

The gut and the liver communicate *via* a tight bidirectional crosstalk through the biliary tract, portal vein, and systemic circulation. This bidirectional crosstalk is termed the gut-liver axis [23]. The liver is intrinsically connected to the intestines: it receives 70% of its blood supply *via* the portal vein and offers primary metabolism for the gastrointestinal luminal contents [24, 25]. In addition, the liver releases bile salts and other bioactive mediators into the biliary tract and systemic circulation. In the intestine, host and microbes metabolize dietary and environmental components, as well as endogenously produced substrates such as bile acids, the products of which translocate to the liver to modulate its function [26]. Therefore, due to the direct connection *via* the portal vein between the intestines and the liver, it is not surprising that the gut microbiota and associated metabolites have been implicated in the pathophysiology of numerous chronic liver conditions such as NAFLD [27]. The liver transports bile salts and antimicrobial molecules to the intestinal lumen through the biliary tract. Bile salts not only serve as emulsifiers, but they also maintain gut homeostasis by controlling unrestricted bacterial overgrowth. Bile acids also act as signaling molecules modulating glucose and lipid metabolism and hepatic bile acid synthesis (further details below). On the other direction, gut luminal products such as microbial-derived metabolites and microbial-associated molecular patterns (MAMPs) translocate to the liver via the portal vein to influence liver functions (**Figure** 5) [28].

5.1 The link between the gut microbiota and NAFLD

The gut microbiome has numerous functions, among which are nutrition, immune modulation, metabolism, and defense against pathogens. Short-chain fatty acids (SCFA), including acetate, propionate, and butyrate, are the main bacterial metabolites produced upon carbohydrate fermentation and are of major importance for the maintenance of gut immune and metabolic homeostasis [29]. In addition, the gut microbiota affects hepatic carbohydrate and lipid metabolism and impacts the balance between pro-inflammatory and anti-inflammatory mediators in the liver. Therefore, perturbations in the composition and function of the gut microbiota, termed dysbiosis, are likely to have an impact on NAFL and progression to NASH [1]. This impairment of the gut microbiota triggers intestinal inflammation and consequently disrupts gut barrier integrity. Microbial products can then reach the liver to induce hepatic inflammation and liver damage (**Figure** 5) [30]. The transmissibility of an obesogenic gut microbiome has been elegantly demonstrated in germ-free

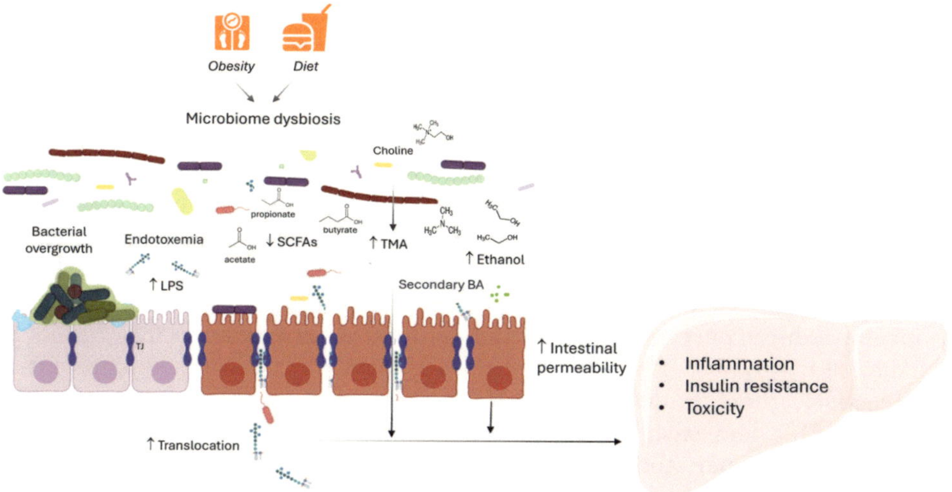

Figure 5.
Role of the gut microbiome and microbiota-derived compounds on the development and progression of NAFL/NASH. The pathogenesis of NAFLD is not fully understood but involves complex interactions among genetic susceptibility variants and environmental factors, such as obesity and a high-fat diet, which will induce intestinal microbial dysbiosis and increase intestinal permeability. The mechanisms by which the gut microbiota and its metabolites contribute to disease include alterations in SCFAs and choline metabolism, endogenous ethanol production, release of pro-inflammatory mediators, endotoxemia, and bile acid metabolism. These will in turn contribute to liver inflammation, toxicity, and insulin resistance. BA: bile acids; LPS: lipopolysaccharides; SCFAs: short-chain fatty acids; TMA: trimethylamine.

animals: mice receiving cecal microbiome from obese (*ob/ob*) mice had a greater increase in body fat over time when compared to mice colonized with microbiota collected from lean donors [31]. In addition, germ-free mice inoculated with stools from NASH patients suffered from aggravated hepatic steatosis and inflammation when fed a high-fat diet (HFD), when compared to animals receiving feces from healthy subjects [32]. Altogether, these studies suggest that an altered microbiome in combination with an obesogenic diet can contribute to disease onset and aggravate liver disease.

5.2 Microbiota composition and NAFLD

Accumulating evidence indicates that decreased microbial diversity correlates with obesity and NAFLD [33, 34]. However, microbiota studies in human NASH are scarce, and only a limited number of reports have demonstrated an association between gut dysbiosis and NASH [34]. Recently, *Bacteroides* and *Prevotella* were found to be significantly differently abundant in feces collected from NASH patients [35]. But, whereas *Bacteroides* showed higher abundance, *Prevotella* proportions were lower. This imbalance is likely influenced by the Western diet, rich in fat, animal proteins, and sugar, which favors the growth of *Bacteroides* [36]. In pediatric populations, the results are somewhat contrasting to the adult population. For instance, one study found that Proteobacteria, Enterobacteriaceae, and *Escherichia* were the only phylum, family, and genus significantly higher in NASH patients when compared to healthy controls and obese subjects [37]. Pediatric NASH patients also showed decreased levels of *Alistipes*, *Blautia*, *Coprococcus*, *Eubacterium*, *Oscillospira*, and *Bifidobacterium*. However, in contrast to adults, pediatric patients showed a significant increase in

Prevotella [37]. Another study performed in children with NASH, found decreased levels of *Oscillospira* and, like in adults, an increase in *Ruminococcus* [33]. Other genera that were significantly different in pediatric NASH patients included an increase in *Dorea* and *Blautia* when compared to healthy counterparts [33]. These discrepancies between studies may be partially explained by the small sample size, differences in age (adults *vs* children), diet, and diagnostic criteria [30]. The most consistent finding among different studies is that patients with NASH have an increased abundance of alcohol-producing bacteria, and increased blood ethanol levels, when compared to NAFL patients and healthy subjects, thus suggesting a possible role for alcohol-producing bacteria in the pathogenesis of NASH [37, 38]. However, a role for the insulin-induced decrease in alcohol dehydrogenase activity in the liver cannot be excluded [39].

Collectively, these studies suggest that a correlation between bacterial composition and NAFLD does exist; however, no consistent microbiota signature has, so far, been identified. Human studies are sparse and limited by the lack of reproducibility between cohorts and the absence of mechanistic demonstration of the presence of dysbiosis and its effects on NAFLD [1]. However, some hypotheses have been raised, and most likely, there is no single bacterium, metabolite, or mode of action responsible for disease progression, but a collection of multiple hits that together contribute to pathology.

5.3 Intestinal microbiota and NASH progression

As previously mentioned, as a consequence of gut microbial dysbiosis there is an increase in the translocation of bacterial products and metabolic mediators from the gut lumen into circulation, favoring hepatic inflammation and the development/progression of NAFLD [6]. Small intestinal bacterial overgrowth (SIBO), increased intestinal permeability, and a number of bacterial derived metabolites and endotoxins, have been reported as potential factors contributing to NAFLD progression (**Figure 5**) [40].

5.3.1 Intestinal barrier dysfunction and SIBO

The intestinal epithelial barrier is not a mere static physical barrier, but a place that continuously interacts with the gut microbiome and underlying mucosal immune cells [41]. The intestinal barrier is fundamental to protect the host against the invasion of microorganisms and toxins but also as the site of absorption of fluids and nutrients [42]. Dysregulation of this barrier, with concomitant disruption of tight junction functionality, leads to what is known as "leaky gut", a phenomenon that is accompanied by microbial translocation from the intestinal lumen to the liver and to the bloodstream [43]. Besides tight junctions, the intestinal barrier is further strengthened by several additional lines of defense, and disruption of any of these barrier components compromises gut barrier integrity. These include (i) mucins, protein aggregates that form a barrier between the luminal bacteria and the epithelium [44]; (ii) antibacterial peptides, such as regenerating islet-derived protein III-gamma (REG3γ), produced by intestinal Paneth cells [45, 46]; (iii) immunoglobulins, in particular secretory (s)IgA, produced by plasma cells, aimed to neutralize bacterial enterotoxins and to inhibit pathogen attachment to the gastrointestinal epithelium, thereby preventing bacterial colonization and cell invasion [47]; and (iv) commensal microbes associated with the gut mucosa; they support barrier integrity *via* toll-like receptor (TLR) signaling [46, 48], or by producing metabolites that reinforce tight junctions and inhibit the growth of other microbes. A meta-analysis based on five clinical studies showed that NAFL and NASH patients are more likely to have increased gut permeability. This association is stronger in NASH patients [49]. In animals, increased intestinal permeability induced by dextran sulfate sodium led to systemic translocation of lipopolysaccharide (LPS; also referred to as endotoxin) and thereby worsened liver inflammation and fibrosis in mice receiving HFD, suggesting a role for barrier dysfunction in disease severity and NASH development [50].

Liver damage is associated with small intestinal bacterial overgrowth (SIBO) [51] and microbial dysbiosis of the lower gastrointestinal tract [52]. SIBO is defined as the total bacteria growth of more than 10^5 colony-forming units per milliliter of intestinal fluid [53]. SIBO occurs with high incidence in patients with NAFLD, ranging from 50% to 78% [51, 54, 55], which is higher when compared to healthy subjects (21%). SIBO is accompanied by significantly higher endotoxin levels [56], elevated concentrations of pro-inflammatory cytokines such as IL-8, and disrupted metabolic activity of the intestinal microbiota [55], which may affect intestinal barrier function and lead to microbial translocation [57]. Thus, compromised intestinal permeability and SIBO result in increased bacterial translocation into the portal circulation. In turn, microbe-associated molecular patterns (MAMPs) induce hepatic inflammation through pattern recognition receptors on Kupffer cells and hepatic stellate cells (HSCs). For instance, LPS is a Gram-negative bacterial cell wall component that can translocate, upon barrier disruption, from the gut lumen to the portal vein and liver. Although it is not clear whether altered permeability is a cause or consequence of endotoxin exposure, once in the liver, LPS is recognized by TLR4 and its co-receptors, thereby activating a downstream pro-inflammatory cascade [30]. Consistently, systemic LPS levels are significantly elevated in NAFLD in both human and animal models [58–61]. TLR4 signaling also leads to increased production of ROS and TNFα, which in turn promote the recruitment of inflammatory cells and activation of HSCs, the major contributors to fibrosis. This results in the expression of inflammatory cytokines, oxidative and endoplasmic reticulum (ER) stress, and subsequent liver damage. Other TLRs have also been implicated in the development of NASH, including TLR9 [62] and TLR2 [63], which recognize bacterial DNA and peptidoglycan (a surface component of Gram-positive bacteria), respectively. In contrast, other TLRs, such as TLR5, which recognizes bacterial flagellin, have been shown to be protective [64, 65]. For instance, TLR5 knock-out mice exhibited hyperphagia and developed hallmark features of metabolic syndrome, including hyperlipidemia, hypertension, insulin resistance, and increased adiposity [65]. Moreover, mice lacking TLR5 on hepatocytes showed exacerbated disease upon methionine- and choline-deficient diet and HFD [64]. In addition, a recent study associated SIBO with significantly higher steatosis and fibrosis grade, as well as lobular and portal inflammation [66]. Due to the technical difficulty of sampling the small intestinal microbiota and associated metabolites, the exact composition and metabolism of microbiota overgrowing in the small intestine of NAFLD patients, which could contribute to disease progression, have not been established so far. Nevertheless, it is known that the energy metabolism of small intestinal bacteria is dominated by carbohydrate metabolism [67]. Increased fructose consumption, which has become increasingly dominant in the Western diet, is associated with DNL, and this has been proposed to be further enhanced by bacterial small intestinal turnover of fructose into acetate, a precursor of lipogenic acetyl-CoA [68]. In addition, metabolization of fructose in the small intestine has also been linked to intestinal epithelial barrier deterioration [69]. Therefore, the role of small intestinal bacteria, whether associated with SIBO or not, is certainly of relevance in NAFLD but remains largely unexplored.

5.3.2 Gut microbiota-derived metabolites and NAFLD

Inflammation is a distinctive feature of NASH pathogenesis, and it is most likely resulting from numerous triggers including visceral ethanol production, and release of toxins and inflammatory mediators. Well-described products from microbial intestinal metabolism include SCFAs, tryptophan catabolites (e.g., indole, tryptamine), and secondary bile acids [70]. In this regard, dysbiosis can tip the balance to an increase in the production of harmful metabolites, which in turn will promote inflammation and hepatic lipid accumulation. Among the intestinal metabolic changes that presumably promote NASH pathology, an increase in ethanol, endotoxins, phenylacetic acid (PAA), and the choline and L-carnitine degradation by-product trimethylamine (TMA) have been described. In contrast, a NAFLD gut microbial dysbiotic state has been associated with a diminished catabolism of tryptophan into beneficial by-products (**Table 1**) [71–73].

Type	Metabolites	Effect on the host
Choline metabolites	TMA → TMAO	Liver triglycerides accumulation Lipogenesis Cardiovascular disease
	Choline	Export of hepatic VLDL
Toxins	Ethanol and LPS	Impaired gut barrier ROS and hepatic inflammation
Amino acids	PAA, BCAA	Hepatic steatosis
Bile acids	DCA, LCA	Bile acid and lipid homeostasis GLP-1 secretion and insulin release Glucose homeostasis
Tryptophan catabolites	IAA, IPA	Decrease lipid synthesis Improve gut barrier Decrease hepatic inflammation
SCFA	Acetate, propionate, butyrate	Improve gut barrier Decrease inflammation and immunomodulation GLP-1 secretion and insulin release PYY release Gluconeogenesis Lipogenesis Energy harvest

Legend: BCAA: branched-chain amino acids; DCA: deoxycholic acid; GLP-1: Glucagon-like peptide 1; IAA: indoleacetic acid; IPA: indolepropionic acid; LCA: lithocholic acid; LPS: lipopolysaccharides; PAA: phenylacetic acid; PYY: peptide YY; ROS: reactive oxygen species; SCFA: short-chain fatty acids; TMA: trimethylamine; TMAO: trimethylamine N-oxide; VLDL: very-low-density lipoprotein.

Table 1.
The role of gut microbiota-derived metabolites in NAFLD. NAFLD is characterized by an increase in deleterious metabolites and toxins such as ethanol, LPS, PAA, and TMA. In contrast, beneficial metabolites such as choline are decreasing (due to higher conversion into TMA), as well as beneficial products of tryptophan catabolism such as IAA and IPA, bile acids, and SCFAs.

5.3.3 The dual role of short-chain fatty acids in NAFLD

Complex carbohydrates, such as fibers and resistant starches, are metabolized by numerous gut bacterial species resulting in the production of SCFAs, such as butyrate, propionate, and acetate. These can have numerous fates: they may be used by other bacteria during cross-feeding or be absorbed by colonic epithelial cells to produce energy (e.g., butyrate). They may also be transported *via* the portal vein to be metabolized by hepatocytes. Small amounts of SCFAs can bypass the liver and be found at low concentrations in systemic circulation. Besides their role as a source of nutrients and energy, SCFAs are also precursors for lipogenesis and gluconeogenesis [74]. Acetate can be oxidized in the Krebs cycle or be used as substrate for the synthesis of cholesterol, ketone bodies, and long-chain fatty acids; butyrate is presumed to participate in mitochondrial FAO and the resultant acetyl-CoA may be used in similar pathways as acetate; propionate, on the other hand, is a well-known precursor for gluconeogenesis in the liver [75, 76]. Despite these unwanted effects, SCFAs have also demonstrated health benefits, such as promoting the production of anorexigenic (i.e., satiety-inducing) hormones such as Peptide YY (PYY) and Glucagon-like peptide 1 (GLP-1) and decreasing intestinal barrier permeability and inflammatory responses. For example, butyrate and propionate have long-described anti-inflammatory effects in the intestine [77]. In contrast, colonic inflammation negatively impacts the abundance of SCFA-producing bacteria; for instance, a reduction in *Faecalibacterium,* a genus containing species capable of producing butyrate, has been described in NASH patients [78]. Moreover, sodium butyrate has been shown to reduce HFD-induced NASH in mice, possibly by restoring gut microbial eubiosis and enhancing the gastrointestinal barrier [79]. Interestingly, overweight and obese people have higher stool levels of propionate, suggesting that either propionate is overly produced or absorption is impaired [80]. Nonetheless, in overweight human adults, propionate has been shown to prevent weight gain and improve insulin resistance [81]. SCFAs exert their biological functions mainly *via* the activation of G-protein coupled receptors 41 and 43 (GPR41, GPR43). These are well expressed not only in the intestine but also in the liver, and their activation has been shown to attenuate insulin resistance in murine models [71]. Through its inhibitory activity on histone deacetylases, SCFAs suppress inflammation [82–84], an effect which may be of benefit in steatohepatitis; in addition, SCFAs could also improve liver health by downregulating insulin signaling in adipocytes. Thus, the apparently opposing roles of SCFAs in liver health could result from imbalanced caloric intake and energy expenditure associated with modern lifestyles. This hypothesis postulates that if a balance between caloric intake and energy expenditure is preserved, SCFAs will benefit liver function. Thus, in conclusion, increasing intestinal microbial SCFA production to beneficial levels can prevent the progression of steatosis to hepatic inflammation.

5.3.4 The detrimental effects of endogenous ethanol production

NASH patients and *ob/ob* mice devoid of alcohol consumption, do show higher levels of ethanol in the blood and breath, a phenomenon accompanied by the upregulation of the enzymes aldehyde dehydrogenase and Cytochrome P450 2E1 (CYP2E1) [85]. This suggests that endogenous ethanol may be involved in NASH pathogenesis. Endogenous ethanol is produced by gut bacteria upon carbohydrate fermentation, and this will stimulate hepatic oxidative stress and inflammation [37, 86]. *Escherichia coli*, *Enterobacteriaceae* spp., and *Klebsiella pneumonia* are alcohol-producing bacteria found to be relatively abundant in NASH patients [37, 87]. In addition, alcohol can be further metabolized into acetaldehyde, which promotes hepatic injury [88] and induces an increase in intestinal permeability, with ensuing endotoxemia, thus further exacerbating hepatic inflammation [89]. Although the exact effects of endogenously produced ethanol in NASH progression are not fully elucidated, these findings indicate that it may play a pivotal role in disease pathogenesis.

5.3.5 Imbalanced amino acids metabolism in NAFLD

Amino acid imbalance has been described in NAFLD [90, 91]. The ratio of branched-chain amino acids (BCAAs) to aromatic amino acids (AAA) is a diagnostic marker of liver dysfunction, with a declining ratio indicative of liver impairment [92]. For instance, phenylacetic acid (PAA) is an AAA-derived metabolite produced by gut bacteria. This has been described to promote hepatic steatosis by inhibiting AKT/Protein Kinase B phosphorylation [90]. Interestingly, *Bacteroides* spp. are likely the major contributors to microbial-mediated PAA production from phenylalanine in humans [93]. Despite some reports that BCAA can inhibit hepatic TG deposition, reduce ER stress, and enhance gut barrier function [90], others suggest that they can also cause hepatic damage due to abnormal lipolysis [94]. *Prevotella copri* and *Bacteroides vulgatus* were suggested to be the leading species fueling the association between the synthesis of BCAAs and insulin resistance in mice. *Prevotella copri* was shown to induce insulin resistance, aggravate glucose intolerance, and augment circulating levels of BCAAs [95]. It is possible, that similarly to SCFAs, an overproduction of BCAAs will tip the balance to a pathogenic outcome.

In contrast to phenylalanine, numerous tryptophan catabolites have been associated with positive outcomes in liver inflammation and lipogenesis [96]. Indole derivatives including indoleacrylic acid, indoleacetic acid, indolealdehyde, indolelactic acid, and indolepropionic acid, constitute, along with tryptamine, the main tryptophan catabolites produced by gut bacteria, including *Bacteroides* spp., *Eubacterium* spp., and *Clostridium* spp. [97, 98]. Among these, indoleacetic acid and tryptamine were found to be depleted in mice upon HFD intake, and whereas both catabolites were able to attenuate markers of inflammation, indoleacetic acid was also able to decrease cytokine-mediated lipogenesis in hepatocytes [96]. This was shown to be mediated by a reduction in hepatic fatty acid synthase (FAS) and the transcription factor SREBP1c (both regulators of lipogenesis) *via* binding to the aryl hydrocarbon receptor. A low abundance of indolepropionic acid has also been reported in obese patients, and its supplementation led to a reduction in weight gain in an animal model of antibiotic-induced dysbiosis [99]. In addition, indolepropionic acid was shown to improve intestinal barrier function *via* Pregnane X receptor, which in turn inhibited endotoxin-induced TLR4 signaling and improved tissue inflammation [100, 101]. Importantly, Ritze et al. [102] reported that tryptophan supplementation significantly reduced hepatic lipid accumulation, while it increased the expression of occludin in a mouse model of NAFLD. In addition, Bansal and colleagues [103] showed that indole reduced TNFα-induced NF-κB and IL-8, while it promoted IL-10 production and increased tight junction expression. Altogether, these studies suggest that tryptophan-derived metabolites of microbial origin are potential therapeutic targets in NAFLD.

5.3.6 The dual fate of choline in NAFLD

Choline is an essential nutrient that can be metabolized to phosphatidylcholine, which is required for VLDL assembly and hepatic lipid export.

Most phosphatidylcholine is derived from dietary choline, and therefore, choline deficiency affects lipid metabolism [104]. Choline-deficient diets are thus commonly used to induce NAFLD in animals. These animals display decreased VLDL levels and β-oxidation, resulting in cholesterol and fatty acids accumulation in the liver, with a concomitant increase in oxidative stress and inflammation. However, choline may also be metabolized to trimethylamine (TMA) by bacterial species such as *Proteus penneri*, *Escherichia fergusonii*, and *Proteus mirabilis*, which can cleave the C-N bond of choline [105]. TMA is subsequently transported to the liver to be oxidized by hepatic flavin-containing monooxygenases into trimethylamine-N-oxide (TMAO). TMAO has been described to contribute to various metabolic diseases, such as cardiovascular disease, T2DM, and NAFLD [106]. Previous studies reported that NAFLD patients exhibit elevated TMAO serum levels, which were positively correlated with the pathological progression of NAFLD [107]. In addition, a dysbiotic microbiota that promotes conversion of choline to methylamines such as TMA can result in choline deficiency and thereby contribute to NASH. Actually, it has been shown that NAFLD is associated with reduced phosphatidylcholine and higher circulating levels of TMA, implicating a role for the gut microbiota in imbalanced choline metabolic flux [108].

5.3.7 Bile acids as important signaling molecules in NAFLD

Bile acids are derived from cholesterol and are synthesized in the liver through a series of reaction steps involving at least 17 different enzymes [109]. The hepatic synthesis of bile acids can be done *via* two pathways: the classical (or neutral) pathway, which accounts for about 90% of the bile acid pool in humans, and the alternative (or acidic) pathway, which, under normal conditions, contributes to about 10% of the bile acid pool. The classical pathway is initiated by 7α-hydroxylation of cholesterol, a reaction catalyzed by cholesterol 7α-hydroxylase (CYP7A1). The alternative pathway is initiated by sterol-27-hydroxylase (CYP27A1); the intermediary 27-hydroxycholesterol is then further hydroxylated by oxysterol 7α-hydroxylase (CYP7B1). All these enzymes have been shown to be regulated by gut microbes (reviewed in Ref. [109]). While the alternative pathway mainly generates chenodeoxycholic acid (CDCA), the classical pathway produces both cholic acid (CA) and CDCA. The ratio between these two primary bile acids is established by the enzyme sterol 12α-hydroxylase (CYP8B1), required for CA synthesis; this enzyme has been shown not to be under microbial regulation [110]. Following synthesis, the liver conjugates bile acids with glycine or taurine in a two-step reaction mediated by the enzymes bile acid CoA-ligase (BAL) and bile acid CoA: amino acid N-acyltransferase (BAT). Conjugated bile acids are then referred to as bile salts, and this process facilitates solubility and transport. Conjugated bile acids are actively transported into bile and stored in the gallbladder; they are then released in the duodenum upon meal ingestion. This will facilitate emulsification and absorption of dietary lipids and fat-soluble vitamins. Approximately 95% of bile acids are reabsorbed from the intestine, predominantly in conjugated forms in the distal ileum, and recirculated *via* the portal vein back to the liver. This process is denominated enterohepatic circulation and occurs about six times a day in humans. In the small and large intestines, the remaining conjugated bile acids can be rapidly deconjugated by bacterial bile salt hydrolases (BSHs). Deconjugation, that is, removal of glycine or taurine conjugates averts the re-uptake from the intestine, and it is accomplished by bacteria possessing BSH activity. This feature is functionality present in all major bacterial divisions, including members of *Lactobacillus*, *Bifidobacterium*, *Clostridium,* and *Bacteroides*. After deconjugation, primary bile acids can be subjected to further modifications mediated by anaerobes in the large intestine. The formation of secondary bile acids occurs through dehydroxylation, oxidation, and epimerization of hydroxyl groups. Removal of the 7α-hydroxyl group of CA and CDCA results in the production of deoxycholic acid (DCA) and lithocholic acid (LCA), respectively. Species able to produce secondary bile acids have been identified in *Clostridium* (clusters XIVa and XI) and in *Eubacterium*. Other major bile acid conversions taking place in the large intestine include oxidation and epimerization. Epimerization is mediated by two distinct hydroxysteroid dehydrogenase enzymes (HSDH). In humans, CDCA is oxidized by 7α-HSDH into 7-oxo-LCA, which is then reduced to ursodeoxycholic acid (UDCA) by 7β-HSDH; 7α-HSDHs are broadly present in species belonging to the genera *Clostridium*, *Eubacterium*, *Bacteroides*, *Bifidobacterium,* and *Pseudomonas*. However, only limited members of *Clostridia* are described to possess 7β-HSDH activity (reviewed in Refs. [109, 111]). Once transported back to the liver, secondary bile acids can be further processed by conjugation with taurine or glycine. In NAFLD, the abundance of bacteria that convert primary to secondary bile acids is diminished [112]. This could result in decreased stimulation and signaling *via* bile acid receptors, but also further disturb the gut microbial environment.

Bile acids can have direct effects on intestinal bacteria by triggering membrane disruption, due to their detergent-like nature. Hence, it is reasonable to expect that NASH patients have altered bile acid profiles. Patients with non-cirrhotic NASH have increased total serum bile acid concentrations, especially taurine and glycine-conjugated primary and secondary bile acids [113]. One study reported that plasma bile acids are only elevated in NASH patients who display significant insulin resistance [114]. Another clinical study further demonstrated that an increase in specific bile salts was significantly associated with higher scores of hepatic steatoses (taurocholic acid, TCA), lobular inflammation (glycocholic acid, GCA), portal inflammation (taurolithocholic acid, TLCA), and hepatocyte ballooning (TCA) [115]. These results suggest a relationship between specific bile acids and histopathological features of NASH. In addition to their emulsifying and antimicrobial functions, bile acids are also signaling molecules with beneficial effects. At the molecular level, individual bile acids act either as agonists or antagonists of the Takeda G-protein-coupled receptor 5 (TGR5) and Farnesoid X receptor (FXR). FXR-mediated signaling has demonstrated beneficial effects on hepatic lipid and carbohydrate metabolism, whereas TGR5 is essential for glucose metabolism while having also a role in inflammatory responses. In addition, both receptors are involved in bile acid homeostasis and liver regeneration.

FXR is a member of the nuclear receptor superfamily, and it is expressed mainly in the liver, kidney, intestinal villi, and adrenal cortex. Although bile acids have confirmed beneficial effects, their production must be fine-tuned to avoid excess and bile acid-induced hepatotoxicity. FXR is a pivotal sensor of bile acids, regulating their production by the liver. Among its most potent ligands are the primary bile acids CDCA and CA. Recently, even more potent FXR agonists resulting from gut microbiota-mediated conjugation of CA have been reported: phenylalanocholic acid, tyrosocholic acid, and leucocholic acid [116]. The major FXR target in the gut is fibroblast growth factor 19 (FGF19; FGF15 in mice), which is an endocrine-acting protein produced in the ileum (enterokine) that is secreted into the portal vein upon bile acid stimulation. When reaching the liver, FGF19/15 activates the duo FGF receptor (R)4/β-Klotho on hepatocytes thereby triggering a signaling cascade that leads to the repression of CYP7A1, the rate-limiting enzyme in bile acid synthesis [117].

The downregulation of bile acid synthesis by FXR-FGF19/15 is crucial to protect the liver from cholestatic injury and bile acid-induced hepatotoxicity. The activation of this pathway is also important for liver growth and regeneration [118]. A previous study performed in NAFLD patients has observed an increase in DCA and a decrease in CDCA; in addition, the serum levels of FGF19 were also diminished in these patients, thus suggesting that suppression of the FXR-FGF19 pathway could contribute to disease progression [119]. Another study reported that UDCA combined with a low-calorie diet has therapeutic effects in steatohepatitis in rats [120]. Besides its role in bile acid homeostasis, FXR is also critical in the regulation of hepatic lipid accumulation (reviewed in Ref. [121]). As previously described, liver steatosis results from hepatic lipid acquisition (i.e., FFA uptake and DNL) exceeding lipid removal (i.e., FAO and export as VLDL particles). Hepatic FXR and intestine-imported FGF19 also contribute to hepatic lipid regulation by repressing lipogenesis and reducing FFA uptake, and by promoting FAO and TG clearance [121]. In obese and insulin-resistant *ob/ob* mice, the hepatic expression of both SREBP-1c and ChREBP are markedly increased, and a decrease in either of these two factors ameliorates steatosis [122]. In addition, FXR-deficient mice exhibit a prominent induction of lipogenic genes such as FAS, SREBP-1c, and Stearoyl-CoA desaturase 1 (SCD1) [123], thereby suggesting that FXR is critical for downregulating lipogenesis. Importantly, treatment with CDCA decreased serum TG levels in patients with hypertriglyceridemia [124], and in primary hepatocytes *in vitro,* CDCA was shown to lower the expression of SREBP-1c and its target genes [125]. Thus, it is not surprising that synthetic ligands have been developed to target FXR. These have been shown to improve insulin sensitivity and to exhibit anti-inflammatory and anti-fibrotic effects in mouse models of NASH and in human tissues [126, 127].

TGR5 is a G-protein coupled receptor (GPCR), which, upon ligand binding, transduces the extracellular signal to intracellular downstream cascades by activating multiple effector pathways. TGR5 is expressed in several tissues such as the small intestine, stomach, liver, lung, placenta, and spleen, and its endogenous natural agonists are bile acids. TLCA, LCA, DCA, CDCA, and CA can dose-dependently induce TGR5-mediated signaling in human TGR5-transfected Chinese hamster ovary (CHO) cells (reviewed in Ref. [128]). Upon bile acid binding, TGR5 induces cyclic adenosine monophosphate (cAMP) production, to regulate important cell signaling pathways such as NF-κB, AKT, and ERK. Therefore, TGR5 agonists are potential drugs for the treatment of metabolic, inflammation, and digestive disorders [129, 130]. TGR5 has been shown to promote GLP-1 secretion in intestinal L-cells, thereby stimulating pancreatic β-cells to produce insulin, in a process dependent on cAMP [131, 132]. These results fueled the interest to explore the potential treatment of T2DM by activation of TGR5, and therefore a few synthetic ligands and plant-derived agonists have been isolated [128]. In addition, the protective role of TGR5 in thermogenesis, inflammation, and liver regeneration, has also raised interest in the use of TGR5 agonists in obesity and NAFLD [109, 128].

5.4 Intestinal and liver targets for the management of NAFLD

Modulation of the gut microbiota is considered a potentially effective therapeutic option for the treatment of NAFLD and to slow down disease progression [133, 134]. In the last years, basic and animal researches have been translated into therapeutic and/or preventive drugs targeting human liver disease, which exploit intestinal-related molecular pathways. The best example is the development of *bile acid*-mimicking drugs, or drugs modulating enterokine signaling. Several mechanisms that have the gut microbiome at its genesis can be targeted to treat or prevent NAFLD. For instance, microbial eubiosis can be restored by improving microbial ecological networks, aimed to reduce specific luminal-derived metabolites that are known to contribute to NAFL and NASH progression. Among these are endogenously produced ethanol, TMA, or PAA. In addition, decreasing the load of microbial- and pathogen-associated molecular patterns (MAMPs and PAMPs) is of interest as they can activate innate immune responses and thereby contribute to inflammation (**Figure 6**). At the level of the gut epithelium, numerous processes may also be targeted, namely, strengthening of the epithelial barrier, decreasing pro-inflammatory mediators, or modulation of the bile acid pool, so to promote the activation of the two bile acid receptors FXR and TGR5 (**Figure 6**). This approach is currently being explored with the development of both FXR synthetic agonists and GLP-1 receptor agonists (reviewed in Ref. [134]). The prototype of FXR agonists is obeticholic acid (OCA) (Intercept Pharmaceuticals), a steroidal semisynthetic bile acid derivative. This has already been tested in a human NASH trial with positive outcomes, that is, improvement of histological NAFLD score, and reduced liver fibrosis (the FLINT trial) [135]. However, it has raised safety concerns as some OCA-treated subjects

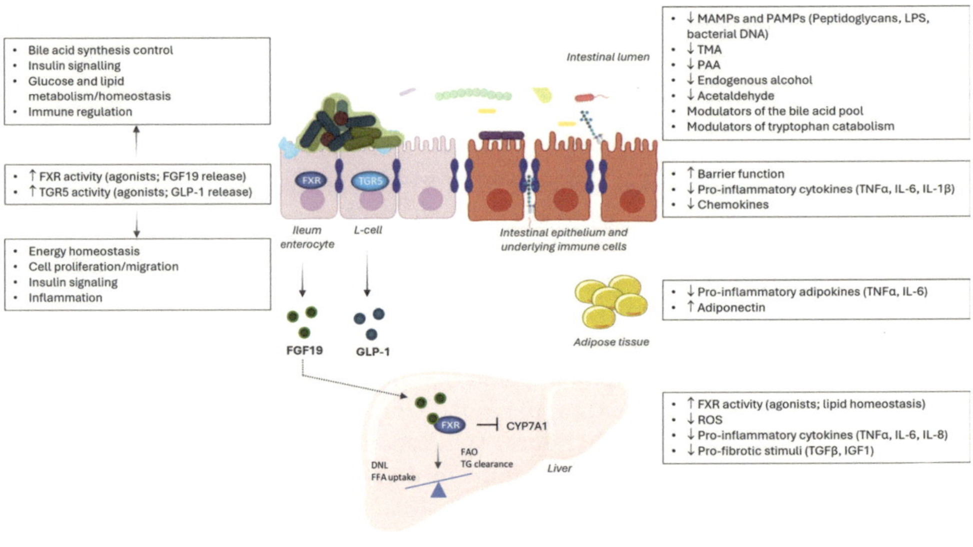

Figure 6.
Potential microbiome-related therapeutic targets within the gut-liver axis for the management of NAFLD. NAFLD-associated microbiome eubiosis may be restored by targeting the production of numerous metabolites of microbial origin known to contribute to disease, such as TMA, PAA, acetaldehyde, and alcohol. In addition, the bile acid pool and tryptophan catabolism can be fine-tuned to increase the production of favorable by-products. Host-related processes may also be influenced by gut microbes in the local gut environment such as barrier function and inflammation, but also in extra-intestinal tissues such as white adipose tissue and liver. In adipose tissue, the adipokine profile can be changed into a beneficial one, that is, a reduction in pro-inflammatory adipokines and increase in adiponectin. In addition, the release of gut hormones such as FGF19 and GLP-1 are directly influenced by bile acids, and therefore, FXR and TGR5 agonists can be used to ameliorate disease. Finally, in the liver, disease progression can be delayed by targeting FXR, ROS, and pro-inflammatory and pro-fibrotic stimuli. CYP7A1: cholesterol 7α-hydroxylase; DNL: de novo *lipogenesis; FAO: fatty acid oxidation; FFA: free-fatty acids; FGF19: fibroblast growth factor 19; FXR: farnesoid X nuclear receptor; GLP-1: glucagon-like protein 1; IGF1: insulin-like growth factor 1; IL: interleukin; LPS: lipopolysaccharides; MAMPs: microbial associated molecular patterns; PAA: phenylacetic acid; PAMPs: pathogen associated molecular patterns; ROS: reactive oxygen species; TG: triglycerides; TGFβ: transforming growth factor beta; TGR5: Takeda G-protein coupled receptor 5; TMA: trimethylamine; TNFα: tumor necrosis factor-alpha.*

displayed pruritus, and an increase in low-density lipoprotein (LDL)- and a decrease in high-density lipoprotein (HLD)-cholesterol (reviewed in Refs. [134, 136]). Therefore, the results from the FLINT trial have encouraged the search for more efficient and safer FXR agonists than OCA [134]. A recent animal study testing an intestine-specific FXR agonist (Fexaramine) led to the activation of ileal FXR, thereby resulting in lesser weight gain, reduced insulin resistance, and diminished hepatic steatosis in mice fed HFD [137]. These results suggest that the intestine is the optimal target tissue to treat liver disease [134]. However, contrasting findings have also been described in the literature, and FXR has been shown to inhibit SCFA-induced GLP-1 secretion by regulating GPR43. This has been shown in murine models *in vivo, ex vivo*, and *in vitro*, in human cells [138]. FXR activity in the ileum results in the release of FGF19, an endocrine hormone that regulates bile acid synthesis and promotes hepatic glycogen storage and FAO [139]. Therefore, FGF19 mimetics have been engineered and are currently under test. However, the potential carcinogenic effects of FGF19 have raised some concerns: by binding to FGFR4, FGF19 not only inhibits CYP7A1 but also promotes hepatic cell proliferation. In this context, overexpression of FGF19 has been associated with HCC in animal models [140]. Actually, the FXR-FGF19 pathway is considered a novel and important *hepatostat* [118], a mechanism essential for liver regeneration but that must be tightly controlled in order to prevent excessive liver growth. Thus, the FXR-FGF19 pathway seems to be important for the regulation of hepatocyte mass and liver size [141]. In line with these findings, Degirolamo and colleagues (2015) have shown that the reactivation of the FXR-FGF15 axis reduced circulating bile acid levels to normal and prevented spontaneous proliferation and HCC in FXR-null mice [142].

Bile acids are the common language of communication along the gut-liver axis. As described above, bile acids stimulate GLP-1 release via TGR5 activation. GLP-1 is an incretin hormone that induces insulin release by pancreatic β-cells. It also inhibits glucagon release, slows down nutrient absorption by reducing gastric emptying, and reduces food intake. Liraglutide (Saxenda, Novo Nordisk), a GLP-1 analog, was shown to reduce NAFLD activity score and fibrosis in a diet-induced obese mouse model of NASH [143]. In addition, liraglutide was able to deactivate HSCs, exert anti-fibrotic effects, and improve sinusoidal microvascular dysfunction in rats and human liver slices. However, HSCs do not express the GLP-1 receptor (GLP-1R), indicating that GLP-1 has potential and important off-target effects [144]. In humans, liraglutide was shown to be safe, well tolerated, and led to histological resolution of NASH, but the anti-fibrotic effects were rather disappointing, possibly owing to the small number of participants [145]. Nonetheless, both liraglutide and semaglutide (Ozempic, Novo Nordisk), another GLP-1R agonist, have been approved for the management of weight gain in diabetes patients, being semaglutide very effective at lowering blood glucose levels and reducing the risk of health complications in patients with T2DM [146]. Interestingly, results obtained with sitagliptin (Januvia, Merck, and Co.), an inhibitor of dipeptidyl peptidase 4, an enzyme that degrades GLP-1, have also been disappointing [147]. Although safe, sitagliptin was not better than placebo at reducing liver fat in pre-diabetic and diabetic patients with NAFLD. Nonetheless, stimulation of the local release of GLP-1 by bile acids or TGR5 analogs has been suggested to be superior to exogenous administration of GLP-1 receptor agonists for controlling obesity and T2DM [148]. However, although modulation of TGR5 activity in the intestine by bile acids is a potentially valid approach, this is yet to be demonstrated. Finally, approaches that reduce hepatic inflammation and oxidative stress may ultimately prevent progression to fibrosis, and therefore these are also valid targets for the management of NAFLD, and may be explored by live biotherapeutic products [149]. In this context, various probiotic formulations have been tested in human trials, but with variable outcomes, which may be related to the bacterial species tested, dosage and duration of treatment, and trial design (reviewed in Ref. [150]). Therefore, despite the observed improvements in lipids profile and liver enzymes, the long-term benefits of probiotics remain to be evaluated.

6. Conclusion

NAFLD, the hepatic expression of the metabolic syndrome, is the most common liver disease worldwide. NAFLD incidence is increasing owing to the Westernization of societies and changes in lifestyle, where Western diet, sedentarism, and obesity are alarmingly increasing. The gut microbiome is recognized as one of the factors contributing to pathology. An imbalanced microbial community, characterized by altered functionalities not only contributes to increased intestinal permeability and concomitant translocation of toxic and inflammatory mediators to the liver, but it is also depleted of key functions described to promote immune and metabolic homeostasis, such as the production of SCFA and other beneficial metabolites. The growth of unwanted bacterial species contributes to an increase in toxic mediators, such as ethanol, LPS, PAA, and TMA, with demonstrated negative effects. Therefore, treatments aimed to modulate and restore the gut microbiome ecological balance should be considered during early-stage NAFLD.

Author details

Iris Pinheiro
MRM Health NV, Ghent, Belgium

*Address all correspondence to: iris.pinheiro@mrmhealth.com

References

[1] Kolodziejczyk AA, Zheng D, Shibolet O, Elinav E. The role of the microbiome in NAFLD and NASH. EMBO Molecular Medicine. 2019;**11**:e9302

[2] Leung C, Rivera L, Furness JB, Angus PW. The role of the gut microbiota in NAFLD. Nature Reviews. Gastroenterology & Hepatology. 2016;**13**:412-425

[3] Younossi ZM, Koenig AB, Abdelatif D, Fazel Y, Henry L, Wymer M. Global epidemiology of nonalcoholic fatty liver disease-meta-analytic assessment of prevalence, incidence, and outcomes. Hepatology. 2016;**64**:73-84

[4] Estes C, Anstee QM, Arias-Loste MT, Bantel H, Bellentani S, Caballeria J, et al. Modeling NAFLD disease burden in China, France, Germany, Italy, Japan, Spain, United Kingdom, and United States for the period 2016-2030. Journal of Hepatology. 2018;**69**:896-904

[5] Milosevic I, Vujovic A, Barac A, Djelic M, Korac M, Radovanovic Spurnic A, et al. Gut-liver axis, gut microbiota, and its modulation in the management of liver diseases: A review of the literature. International Journal of Molecular Sciences. 2019;**20**:395

[6] Chu H, Williams B, Schnabl B. Gut microbiota, fatty liver disease, and hepatocellular carcinoma. Liver Research. 2018;**2**:43-51

[7] Tiniakos DG, Vos MB, Brunt EM. Nonalcoholic fatty liver disease: Pathology and pathogenesis. Annual Review of Pathology: Mechanisms of Disease. 2010;**5**:145-171

[8] Gentric G, Maillet V, Paradis V, Couton D, L'Hermitte A, Panasyuk G, et al. Oxidative stress promotes pathologic polyploidization in nonalcoholic fatty liver disease. The Journal of Clinical Investigation. 2015;**125**:981-992

[9] Buzzetti E, Pinzani M, Tsochatzis EA. The multiple-hit pathogenesis of non-alcoholic fatty liver disease (NAFLD). Metabolism. 2016;**65**:1038-1048

[10] Benedict M, Zhang X. Non-alcoholic fatty liver disease: An expanded review. World Journal of Hepatology. 2017;**9**:715-732

[11] Ding Y, Yanagi K, Cheng C, Alaniz RC, Lee K, Jayaraman A. Interactions between gut microbiota and non-alcoholic liver disease: The role of microbiota-derived metabolites. Pharmacological Research. 2019;**141**:521-529

[12] Ma KL, Ruan XZ, Powis SH, Chen Y, Moorhead JF, Varghese Z. Inflammatory stress exacerbates lipid accumulation in hepatic cells and fatty livers of apolipoprotein E knockout mice. Hepatology. 2008;**48**:770-781

[13] Yu J, Marsh S, Hu J, Feng W, Wu C. The pathogenesis of nonalcoholic fatty liver disease: Interplay between diet, gut microbiota, and genetic background. Gastroenterology Research and Practice. 2016;**2016**:2862173

[14] Younossi Z, Anstee QM, Marietti M, Hardy T, Henry L, Eslam M, et al. Global burden of NAFLD and NASH: Trends, predictions, risk factors and prevention. Nature Reviews. Gastroenterology & Hepatology. 2018;**15**:11-20

[15] Cohen JC, Horton JD, Hobbs HH. Human fatty liver disease: Old

questions and new insights. Science. 2011;**332**:1519-1523

[16] Hansen HH, Feigh M, Veidal SS, Rigbolt KT, Vrang N, Fosgerau K. Mouse models of nonalcoholic steatohepatitis in preclinical drug development. Drug Discovery Today. 2017;**22**:1707-1718

[17] Vacca M, Allison M, Griffin JL, Vidal-Puig A. Fatty acid and glucose sensors in hepatic lipid metabolism: Implications in NAFLD. Seminars in Liver Disease. 2015;**35**:250-261

[18] Lorbek G, Rozm D. Cholesterol and inflammation at the crossroads of non-alcoholic fatty liver disease (NAFLD) and atherogenesis. In: Parthasarathy S, editor. Atherogenesis. United States of America: IntechOpen; 2012

[19] Yamaguchi K, Yang L, McCall S, Huang J, Yu XX, Pandey SK, et al. Inhibiting triglyceride synthesis improves hepatic steatosis but exacerbates liver damage and fibrosis in obese mice with nonalcoholic steatohepatitis. Hepatology. 2007;**45**:1366-1374

[20] Bass NM. Lipidomic dissection of nonalcoholic steatohepatitis: Moving beyond foie gras to fat traffic. Hepatology. 2010;**51**:4-7

[21] Malhi H, Gores GJ. Molecular mechanisms of lipotoxicity in nonalcoholic fatty liver disease. Seminars in Liver Disease. 2008;**28**:360-369

[22] Rosso N, Chavez-Tapia NC, Tiribelli C, Bellentani S. Translational approaches: From fatty liver to non-alcoholic steatohepatitis. World Journal of Gastroenterology. 2014;**20**:9038-9049

[23] Safari Z, Gérard P. The links between the gut microbiome and non-alcoholic fatty liver disease (NAFLD). Cellular and Molecular Life Sciences. 2019;**76**:1541-1558

[24] Rai R, Saraswat VA, Dhiman RK. Gut microbiota: Its role in hepatic encephalopathy. Journal of Clinical and Experimental Hepatology. 2015;**5**:S29-S36

[25] Szabo G. Gut–liver axis in alcoholic liver disease. Gastroenterology. 2015;**148**:30-36

[26] Peter Stärkel BS. Bidirectional communication between liver and gut during alcoholic liver disease. Seminars in Liver Disease. 2016;**36**:331-339

[27] Suk KT, Kim DJ. Gut microbiota: Novel therapeutic target for nonalcoholic fatty liver disease. Expert Review of Gastroenterology & Hepatology. 2019;**13**:193-204

[28] Tripathi A, Debelius J, Brenner DA, Karin M, Loomba R, Schnabl B, et al. The gut-liver axis and the intersection with the microbiome. Nature Reviews. Gastroenterology & Hepatology. 2018;**15**:397-411

[29] Tan J, McKenzie C, Potamitis M, Thorburn AN, Mackay CR, Macia L. The role of short-chain fatty acids in health and disease. Advances in Immunology. 2014;**121**:91-119

[30] Brandl K, Schnabl B. Intestinal microbiota and nonalcoholic steatohepatitis. Current Opinion in Gastroenterology. 2017;**33**:128-133

[31] Turnbaugh PJ, Ley RE, Mahowald MA, Magrini V, Mardis ER, Gordon JI. An obesity-associated gut microbiome with increased capacity for energy harvest. Nature. 2006;**444**:1027-1031

[32] Chiu C-C, Ching Y-H, Li Y-P, Liu J-Y, Huang Y-T, Huang Y-W, et al. Nonalcoholic fatty liver disease is exacerbated in high-fat diet-fed

gnotobiotic mice by colonization with the gut microbiota from patients with nonalcoholic steatohepatitis. Nutrients. 2017;**9**:1220

[33] Del Chierico F, Nobili V, Vernocchi P, Russo A, De SC, Gnani D, et al. Gut microbiota profiling of pediatric nonalcoholic fatty liver disease and obese patients unveiled by an integrated meta-omics-based approach. Hepatology. 2017;**65**:451-464

[34] Kallus S, Brandt L. The intestinal microbiota and obesity. Journal of Clinical Gastroenterology. 2012;**46**:16-24

[35] Boursier J, Mueller O, Barret M, Machado M, Fizanne L, Araujo-Perez F, et al. The severity of nonalcoholic fatty liver disease is associated with gut dysbiosis and shift in the metabolic function of the gut microbiota. Hepatology. 2016;**63**:764-775

[36] Jegatheesan P, Beutheu S, Freese K, Waligora-Dupriet A-J, Nubret E, Butel M-J, et al. Preventive effects of citrulline on Western diet-induced non-alcoholic fatty liver disease in rats. The British Journal of Nutrition. 2016;**116**:191-203

[37] Zhu L, Baker SS, Gill C, Liu W, Alkhouri R, Baker RD, et al. Characterization of gut microbiomes in nonalcoholic steatohepatitis (NASH) patients: A connection between endogenous alcohol and NASH. Hepatology. 2013;**57**:601-609

[38] Volynets V, Küper MA, Strahl S, Maier IB, Spruss A, Wagnerberger S, et al. Nutrition, intestinal permeability, and blood ethanol levels are altered in patients with nonalcoholic fatty liver disease (NAFLD). Digestive Diseases and Sciences. 2012;**57**:1932-1941

[39] Engstler AJ, Aumiller T, Degen C, Dürr M, Weiss E, Maier IB, et al. Insulin resistance alters hepatic ethanol metabolism: Studies in mice and children with non-alcoholic fatty liver disease. Gut. 2016;**65**:1564-1571

[40] Mokhtari Z, Gibson DL, Hekmatdoost A. Nonalcoholic fatty liver disease, the gut microbiome, and diet. Advances in Nutrition. 2017;**8**:240-252

[41] Honda K, Littman DR. The microbiome in infectious disease and inflammation. Annual Review of Immunology. 2012;**30**:759-795

[42] Peterson LW, Artis D. Intestinal epithelial cells: Regulators of barrier function and immune homeostasis. Nature Reviews. Immunology. 2014;**14**:141-153

[43] Dai X, Wang B. Role of gut barrier function in the pathogenesis of nonalcoholic fatty liver disease. Gastroenterology Research and Practice. 2015;**2015**:287348

[44] Turner JR. Intestinal mucosal barrier function in health and disease. Nature Reviews. Immunology. 2009;**9**:799-809

[45] Abreu MT. Toll-like receptor signalling in the intestinal epithelium: How bacterial recognition shapes intestinal function. Nature Reviews. Immunology. 2010;**10**:131-144

[46] Gallo RL, Hooper LV. Epithelial antimicrobial defence of the skin and intestine. Nature Reviews. Immunology. 2012;**12**:503-516

[47] Mantis NJ, Rol N, Corthesy B. Secretory IgA's complex roles in immunity and mucosal homeostasis in the gut. Mucosal Immunology. 2011;**4**:603-611

[48] Rakoff-Nahoum S, Paglino J, Eslami-Varzaneh F, Edberg S, Medzhitov R.

Recognition of commensal microflora by toll-like receptors is required for intestinal homeostasis. Cell. 2004;**118**:229-241

[49] Luther J, Garber JJ, Khalili H, Dave M, Bale SS, Jindal R, et al. Hepatic injury in nonalcoholic steatohepatitis contributes to altered intestinal permeability. Cellular and Molecular Gastroenterology and Hepatology. 2015;**1**:222-232

[50] Gäbele E, Dostert K, Hofmann C, Wiest R, Schölmerich J, Hellerbrand C, et al. DSS induced colitis increases portal LPS levels and enhances hepatic inflammation and fibrogenesis in experimental NASH. Journal of Hepatology. 2011;**55**:1391-1399

[51] Wigg AJ, Roberts-Thomson IC, Dymock RB, McCarthy PJ, Grose RH, Cummins AG. The role of small intestinal bacterial overgrowth, intestinal permeability, endotoxaemia, and tumour necrosis factor α in the pathogenesis of non-alcoholic steatohepatitis. Gut. 2001;**48**:206-211

[52] Philips CA, Pande A, Shasthry SM, Jamwal KD, Khillan V, Chandel SS, et al. Healthy donor fecal microbiota transplantation in steroid-ineligible severe alcoholic hepatitis: A pilot study. Clinical Gastroenterology and Hepatology. 2017;**15**:600-602

[53] Sabaté J-M, Jouët P, Harnois F, Mechler C, Msika S, Grossin M, et al. High prevalence of small intestinal bacterial overgrowth in patients with morbid obesity: A contributor to severe hepatic steatosis. Obesity Surgery. 2008;**18**:371-377

[54] Miele L, Valenza V, La Torre G, Montalto M, Cammarota G, Ricci R, et al. Increased intestinal permeability and tight junction alterations in nonalcoholic fatty liver disease. Hepatology. 2009;**49**:1877-1887

[55] Shanab AA, Scully P, Crosbie O, Buckley M, O'Mahony L, Shanahan F, et al. Small intestinal bacterial overgrowth in nonalcoholic steatohepatitis: Association with toll-like receptor 4 expression and plasma levels of interleukin 8. Digestive Diseases and Sciences. 2011;**56**:1524-1534

[56] Kapil S, Duseja A, Sharma BK, Singla B, Chakraborti A, Das A, et al. Small intestinal bacterial overgrowth and toll-like receptor signaling in patients with non-alcoholic fatty liver disease. Journal of Gastroenterology and Hepatology. 2016;**31**:213-221

[57] Ilan Y. Leaky gut and the liver: A role for bacterial translocation in nonalcoholic steatohepatitis. World Journal of Gastroenterology. 2012;**18**:2609-2618

[58] Bergheim I, Weber S, Vos M, Krämer S, Volynets V, Kaserouni S, et al. Antibiotics protect against fructose-induced hepatic lipid accumulation in mice: Role of endotoxin. Journal of Hepatology. 2008;**48**:983-992

[59] Harte AL, da Silva NF, Creely SJ, McGee KC, Billyard T, Youssef-Elabd EM, et al. Elevated endotoxin levels in non-alcoholic fatty liver disease. Journal of Inflammation. 2010;**7**:15

[60] Sharifnia T, Antoun J, Verriere TGC, Suarez G, Wattacheril J, Wilson KT, et al. Hepatic TLR4 signaling in obese NAFLD. American Journal of Physiology-Gastrointestinal and Liver Physiology. 2015;**309**:G270-G278

[61] Yang SQ, Lin HZ, Lane MD, Clemens M, Diehl AM. Obesity increases sensitivity to endotoxin liver injury: Implications for the pathogenesis

of steatohepatitis. Proceedings of the National Academy of Sciences of the United States of America. 1997;**94**:2557-2562

[62] Miura K, Kodama Y, Inokuchi S, Schnabl B, Aoyama T, Ohnishi H, et al. Toll-like receptor 9 promotes steatohepatitis by induction of interleukin-1beta in mice. Gastroenterology. 2010;**139**:323-34.e7

[63] Szabo G, Dolganiuc A, Mandrekar P. Pattern recognition receptors: A contemporary view on liver diseases. Hepatology. 2006;**44**:287-298

[64] Etienne-Mesmin L, Vijay-Kumar M, Gewirtz AT, Chassaing B. Hepatocyte toll-like receptor 5 promotes bacterial clearance and protects mice against high-fat diet-induced liver disease. Cellular and Molecular Gastroenterology and Hepatology. 2016;**2**:584-604

[65] Vijay-Kumar M, Aitken JD, Carvalho FA, Cullender TC, Mwangi S, Srinivasan S, et al. Metabolic syndrome and altered gut microbiota in mice lacking Toll-like receptor 5. Science. 2010;**328**:228-231

[66] Mikolasevic I, Delija B, Mijic A, Stevanovic T, Skenderevic N, Sosa I, et al. Small intestinal bacterial overgrowth and non-alcoholic fatty liver disease diagnosed by transient elastography and liver biopsy. International Journal of Clinical Practice. 2021;**75**:e13947

[67] Zoetendal EG, Raes J, van den Bogert B, Arumugam M, Booijink CCGM, Troost FJ, et al. The human small intestinal microbiota is driven by rapid uptake and conversion of simple carbohydrates. The ISME Journal. 2012;**6**:1415-1426

[68] Zhao S, Jang C, Liu J, Uehara K, Gilbert M, Izzo L, et al. Dietary fructose feeds hepatic lipogenesis via microbiota-derived acetate. Nature. 2020;**579**:586-591

[69] Febbraio MA, Karin M. "Sweet death": Fructose as a metabolic toxin that targets the gut-liver axis. Cell Metabolism. 2021;**33**:2316-2328

[70] Postler TS, Ghosh S. Understanding the holobiont: How microbial metabolites affect human health and shape the immune system. Cell Metabolism. 2017;**26**:110-130

[71] Chen YH, Wu WK, Wu MS. Microbiota-associated therapy for non-alcoholic steatohepatitis-induced liver cancer: A review. International Journal of Molecular Sciences. 2020;**21**:1-20

[72] Hu H, Lin A, Kong M, Yao X, Yin M, Xia H, et al. Intestinal microbiome and NAFLD: Molecular insights and therapeutic perspectives. Journal of Gastroenterology. 2020;**55**:142-158

[73] Parekh PJ, Arusi E, Vinik AI, Johnson DA. The role and influence of gut microbiota in pathogenesis and management of obesity and metabolic syndrome. Frontiers in Endocrinology. 2014;**5**:1-7

[74] Arslan N. Obesity, fatty liver disease and intestinal microbiota. World Journal of Gastroenterology. 2014;**20**:16452-16463

[75] Alves-Bezerra M, Cohen DE. Triglyceride metabolism in the liver. Comprehensive Physiology. 2017;**8**:1-8

[76] den Besten G, Lange K, Havinga R, van Dijk TH, Gerding A, van Eunen K, et al. Gut-derived short-chain fatty acids are vividly assimilated into host carbohydrates and lipids. American Journal of Physiology-Gastrointestinal and Liver Physiology. 2013;**305**:G900-G910

[77] Ferreira CM, Vieira AT, Vinolo MAR, Oliveira FA, Curi R, Martins F d S. The central role of the gut microbiota in chronic inflammatory diseases. Journal of Immunology Research. 2014;**2014**:689492

[78] Wong VW-S, Tse C-H, Lam TT-Y, Wong GL-H, Chim AM-L, Chu WC-W, et al. Molecular characterization of the fecal microbiota in patients with nonalcoholic steatohepatitis—A longitudinal study. PLoS One. 2013;**8**:e62885

[79] Zhou D, Pan Q, Xin FZ, Zhang RN, He CX, Chen GY, et al. Sodium butyrate attenuates high-fat diet-induced steatohepatitis in mice by improving gut microbiota and gastrointestinal barrier. World Journal of Gastroenterology. 2017;**23**:60-75

[80] Schwiertz A, Taras D, Schäfer K, Beijer S, Bos NA, Donus CHP. Microbiota and SCFA in lean and overweight healthy subjects. Obesity. 2010;**18**:190-195

[81] Chambers ES, Viardot A, Psichas A, Morrison DJ, Murphy KG, Zac-Varghese SEK, et al. Effects of targeted delivery of propionate to the human colon on appetite regulation, body weight maintenance and adiposity in overweight adults. Gut. 2015;**64**:1744-1754

[82] Lin MY, De Zoete MR, Van Putten JPM, Strijbis K. Redirection of epithelial immune responses by short-chain fatty acids through inhibition of histone deacetylases. Frontiers in Immunology. 2015;**6**:1-11

[83] Li M, van Esch BCAM, Wagenaar GTM, Garssen J, Folkerts G, Henricks PAJ. Pro- and anti-inflammatory effects of short chain fatty acids on immune and endothelial cells. European Journal of Pharmacology. 2018;**831**:52-59

[84] Corrêa-Oliveira R, Fachi JL, Vieira A, Sato FT, Vinolo MAR. Regulation of immune cell function by short-chain fatty acids. Clinical & Translational Immunology. 2016;**5**:1-8

[85] Cope K, Risby T, Diehl AM. Increased gastrointestinal ethanol production in obese mice: Implications for fatty liver disease pathogenesis. Gastroenterology. 2000;**119**:1340-1347

[86] Fuster D, Samet JH. Alcohol use in patients with chronic liver disease. The New England Journal of Medicine. 2018;**379**:1251-1261

[87] Yuan J, Chen C, Cui J, Lu J, Yan C, Wei X, et al. Fatty liver disease caused by high-alcohol-producing *Klebsiella pneumoniae*. Cell Metabolism. 2019;**30**:675-688.e7

[88] Baker SS, Baker RD, Liu W, Nowak NJ, Zhu L. Role of alcohol metabolism in non-alcoholic steatohepatitis. PLoS One. 2010;**5**:e9570

[89] Ghoshal UC, Goel A, Quigley EMM. Gut microbiota abnormalities, small intestinal bacterial overgrowth, and non-alcoholic fatty liver disease: An emerging paradigm. Indian Journal of Gastroenterology: Official Journal of the Indian Society of Gastroenterology. 2020;**39**:9-21

[90] Hoyles L, Fernández-Real J-M, Federici M, Serino M, Abbott J, Charpentier J, et al. Molecular phenomics and metagenomics of hepatic steatosis in non-diabetic obese women. Nature Medicine. 2018;**24**:1070-1080

[91] Iida A, Kuranuki S, Yamamoto R, Uchida M, Ohta M, Ichimura M, et al. Analysis of amino acid profiles of blood over time and biomarkers associated with non-alcoholic steatohepatitis in STAM mice. Experimental Animals. 2019;**68**:417-428

[92] Campollo O, Sprengers D, McIntyre N. The BCAA/AAA ratio of plasma amino acids in three different groups of cirrhotics. Revista de Investigacion Clinica; Organo del Hospital de Enfermedades de la Nutricion. 1992;**44**:513-518

[93] Delzenne NM, Bindels LB. Microbiome metabolomics reveals new drivers of human liver steatosis. Nature Medicine. 2018;**24**:906-907

[94] Zhang F, Zhao S, Yan W, Xia Y, Chen X, Wang W, et al. Branched chain amino acids cause liver injury in obese/diabetic mice by promoting adipocyte lipolysis and inhibiting hepatic autophagy. eBioMedicine. 2016;**13**:157-167

[95] Pedersen HK, Gudmundsdottir V, Nielsen HB, Hyotylainen T, Nielsen T, Jensen BAH, et al. Human gut microbes impact host serum metabolome and insulin sensitivity. Nature. 2016;**535**:376-381

[96] Krishnan S, Ding Y, Saedi N, Choi M, Sridharan GV, Sherr DH, et al. Gut microbiota-derived tryptophan metabolites modulate inflammatory response in hepatocytes and macrophages. Cell Reports. 2019;**28**:3285

[97] Agus A, Planchais J, Sokol H. Gut microbiota regulation of tryptophan metabolism in health and disease. Cell Host & Microbe. 2018;**23**:716-724

[98] Roager HM, Licht TR. Microbial tryptophan catabolites in health and disease. Nature Communications. 2018;**9**:1-10

[99] Konopelski P, Konop M, Gawrys-Kopczynska M, Podsadni P, Szczepanska A, Ufnal M. Indole-3-propionic acid, a tryptophan-derived bacterial metabolite, reduces weight gain in rats. Nutrients. 2019;**11**:591

[100] Jennis M, Cavanaugh CR, Leo GC, Mabus JR, Lenhard J, Hornby PJ. Microbiota-derived tryptophan indoles increase after gastric bypass surgery and reduce intestinal permeability in vitro and in vivo. Neurogastroenterology & Motility. 2017;**30**:e13178

[101] Venkatesh M, Mukherjee S, Wang H, Li H, Sun K, Benechet AP, et al. Symbiotic bacterial metabolites regulate gastrointestinal barrier function via the xenobiotic sensor PXR and Toll-like receptor 4. Immunity. 2014;**41**:296-310

[102] Ritze Y, Bárdos G, Hubert A, Böhle M, Bischoff SC. Effect of tryptophan supplementation on diet-induced non-alcoholic fatty liver disease in mice. The British Journal of Nutrition. 2014;**112**:1-7

[103] Bansal T, Alaniz RC, Wood TK, Jayaraman A. The bacterial signal indole increases epithelial-cell tight-junction resistance and attenuates indicators of inflammation. Proceedings of the National Academy of Sciences of the United States of America. 2010;**107**:228-233

[104] Smallwood T, Allayee H, Bennett BJ. Choline metabolites: Gene by diet interactions. Current Opinion in Lipidology. 2016;**27**:33-39

[105] Zhou D, Fan JG. Microbial metabolites in non-alcoholic fatty liver disease. World Journal of Gastroenterology. 2019;**25**:2019-2028

[106] Bennett BJ, de Aguiar Vallim TQ, Wang Z, Shih DM, Meng Y, Gregory J, et al. Trimethylamine-N-oxide, a metabolite associated with atherosclerosis, exhibits complex genetic and dietary regulation. Cell Metabolism. 2013;**17**: 49-60

[107] Chen Y, Liu Y, Zhou R, Chen X, Wang C, Tan X, et al. Associations

of gut-flora-dependent metabolite trimethylamine-N-oxide, betaine and choline with non-alcoholic fatty liver disease in adults. Scientific Reports. 2016;**6**:19076

[108] Dumas M-E, Barton RH, Toye A, Cloarec O, Blancher C, Rothwell A, et al. Metabolic profiling reveals a contribution of gut microbiota to fatty liver phenotype in insulin-resistant mice. Proceedings of the National Academy of Sciences of the United States of America. 2006;**103**:12511-12516

[109] Wahlström A, Sayin SI, Marschall H-U, Bäckhed F. Intestinal crosstalk between bile acids and microbiota and its impact on host metabolism. Cell Metabolism. 2016;**24**:41-50

[110] Sayin SII, Wahlström A, Felin J, Jäntti S, Marschall H-UU, Bamberg K, et al. Gut microbiota regulates bile acid metabolism by reducing the levels of tauro-beta-muricholic acid, a naturally occurring FXR antagonist. Cell Metabolism. 2013;**17**:225-235

[111] Van den Bossche L. Bile acids as novel therapeutic agents for inflammatory bowel disease. In: Thesis Submitted in Fulfilment of the Requirements for the Degree of Doctor in Health Sciences, Faculty of Medicine and Health Sciences of the University of Ghent. Ghent: University of Ghent; 2017

[112] Chen J, Thomsen M, Vitetta L. Interaction of gut microbiota with dysregulation of bile acids in the pathogenesis of nonalcoholic fatty liver disease and potential therapeutic implications of probiotics. Journal of Cellular Biochemistry. 2019;**120**:2713-2720

[113] Ferslew BC, Xie G, Johnston CK, Su M, Stewart PW, Jia W, et al. Altered bile acid metabolome in patients with nonalcoholic steatohepatitis. Digestive Diseases and Sciences. 2015;**60**:3318-3328

[114] Grzych G, Chávez-Talavera O, Descat A, Thuillier D, Verrijken A, Kouach M, et al. NASH-related increases in plasma bile acid levels depend on insulin resistance. JHEP Reports: Innovation in Hepatology. 2021;**3**:100222

[115] Puri P, Daita K, Joyce A, Mirshahi F, Santhekadur PK, Cazanave S, et al. The presence and severity of nonalcoholic steatohepatitis is associated with specific changes in circulating bile acids. Hepatology. 2018;**67**:534-548

[116] Quinn RA, Melnik AV, Vrbanac A, Fu T, Patras KA, Christy MP, et al. Global chemical effects of the microbiome include new bile-acid conjugations. Nature. 2020;**579**:123-129

[117] Inagaki T, Choi M, Moschetta A, Peng L, Cummins CL, McDonald JG, et al. Fibroblast growth factor 15 functions as an enterohepatic signal to regulate bile acid homeostasis. Cell Metabolism. 2005;**2**:217-225

[118] Avila MA, Moschetta A. The FXR-FGF19 gut-liver axis as a novel "hepatostat.". Gastroenterology. 2015;**149**:537-540

[119] Jiao N, Baker SS, Chapa-Rodriguez A, Liu W, Nugent CA, Tsompana M, et al. Suppressed hepatic bile acid signalling despite elevated production of primary and secondary bile acids in NAFLD. Gut. 2018;**67**:1881-1891

[120] Fan J-G, Zhong L, Tia L-Y, Xu Z-J, Li M-S, Wang G-L. Effects of ursodeoxycholic acid and/or low-calorie diet on steatohepatitis in rats with obesity and hyperlipidemia. World Journal of Gastroenterology. 2005;**11**:2346-2350

[121] Xi Y, Li H. Role of farnesoid X receptor in hepatic steatosis in nonalcoholic fatty liver disease. Biomedicine & Pharmacotherapy. 2020;**121**:109609

[122] Dentin R, Benhamed F, Hainault I, Fauveau V, Foufelle F, Dyck JRB, et al. Liver-specific inhibition of ChREBP improves hepatic steatosis and insulin resistance in ob/ob mice. Diabetes. 2006;**55**:2159-2170

[123] Ma K, Saha PK, Chan L, Moore DD. Farnesoid X receptor is essential for normal glucose homeostasis. The Journal of Clinical Investigation. 2006;**116**:1102-1109

[124] Massafra V, van Mil SWC. Farnesoid X receptor: A "homeostat" for hepatic nutrient metabolism. Biochimica et Biophysica Acta - Molecular Basis of Disease. 2018;**1864**:45-59

[125] Watanabe M, Houten SM, Wang L, Moschetta A, Mangelsdorf DJ, Heyman RA, et al. Bile acids lower triglyceride levels via a pathway involving FXR, SHP, and SREBP-1c. The Journal of Clinical Investigation. 2004;**113**:1408-1418

[126] Kong B, Luyendyk JP, Tawfik O, Guo GL. Farnesoid X receptor deficiency induces nonalcoholic steatohepatitis in low-density lipoprotein receptor-knockout mice fed a high-fat diet. The Journal of Pharmacology and Experimental Therapeutics. 2009;**328**:116-122

[127] Mudaliar S, Henry RR, Sanyal AJ, Morrow L, Marschall H-U, Kipnes M, et al. Efficacy and safety of the farnesoid X receptor agonist obeticholic acid in patients with type 2 diabetes and nonalcoholic fatty liver disease. Gastroenterology. 2013;**145**:574-82.e1

[128] Guo C, Chen WD, Wang YD. TGR5, not only a metabolic regulator. Frontiers in Physiology. 2016;**7**:1-9

[129] Broeders EPM, Nascimento EBM, Havekes B, Brans B, Roumans KHM, Tailleux A, et al. The bile acid chenodeoxycholic acid increases human brown adipose tissue activity. Cell Metabolism. 2015;**22**:418-426

[130] Kumar DP, Rajagopal S, Mahavadi S, Mirshahi F, Grider JR, Murthy KS, et al. Activation of transmembrane bile acid receptor TGR5 stimulates insulin secretion in pancreatic β cells. Biochemical and Biophysical Research Communications. 2012;**427**:600-605

[131] Thomas C, Gioiello A, Noriega L, Strehle A, Oury J, Rizzo G, et al. TGR5-mediated bile acid sensing controls glucose homeostasis. Cell Metabolism. 2009;**10**:167-177

[132] Katsuma S, Hirasawa A, Tsujimoto G. Bile acids promote glucagon-like peptide-1 secretion through TGR5 in a murine enteroendocrine cell line STC-1. Biochemical and Biophysical Research Communications. 2005;**329**:386-390

[133] Mouzaki M, Bandsma R. Targeting the gut microbiota for the treatment of non-alcoholic fatty liver disease. Current Drug Targets. 2015;**16**:1324-1331

[134] Wiest R, Albillos A, Trauner M, Bajaj JS, Jalan R. Targeting the gut-liver axis in liver disease. Journal of Hepatology. 2017;**67**:1084-1103

[135] Neuschwander-Tetri BA, Loomba R, Sanyal AJ, Lavine JE, Van Natta ML, Abdelmalek MF, et al. Farnesoid X nuclear receptor ligand obeticholic acid for non-cirrhotic, non-alcoholic steatohepatitis (FLINT): A multicentre, randomised, placebo-controlled trial. Lancet. 2015;**385**:956-965

[136] Friedman SL, Neuschwander-Tetri BA, Rinella M, Sanyal AJ. Mechanisms of NAFLD development and therapeutic strategies. Nature Medicine. 2018;**24**:908-922

[137] Fang S, Suh JM, Reilly SM, Yu E, Osborn O, Lackey D, et al. Intestinal FXR agonism promotes adipose tissue browning and reduces obesity and insulin resistance. Nature Medicine. 2015;**21**:159-165

[138] Ducastel S, Touche V, Trabelsi MS, Boulinguiez A, Butruille L, Nawrot M, et al. The nuclear receptor FXR inhibits glucagon-like peptide-1 secretion in response to microbiota-derived short-chain fatty acids. Scientific Reports. 2020;**10**:1-10

[139] Arab JP, Karpen SJ, Dawson PA, Arrese M, Trauner M. Bile acids and nonalcoholic fatty liver disease: Molecular insights and therapeutic perspectives. Hepatology. 2017;**65**:350-362

[140] Nicholes K, Guillet S, Tomlinson E, Hillan K, Wright B, Frantz GD, et al. A mouse model of hepatocellular carcinoma: Ectopic expression of fibroblast growth factor 19 in skeletal muscle of transgenic mice. The American Journal of Pathology. 2002;**160**:2295-2307

[141] Naugler WE, Tarlow BD, Fedorov LM, Taylor M, Pelz C, Li B, et al. Fibroblast growth factor signaling controls liver size in mice with humanized livers. Gastroenterology. 2015;**149**:728-40.e15

[142] Degirolamo C, Modica S, Vacca M, Di Tullio G, Morgano A, D'Orazio A, et al. Prevention of spontaneous hepatocarcinogenesis in farnesoid X receptor-null mice by intestinal-specific farnesoid X receptor reactivation. Hepatology. 2015;**61**:161-170

[143] Tølbøl KS, Kristiansen MN, Hansen HH, Veidal SS, Rigbolt KT, Gillum MP, et al. Metabolic and hepatic effects of liraglutide, obeticholic acid and elafibranor in diet-induced obese mouse models of biopsy-confirmed nonalcoholic steatohepatitis. World Journal of Gastroenterology. 2018;**24**:179-194

[144] de Mesquita FC, Guixé-Muntet S, Fernández-Iglesias A, Maeso-Díaz R, Vila S, Hide D, et al. Liraglutide improves liver microvascular dysfunction in cirrhosis: Evidence from translational studies. Scientific Reports. 2017;**7**:3255

[145] Armstrong MJ, Gaunt P, Aithal GP, Barton D, Hull D, Parker R, et al. Liraglutide safety and efficacy in patients with non-alcoholic steatohepatitis (LEAN): A multicentre, double-blind, randomised, placebo-controlled phase 2 study. Lancet. 2016;**387**:679-690

[146] Jahagirdar D, Mahood Q. Semaglutide for type 2 diabetes (2 mg). CADTH Health Technology Review. 2023;**3**:1-18

[147] Cui J, Philo L, Nguyen P, Hofflich H, Hernandez C, Bettencourt R, et al. Sitagliptin vs. placebo for non-alcoholic fatty liver disease: A randomized controlled trial. Journal of Hepatology. 2016;**65**:369-376

[148] Knop FK. Bile-induced secretion of glucagon-like peptide-1: Pathophysiological implications in type 2 diabetes? American Journal of Physiology-Endocrinology and Metabolism. 2010;**299**:E10-E13

[149] Pinheiro I, Barberá A, Raurell I, Estrella F, de Leeuw M, Bolca S, et al. A nine-strain bacterial consortium improves portal hypertension and insulin signaling and delays NAFLD progression in vivo. Biomedicine. 2022;**10**:1-20

[150] Cao C, Shi M, Wang X, Yao Y, Zeng R. Effects of probiotics on non-alcoholic fatty liver disease: A review of human clinical trials. Frontiers in Nutrition. 2023;**10**:1155306

Chapter 4

Principles of Nutrition in Patients with Non-alcoholic Fatty Liver Disease

Narges Mobasheri, Leila Ghahremani and Mahin Nazari

Abstract

This chapter will comprehensively address the nutritional principles essential for managing nonalcoholic fatty liver disease (NAFLD). It will explore the critical role of diet in the prevention and treatment of NAFLD, providing evidence-based dietary recommendations to improve liver health and the overall well-being of patients. Key topics will include the importance of balanced macronutrient intake, the role of specific nutrients and food groups (e.g., antioxidants, fiber, and healthy fats), and the impact of dietary patterns such as the Mediterranean and Dietary Approaches to Stop Hypertension (DASH) diet on liver fat reduction and inflammation. Additionally, the chapter will discuss the significance of weight management, outlining the standard amount of weight loss beneficial for NAFLD patients. Practical guidelines on how to implement these dietary changes, overcome common barriers, and maintain long-term adherence will be provided. This chapter aims to equip healthcare professionals and patients with the knowledge and tools necessary to effectively manage NAFLD through diet, ultimately improving patient outcomes and quality of life.

Keywords: nonalcoholic fatty liver disease, NAFLD, dietary intervention, Mediterranean diet, DASH diet

1. Introduction

Nonalcoholic fatty liver disease (NAFLD) is characterized by excessive hepatic fat accumulation in individuals with minimal or no alcohol consumption. This condition results from a combination of pathological factors and lifestyle choices, often arising primarily from metabolic imbalances and unhealthy habits rather than traditional risk factors. As a metabolic disease, NAFLD is closely linked to poor dietary practices, sedentary behavior, and obesity [1, 2].

Management of NAFLD centers on lifestyle modification, encompassing dietary changes, increased physical activity, and weight reduction. Evidence suggests that a 5–7% weight loss can improve hepatic steatosis, while a loss exceeding 10% is recommended for ameliorating fibrosis and inflammation. Studies indicate that a 7–10% reduction in initial body weight leads to improvements in liver enzymes and histological changes in overweight and obese NAFLD patients [2, 3].

Physical activity plays a crucial role in NAFLD management. Guidelines recommend 150–200 minutes of exercise per week, spread across 3–5 days. Both aerobic and resistance training have shown benefits in improving NAFLD outcomes [1, 2, 4].

Dietary interventions focus on calorie restriction, typically 500–1000 kcal below daily requirements, though some sources suggest a 350–750 kcal reduction may suffice. The diet should minimize high-calorie, processed foods and emphasize vegetables, fruits, whole grains, lean proteins, and healthy fats [1–3, 5].

Understanding the specific contributions of macronutrients is essential for developing effective dietary strategies for NAFLD. The following sections delve into the recommended intake and key considerations for macronutrients in the context of NAFLD management. This detailed examination of macronutrients provides the foundation for understanding specific dietary approaches that have shown promise in NAFLD treatment.

We will then explore two dietary patterns that have demonstrated particular efficacy in managing NAFLD, integrating the principles of macronutrient balance with practical dietary recommendations. These dietary approaches offer comprehensive strategies for improving liver health through nutritional interventions, addressing both the quantity and quality of food intake.

While lifestyle modifications including physical activity and weight management can complement dietary interventions, the primary focus of this chapter will be on the crucial role of diet in NAFLD management, providing evidence-based nutritional strategies for improving liver health.

2. Carbohydrates consumption guidelines for NAFLD patients

The consumption of carbohydrates plays a significant role in the management and outcomes of NAFLD. The American Heart Association recommends that adults obtain 45–65% of their daily caloric intake from carbohydrates. In contrast, the Academy of Nutrition and Dietetics suggests that adults with NAFLD should derive 45–55% of their daily calories from carbohydrates [6]. For patients with NAFLD, it is essential that the carbohydrates consumed exhibit specific characteristics:

2.1 Low glycemic index (GI) and glycemic load (GL)

Carbohydrates with a low glycemic index (GI) and glycemic load (GL) lead to a slower, more gradual increase in blood glucose, as illustrated in **Figure 1**. This figure demonstrates how foods with different GI and GL values impact blood glucose and insulin levels over time. The glycemic index reflects how rapidly a food raises blood glucose, while the glycemic load considers both the quality (GI) and quantity of carbohydrates, providing a fuller picture of its effect. High-GI (≥70) and high-GL (≥20) foods, shown by the red curve, cause a sharp rise in blood glucose, peaking around 30 minutes post-ingestion. This rapid increase triggers a significant insulin response, which then quickly lowers glucose levels, sometimes below baseline, potentially causing reactive hypoglycemia. This response is common in refined or processed carbohydrates, which are rapidly absorbed. Medium-GI (56–69) and medium-GL (11–20) foods, represented by the yellow curve, produce a more moderate rise in glucose and insulin levels, with a lower peak and slower return to baseline. This intermediate response is typical of foods with a balanced carbohydrate composition, providing a sustained glucose supply and avoiding extreme fluctuations. Low-GI (≤55) and

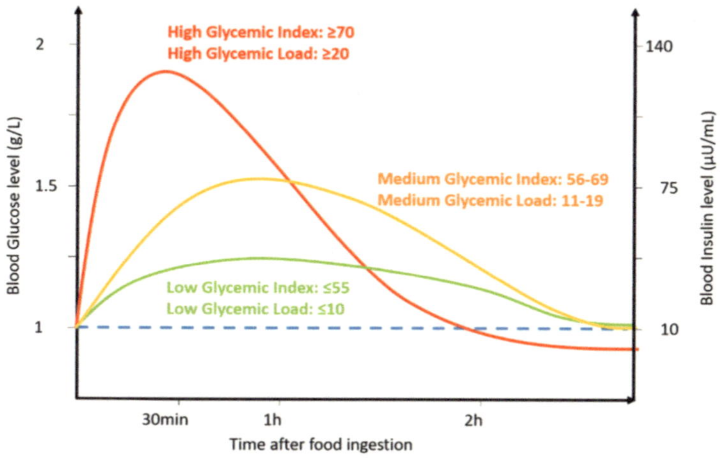

Figure 1.
Blood glucose and insulin responses to foods with varying glycemic indices and glycemic loads. Source: Adapted from Carneiro L, Leloup C. "Mens sana in corpore sano: Does the Glycemic Index Have a Role to Play?" Nutrients, 2020. Reproduced with permission [7].

low-GL (≤10) foods, illustrated by the green curve, minimally impact blood glucose and insulin levels. The gradual increase and prolonged glucose availability are characteristic of high-fiber and complex carbohydrate foods, which help stabilize blood glucose and minimize excessive insulin release, supporting metabolic health [7].

To achieve these benefits, it is recommended to choose whole grains over refined grains, increase intake of vegetables and fruits, use legumes as both protein and carbohydrate sources, and limit consumption of simple sugars and processed foods.

2.2 High-fiber content

Fiber-rich carbohydrates play a crucial role in managing NAFLD by slowing down the digestion and absorption of sugars. This slower digestion process promotes feelings of fullness, which can be beneficial for weight management. Soluble fiber, in particular, is effective in reducing liver fat accumulation. Excellent sources of fiber-rich carbohydrates include oats, barley, fruits, vegetables, and legumes. Incorporating these foods into the diet can support overall health and contribute to better management of NAFLD.

2.3 Complex carbohydrates

Complex carbohydrates are preferable to simple sugars because they provide sustained energy and are less likely to be converted to fat in the liver. This makes them a beneficial choice for individuals seeking to maintain stable energy levels and support liver health. However, it's important to note that the relationship between carbohydrates and liver health is complex and multifaceted. Recent research has shown that carbohydrates are positively correlated with inflammation, which can increase lipid deposition through multiple pathways. This finding may explain why some patients with NAFLD experience worsening conditions after switching to a 'vegetarian' diet that is often high in carbohydrates [8]. Examples of complex carbohydrates include whole grains, brown rice, and quinoa, all of which can be effectively incorporated into a balanced diet to promote overall well-being.

2.4 Minimal added sugars

Reducing the intake of added sugars is crucial for patients with NAFLD, as high sugar consumption is linked to increased liver fat accumulation and inflammation. A significant contributor to this risk is the consumption of foods and beverages sweetened with high-fructose corn syrup (HFCS), which is known to stimulate de novo lipogenesis, leading to the development and progression of NAFLD [1, 9, 10]. Fructose, a component of HFCS, bypasses the major rate-limiting step of glycolysis, promoting hepatic fat accumulation and inflammation [10]. To mitigate these risks, it is advisable to avoid or limit foods with added sugars, such as sodas, candies, and processed snacks, particularly those containing HFCS. By minimizing the consumption of these sugars, individuals with NAFLD can better manage their condition and support liver health [9–11].

2.5 Rich in antioxidants

Carbohydrate sources rich in antioxidants play a crucial role in mitigating oxidative stress and inflammation in the liver, both of which are key factors in the progression of NAFLD. The significance of antioxidants in managing NAFLD is intricately linked to the complex interplay between reactive oxygen species (ROS), inflammation, and lipid metabolism within the liver. ROS are generated from various cellular sources, including the mitochondrial respiratory chain, cytochrome P450 system (CYP450), and NADPH oxidase complex. When present in excess, ROS can lead to oxidative stress. In inflammatory conditions, immune cells release large quantities of reactive oxygen radicals, which can potentially cause chronic inflammation if healthy tissues are not reconstructed in a timely manner. This chronic inflammation, which may be triggered by high intake of starchy carbohydrates, perpetuates the activation of inflammatory mediators such as NF-κB, thereby sustaining the inflammatory cycle. The oxidative stress induced by elevated ROS levels can result in apoptosis and necrosis of liver cells. Moreover, ROS can initiate chain reactions between free radicals and unsaturated fatty acids, forming toxic lipid intermediates that exacerbate liver damage. Additionally, carbohydrates may activate ROS through CYP enzymes, further aggravating lipid metabolism disorders due to oxidative stress. Given these mechanisms, consuming a diet rich in antioxidants is essential for individuals managing NAFLD. Colorful fruits and vegetables are excellent sources of antioxidants that can help alleviate the effects of oxidative stress and support liver health. Incorporating a variety of antioxidant-rich foods into the diet provides a range of beneficial compounds that work through different mechanisms to combat oxidative stress and inflammation. These compounds may include vitamins C and E, carotenoids, flavonoids, and other polyphenols found in fruits, vegetables, nuts, and whole grains [8].

3. Fruits consumption guidelines for NAFLD patients

Fruits play a significant role in the dietary management of NAFLD. When selecting fruits for a food basket aimed at patients with NAFLD, several characteristics should be considered:

3.1 Key characteristics of fruits for NAFLD patients

3.1.1 Low sugar content

While fruits are generally healthy, those with lower sugar levels are preferable for individuals with NAFLD. Excessive sugar intake can exacerbate liver fat accumulation. Fruits like berries (strawberries, blueberries) and citrus fruits (lemons, limes) are lower in sugar compared to tropical fruits like bananas and mangoes. This is particularly important as high fructose intake increases hepatic de novo lipogenesis (DNL), reduces fatty acid β-oxidation (FAO), and leads to fatty acid deposition [12, 13].

3.1.2 High antioxidant content

Fruits rich in antioxidants, such as polyphenols and flavonoids, can help reduce oxidative stress and inflammation associated with NAFLD. Examples include apples, grapes, and cherries, which have been noted for their beneficial phytoconstituents. These antioxidants, including vitamin C, vitamin E, beta-carotene, and polyphenols, neutralize free radicals and mitigate the detrimental effects of oxidative stress on the liver. The anti-inflammatory properties of these compounds are crucial in alleviating NAFLD symptoms, as the condition is frequently accompanied by an inflammatory response [12, 13].

3.1.3 Anti-inflammatory properties

Certain fruits possess anti-inflammatory properties that can be beneficial for liver health. Berries, for example, are known to have compounds that may help modulate inflammatory pathways. The polyphenols and flavonoids found in fruits can reduce the severity of inflammation in the liver. This is particularly important as NAFLD is often associated with chronic inflammation, and inhibiting this inflammation is crucial to managing the condition [12, 13].

3.1.4 Fiber-rich

Fruits that are high in dietary fiber can aid in digestion and help maintain a healthy weight, which is crucial for managing NAFLD. Apples, pears, and raspberries are excellent sources of fiber. Dietary fiber, abundant in fruits, is a type of short-chain fatty acid (SCFA) produced by the fermentation of intestinal microorganisms. These SCFAs have numerous benefits, including maintaining the integrity of the intestinal barrier, reducing inflammatory reactions in the liver, regulating appetite, and maintaining glucose balance at the systemic level. Furthermore, dietary fiber enhances satiety, thus promoting calorie restriction [12].

3.1.5 Bioactive compounds

Fruits containing bioactive compounds such as catechins, resveratrol, and other phytochemicals may help in improving liver health by enhancing lipid metabolism and reducing fat accumulation in the liver. Examples include grapes, berries, apples, citrus fruits, and cherries. These bioactive compounds have been shown to have various beneficial effects on liver health, including improving insulin sensitivity and regulating liver lipid metabolism [12, 13].

3.1.6 Moderation in consumption

While fruits are healthy, moderation is key. Studies suggest that excessive fruit consumption (more than four servings per day) may exacerbate liver steatosis and dyslipidemia in patients with NAFLD. This is because fruits contain natural fructose, and high fructose intake can promote the development of NAFLD. It's important to note that the effects of fruit consumption may vary between individuals and populations. For instance, some studies have found differences in the relationship between fruit intake and NAFLD prevalence between males and females, which may be attributed to differences in dietary patterns and metabolic processes [12, 13].

3.2 Recommended fruits

Berries: Strawberries, blueberries, and blackberries.
Citrus fruits: Oranges, lemons, and grapefruits.
Apples: Particularly with the skin for added fiber.
Pears: High in fiber and low in sugar.
Grapes, Pomegranates: Contain beneficial antioxidants.

4. Vegetable consumption guidelines for NAFLD patients

Vegetable consumption is crucial for individuals with NAFLD due to their rich nutrient profile and low-calorie content. Vegetables provide essential fiber and antioxidants, which help regulate blood sugar, reduce liver fat accumulation, and combat oxidative stress and inflammation. Incorporating a variety of non-starchy vegetables into the diet can significantly support liver health and overall well-being in NAFLD patients. Patients with nonalcoholic fatty liver disease should aim for a daily intake of four to five servings of non-starchy vegetables, totaling at least 500 grams per day [14]. This intake helps manage blood sugar levels, reduces fat accumulation in the liver, and provides essential nutrients [13–15].

4.1 Types of vegetables

4.1.1 Non-starchy vegetables (recommended)

Examples include artichoke, asparagus, baby corn, bell peppers, beets, Brussels sprouts, broccoli, cabbage, carrots, cauliflower, celery, chayote, cucumber, eggplant, leeks, okra, radishes, salad greens, spinach, turnips, tomato, and zucchini. These vegetables are low in calories and carbohydrates but high in essential nutrients and fiber [15].

4.1.2 Starchy vegetables (limit consumption)

Examples: Beans (black, kidney, navy, andpinto), butternut squash, cassava, chickpeas, corn, lentils, peas, sweet potatoes, vegetable juices, white potatoes, and yams.

4.2 Key recommendations

4.2.1 High-fiber vegetables

Leafy greens like spinach, kale, and lettuce are excellent choices for improving digestive health and aiding in weight management, which are crucial factors in NAFLD management [14, 15].

4.2.2 Antioxidant-rich vegetables

Consuming broccoli and other antioxidant-rich vegetables can help reduce inflammation and oxidative stress in the liver, potentially slowing the progression of NAFLD [16].

4.2.3 Preparation methods

To maximize nutrient benefits, it's recommended to eat vegetables in their whole form. This can include raw, roasted, sautéed, grilled, blanched, or in soups. These methods help preserve the nutritional value of the vegetables [16].

4.2.4 Vegetables to avoid

It's advisable to limit or avoid fried vegetables, such as french fries and potato chips. These foods are high in unhealthy fats and can contribute to liver fat accumulation and inflammation, potentially worsening NAFLD [16].

5. Protein consumption guidelines for patients with NAFLD

Managing NAFLD requires careful attention to dietary choices, particularly regarding protein intake. This guide outlines essential recommendations for protein consumption to support liver health and overall well-being.

5.1 Key recommendations

5.1.1 Balanced protein intake

For individuals with NAFLD, a daily protein intake of 1.0 to 1.2 grams per kilogram of ideal body weight is advisable, which can vary based on personal health and activity levels [17]. To calculate daily protein requirements more accurately, several factors should be considered: Age, gender, height, weight, activity level, health goals. Online tools and specialized applications can assist in this calculation by taking these factors into account. These resources provide a more precise estimate of an individual's protein needs, offering valuable guidance for those managing NAFLD or other health conditions.

It is important to note that while these calculators offer helpful insights, they should be used as general guidelines. For personalized nutritional advice, especially for those with NAFLD, consultation with a registered dietitian or healthcare professional is recommended.

5.1.2 Quality of protein sources

Plant-based proteins: Prioritize legumes (beans, lentils, chickpeas), tofu, tempeh, and quinoa. These options are not only rich in protein but also high in fiber, promoting digestive health [17].

Lean animal proteins: Include chicken, turkey, and fish (especially fatty varieties like salmon and mackerel). These sources are lower in saturated fats, making them more suitable for liver health [17, 18].

Dairy: Incorporate low-fat or fat-free dairy products such as yogurt, milk, and cheese, which can also contribute to protein intake [17].

5.1.3 Limit certain proteins

Reduce consumption of red meat and processed meats (like bacon, sausages, and deli meats) due to their high saturated fat content, which can worsen liver inflammation [17].

5.1.4 Balancing nutrients

Ensure protein intake is complemented with healthy fats (from nuts, seeds, avocados, and olive oil) and complex carbohydrates (such as whole grains, fruits, and vegetables) [18–20].

Avoid diets excessively high in protein that may neglect other essential nutrients, as this can place additional stress on the liver [19].

5.1.5 Weight management considerations

For those aiming to lose weight, protein can be beneficial in preserving muscle mass while reducing fat [21]. Additionally, dietary modifications, such as following a Mediterranean diet rich in fruits, vegetables, whole grains, and olive oil, have been associated with improved outcomes in NAFLD patients. Considering the multifactorial nature of NAFLD, personalized dietary approaches tailored to individual preferences and needs are crucial for successful weight management and overall disease management [22].

5.1.6 Avoid excessive protein intake

Extremely high-protein diets, particularly those focusing heavily on animal proteins, should be avoided to prevent increased liver workload and potential health complications [18].

For patients with NAFLD, a balanced approach to protein consumption is crucial. Emphasizing plant-based proteins and lean animal sources while limiting red and processed meats can significantly contribute to liver health. Ongoing research is essential to refine these guidelines and further understand the impact of specific amino acids on NAFLD management.

6. Dairy consumption guidelines for NAFLD patients

The role of dairy products in NAFLD management has been a subject of research, with mixed findings. However, recent studies and guidelines suggest that moderate dairy consumption can be part of a healthy diet for individuals with NAFLD.

6.1 Key recommendations

6.1.1 Type of dairy matters

Research indicates that the type of dairy consumed matters significantly, with full-fat dairy products potentially increasing the risk of metabolic syndrome and NAFLD, while low-fat or fat-free dairy products may offer protective effects [23, 24].

6.1.2 Potential benefits of low-fat dairy

Improved insulin sensitivity: Low-fat dairy products are rich in calcium, magnesium, and high-quality proteins, which can help improve insulin sensitivity, a key factor in NAFLD development and progression [25].

Weight management: Dairy products, especially those low in fat, can help with weight management by increasing satiety and reducing overall calorie intake [26].

Reduced inflammation: fermented dairy products containing probiotics, such as lactic acid bacteria and bifidobacteria, have been associated with various health benefits, including improved glucose homeostasis and inflammatory markers, which are essential for managing conditions like diabetes and obesity [23].

6.1.3 Guidelines and recommendations

The American Association for the Study of Liver Diseases (AASLD) does not have specific dairy recommendations for NAFLD patients but supports a balanced diet that includes low-fat or fat-free dairy products as part of an overall strategy for weight management and metabolic health [27].

The Dietary Approaches to Stop Hypertension (DASH) diet and the Mediterranean diet are two well-known dietary regimens that, in addition to emphasizing the consumption of fruits, vegetables, whole grains, and low-calorie foods, also focus on low-fat dairy products. According to research findings, these diets have resulted in improved liver enzymes and reduced hepatic steatosis (fat accumulation in the liver), and favorable changes in oxidative stress biomarkers in overweight and obese patients with NAFLD [28, 29].

6.2 Individual considerations

When recommending dairy products for patients with NAFLD, it is crucial to consider individual factors such as lactose intolerance, dairy allergies, and personal preferences. Lactose-hydrolyzed dairy products and plant-based milk alternatives are becoming popular options for those with lactose intolerance and dairy allergies, respectively [30, 31]. The development of lactose-free dairy products, like lactose-free albumin from whey, provides alternatives rich in amino acids and high digestibility. Understanding consumer preferences, availability, quality, and health consciousness is essential when making dairy product recommendations [32]. By considering these individual factors and the diverse range of dairy alternatives available, tailored recommendations can be made to meet the specific needs and preferences of each patient with NAFLD.

In conclusion, moderate consumption of low-fat or fat-free dairy products can be part of a healthy diet for individuals with NAFLD, potentially offering benefits for insulin sensitivity, weight management, and inflammation. However, it's essential to tailor dietary recommendations to each patient's specific needs and preferences, and to consider them as part of a comprehensive approach to managing NAFLD, which includes regular physical activity, weight loss if overweight or obese, and management of other metabolic risk factors.

7. Fat consumption guidelines for NAFLD patients

Contrary to common belief, not all dietary fats are detrimental for those with NAFLD. In fact, certain fats can promote liver health. It's important to differentiate between various types of fats and their respective effects on the liver.

7.1 Types of fats and their implications

7.1.1 Saturated fats

Commonly found in animal products like red meat and dairy, as well as some plant oils (e.g., coconut and palm oil), saturated fats can exacerbate liver fat accumulation and inflammation [33, 34]. Moreover, studies highlight the association between the consumption of foods high in saturated fat content and the increasing prevalence of obesity, which is closely related to NAFLD and other metabolic disorders like insulin resistance and fatty liver disease [35, 36]. Therefore, individuals with NAFLD should limit their intake of these fats.

7.1.2 Trans fats

These unhealthy fats are typically present in processed foods and baked goods. Trans fats are produced through hydrogenation and have a negative impact on liver function [6, 37]. It is advisable to eliminate them from the diet entirely.

7.1.3 Monounsaturated fats

Monounsaturated Fats (MUFAs) are present in foods such as olive oil, avocados, nuts, and seeds. These fats can enhance liver enzyme levels and decrease liver fat, making them beneficial additions to your diet [6, 37]. The Mediterranean diet, renowned for its health benefits, emphasizes the consumption of MUFAs. Foods rich in MUFAs, such as olive oil, nuts, and seeds, play a crucial role in providing these healthy fats, which can improve liver enzyme levels and reduce liver fat.

7.1.4 Polyunsaturated fats

Polyunsaturated Fats (PUFAs): Found in fatty fish (like salmon and mackerel), flaxseed oil, and walnuts, PUFAs, especially omega-3 fatty acids, are known for their anti-inflammatory properties and support liver health [6, 37].

7.2 Key recommendations

7.2.1 Minimize saturated and trans fats

Cut back on red meat and processed foods. Opt for lean proteins, such as poultry and fish, to reduce fat intake that can harm liver health [6].

7.2.2 Incorporate MUFAs

Add healthy fats like olive oil, avocados, nuts, and seeds to your meals. Use olive oil for cooking and as a dressing for salads [6].

7.2.3 Focus on omega-3 fatty acids

Aim to eat fatty fish at least twice weekly. If fish is not a regular part of your diet, consider flaxseed oil or algae-based omega-3 supplements [6].

7.2.4 Moderate total fat intake

Recommendations for NAFLD patients suggest that fat intake should be less than 30% of daily calories, with an emphasis on increasing consumption of foods rich in mono- and polyunsaturated fatty acids [6, 17].

7.2.5 Prioritize whole foods

Choose whole, unprocessed foods over refined carbohydrates and sugary beverages, as these can contribute to increased liver fat [6, 38].

8. Beverage selection guidelines for NAFLD patients

The body is mostly composed of water, so staying hydrated is crucial for good health. When selecting beverages for patients with NAFLD, it is important to consider the impact of different types of drinks on liver health. Here are some key points based on recent research:

8.1 Avoid sugar-sweetened beverages (SSBs)

Sugar-sweetened beverages are strongly associated with an increased risk of NAFLD. Studies indicate that each additional serving of SSBs per day can significantly raise the prevalence of NAFLD [39–41].

8.2 Limit artificially sweetened beverages (ASBs)

Multiple studies suggest that limiting the consumption of ASBs is advisable in the context of NAFLD [41]. Additionally, Interestingly, replacing SSBs with ASBs has been associated with a higher prevalence of NAFLD, emphasizing the potential adverse effects of ASBs on liver health [40, 42]. Although further research is recommended in this area, the existing evidence highlights the importance of being mindful of ASB consumption for individuals at risk of or managing NAFLD [41].

8.3 Consider low/No-calorie beverages

These may have a nonlinear association with NAFLD, with moderate consumption potentially being safer, but caution is advised as higher intake levels might not be beneficial [40].

8.4 Include coffee and tea

The consumption of coffee and tea has been extensively studied in relation to NAFLD. Although the results of studies have shown conflicting effects regarding the efficacy of these beverages in reducing the incidence and progression of NAFLD [43, 44], there is overall increasing evidence supporting the protective role of coffee and tea in patients with NAFLD [39, 43, 45].

8.5 Moderate fruit juice intake

The consumption of fruit juice in individuals with NAFLD has been a topic of interest in various studies. Research indicates that a higher intake of sugar–sweetened fruit juices is associated with increased NAFLD prevalence. Conversely, low/no-calorie beverages (LNCB) exhibit a nonlinear relationship with NAFLD, suggesting that higher consumption levels may be linked to an increased risk of developing NAFLD [40, 46]. Additionally, studies have shown that 100% fruit juices do not significantly differ from whole fruits in terms of nutrient content; however, whole fruits, due to their fiber content, can help reduce the risk of overweight, obesity, and metabolic syndrome, which are risk factors for NAFLD [47].

9. Dietary approaches for managing NAFLD

In the field of nutritional interventions for individuals with NAFLD, no specific diet has been introduced exclusively for this condition. However, based on existing studies and the effects of the quantity and quality of macronutrients and micronutrients on liver health, two diets that closely align with the nutritional criteria for managing NAFLD are the Dietary Approaches to Stop Hypertension (DASH) diet and, particularly, the Mediterranean diet. Below, we will further introduce these dietary approaches.

9.1 DASH diet

The DASH (Dietary Approaches to Stop Hypertension) diet, originally developed for blood pressure management, offers benefits for liver health. Rich in vegetables, fruits, and whole grains, it promotes low-fat dairy consumption while limiting saturated and trans fats. This approach aids weight loss, reduces inflammation, and decreases oxidative stress – crucial factors in managing NAFLD [48–49]. The diet's low sodium and saturated fat content improve overall metabolic health. Studies show that adhering to the DASH diet is associated with lower NAFLD prevalence, reduced liver fat, and improved liver function markers, including liver enzymes and insulin resistance [48, 50, 51].

9.2 Mediterranean diet

The Mediterranean diet has gained recognition as an effective nutritional strategy for managing NAFLD. This dietary pattern, rich in plant-based foods, healthy fats, and lean proteins, offers multiple benefits for liver health. Key components of the diet include abundant vegetables, fruits, whole grains, legumes, nuts, and seeds, with olive oil as the primary fat source. Fish and poultry are consumed moderately, while red meat and sweets are limited. Research demonstrates several positive effects of this diet on NAFLD:

- Reduced liver inflammation: High antioxidant and polyphenol content combat oxidative stress [52, 53].
- Improved insulin sensitivity: Balanced nutrients help regulate blood sugar levels [54, 55].
- Decreased liver fat: Studies show significant reductions in liver fat content [54, 55].
- Enhanced lipid profile: Lowers harmful cholesterol and triglycerides [56].
- Improved gut microbiome: High fiber intake promotes digestive health, indirectly benefiting the liver [57].

Implementing the Mediterranean diet involves increasing consumption of plant-based foods, using olive oil for cooking, incorporating fish regularly, and limiting red meat intake. However, this dietary approach should be part of a comprehensive NAFLD management plan, including regular exercise and weight control.

Table 1 provides a concise comparison of the DASH diet and Mediterranean diet in the context NAFLD.

Aspect	Mediterranean diet	DASH diet
Main features	• High intake of fruits, vegetables, whole grains • Olive oil as primary fat source • Moderate consumption of fish, poultry, and low-fat dairy • Limited red meat and sweets • Moderate red wine consumption	• Emphasis on vegetables, fruits, whole grains • Lean proteins like fish and poultry • Limited salt, sugar, and saturated fats • Increased intake of potassium, magnesium, and calcium • Controlled portion sizes
Effect on NAFLD	• Reduces liver inflammation • Improves insulin sensitivity • Decreases liver fat • Improves liver enzymes	• Lowers blood pressure, benefiting liver function • Improves blood lipid profile • Aids in weight loss • Reduces insulin resistance
Dietary composition	• 40–50% carbohydrates • 35–40% fat (primarily from olive oil) • 15–20% protein • High fiber (>25 g/day)	• 55% carbohydrates • 27% fat • 18% protein • Low sodium (<2300 mg/day) • High fiber (>30 g/day)
Anti-inflammatory effect	• Highly effective due to high antioxidant content • Reduces inflammatory markers like CRP and IL-6	• Effective, but possibly less than Mediterranean diet • Reduces inflammatory markers, especially in hypertensive individuals
Weight control	• Supports sustainable weight loss • Improves body composition	• May be slightly more effective due to calorie control focus • Faster short-term weight loss

Aspect	Mediterranean diet	DASH diet
Insulin resistance	• Significant improvement in insulin sensitivity • Reduces risk of type 2 diabetes	• Improves insulin sensitivity • Reduces risk of type 2 diabetes
Flexibility	• Generally, more flexible • Easier to adapt to various lifestyles	• More structured approach • Requires more precise meal planning
Overall impact on NAFLD	• Highly effective • Significant improvement in liver fibrosis and steatosis	• Highly effective • Significant improvement in metabolic and hepatic parameters

Table 1.
Comparison of Mediterranean and DASH diets in managing NAFLD.

9.3 Self-assessment tools for adherence to the DASH diet

Self-assessment tools play a crucial role in monitoring adherence to the Dietary Approaches to Stop Hypertension (DASH) diet. These tools help individuals track their dietary intake and assess how closely they are following the DASH diet recommendations. Several validated instruments have been developed for this purpose:

9.3.1 DASH online questionnaire (OLQ)

The Dietary Approaches to Stop Hypertension Online Questionnaire (DASH OLQ) is a web-based dietary assessment tool designed to evaluate the intake of food servings in alignment with the DASH diet. This tool encompasses 11 food groups corresponding to the DASH diet categories and is administered once weekly over a four-week period. The DASH OLQ has been rigorously validated against the Block Food Frequency Questionnaire (FFQ), demonstrating strong correlations in measuring nutrient intake and DASH food group consumption. It provides a quick and efficient method for assessing adherence to the DASH diet, making it a valuable resource for both clinical and research applications [58].

9.3.2 Dash-q

The DASH-Q is a brief self-report tool aimed at evaluating the quality of diet and adherence to the DASH diet. It includes 11 questions focused on the intake of various food groups. This instrument is part of the Hypertension Self-Care Activity Level Effects (H-SCALE) framework. The DASH-Q has undergone validation to confirm its psychometric properties, ensuring it is both reliable and effective for research purposes. It provides a straightforward scoring system that reflects an individual's adherence to the recommendations of the DASH diet. This accessible measure enables researchers and healthcare professionals to effectively assess compliance with DASH dietary guidelines, which are essential for managing hypertension and enhancing cardiovascular health [59].

9.3.3 Mobile apps

Smartphone applications are emerging as innovative tools for DASH diet self-management. These apps, such as NOOM and DASH To TEN, offer a range of features designed to support dietary adherence. Key functionalities include food logging, goal setting, and access to educational resources. By incorporating behavior change techniques, these apps aim to enhance user engagement and promote long-term dietary modifications. Some applications go further by providing calculations for food servings based on DASH recommendations, offering users precise guidance tailored to their individual needs. As digital health solutions continue to evolve, these mobile apps represent a promising avenue for improving accessibility and effectiveness of DASH diet implementation in daily life [60].

9.4 Self-assessment tools for adherence to the Mediterranean diet

Several self-assessment tools have been developed to measure adherence to the Mediterranean diet. These tools vary in their complexity, components, and scoring systems. Here are some of the most prominent and widely used tools:

9.4.1 14-item Mediterranean diet adherence screener (MEDAS)

This tool, developed in Spain, consists of 14 questions about food consumption and dietary habits. It has been widely validated and used in various countries. The MEDAS can be self-administered or completed by a dietitian, providing immediate feedback on adherence levels [61, 62].

9.4.2 Mediterranean eating pattern for Americans (MEPA)

Developed for use in the USA, MEPA includes food groups typical of the Mediterranean diet but adapted for American dietary patterns. The MEPA-III version has additional components and more detailed food categories. It can be delivered electronically or via phone and has shown good concordance with food frequency questionnaires [4].

9.4.3 Mediterranean lifestyle (MEDLIFE) index

This is the only assessment tool that incorporates dietary behaviors and lifestyle factors along with food intake questions. It aims to capture a more comprehensive picture of the Mediterranean lifestyle [63, 64].

9.4.4 Mediterranean diet score (MDS) by Trichopoulou

One of the earliest and most widely used scoring systems, it's based on population-specific median cut-offs. However, it may have limitations for cross-study comparisons due to these population-specific cut-offs [64].

9.4.5 15-items pyramid based Mediterranean diet score (PyrMDS)

This tool is based on the recommendations of the Mediterranean diet pyramid and is suggested as one of the measurement options [64].

10. Behavioral change guide for improving nutrition in patients with NAFLD

10.1 Setting specific and realistic goals

10.1.1 Short-term, achievable objectives

Establish specific goals, such as losing 0.5 kg per week or engaging in 30 minutes of physical activity daily. These goals should be measurable and realistic to maintain patient motivation.

10.1.2 Long-term goals

Focus on improving liver health and reducing cardiovascular risks through sustainable lifestyle and dietary changes.

10.2 Identifying and managing barriers

10.2.1 Recognizing personal obstacles

Identify barriers such as stress, time constraints, or financial issues that may impede healthy eating and physical activity. Develop strategies to manage these obstacles effectively.

10.2.2 Finding alternative solutions

If time is limited, opt for shorter, more frequent exercise sessions instead of lengthy workouts. To combat stress, explore relaxation techniques like meditation or yoga.

10.3 Leveraging social support

10.3.1 Family and friend support

Engage family members and friends for encouragement and companionship in lifestyle changes.

10.3.2 Participation in support groups

Joining exercise groups or weight loss programs can help maintain motivation and facilitate experience sharing.

10.4 Continuous monitoring and evaluation

10.4.1 Food journaling

Recording daily food intake and physical activities helps individuals better understand their dietary and activity patterns, enabling necessary adjustments.

10.4.2 Regular progress assessment

Utilize self-assessment nutrition tools introduced in the previous section and physical activity self-assessment applications to measure progress in behavior change. This practice helps individuals recognize their achievements and find greater motivation to continue.

10.5 Making healthy nutritional choices

10.5.1 Embracing liver-friendly dietary patterns

Adopt Mediterranean, DASH, or other dietary patterns rich in fruits, vegetables, whole grains, lean proteins, and healthy fats, as explained in the previous section, to improve liver health.

10.5.2 Portion control

Implement portion control techniques such as using smaller plates and accurately measuring food quantities to reduce calorie intake.

10.5.3 Limiting processed foods

Reduce consumption of processed meats, refined carbohydrates, and sweetened beverages to prevent liver condition deterioration.

10.6 Enhancing motivation and persistence

10.6.1 Self-rewarding

After achieving short-term goals, reward oneself. This reward can be an enjoyable activity or a desired purchase.

10.6.2 Embracing small changes

Significant and lasting changes require time. Instead of focusing on sudden changes, gradually improve eating and exercise habits to achieve long-term success.

10.7 Utilizing professional resources

10.7.1 Consultation with a nutritionist

Seeking advice from a nutrition specialist to develop a personalized meal plan tailored to individual needs can be beneficial.

10.7.2 Healthcare team support

Maintain contact with physicians or gastroenterologists to monitor health status and implement necessary medication or further dietary changes as needed.

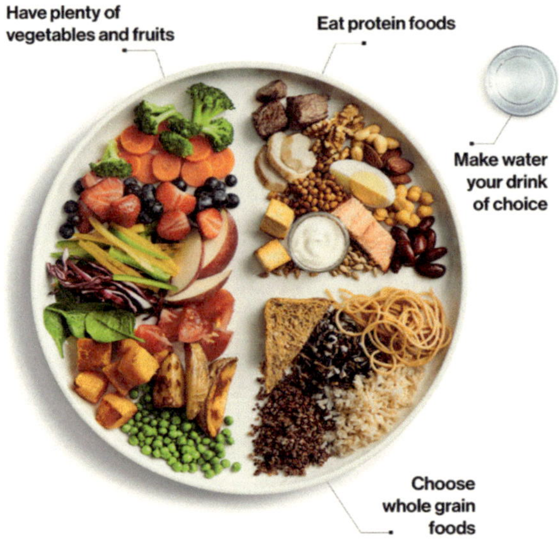
Have plenty of
vegetables and fruits
Eat protein foods
Make water
your drink
of choice
Choose
whole grain
foods

Figure 2.
A healthy plate for managing nonalcoholic fatty liver disease. Source: © All rights reserved. Canada's Food Guide: Snapshot. Health Canada, 2019. Reproduced with permission from the Minister of Health, 2024 [65].

11. Conclusions

Nonalcoholic fatty liver disease is a complex metabolic disorder closely linked to lifestyle factors. Effective management primarily revolves around dietary modifications, increased physical activity, and weight reduction. While overall calorie restriction is crucial, the composition of the diet significantly influences NAFLD outcomes.

This chapter delved into the intricate relationship between macronutrients and NAFLD, emphasizing the importance of carbohydrate quality, fiber intake, and the need to minimize added sugars. The role of fruits and vegetables in providing essential nutrients and antioxidants was highlighted, along with the significance of protein intake for maintaining muscle mass and supporting liver health. The importance of selecting low-fat dairy products and understanding the impact of different fat types on liver health was also discussed. **Figure 2** summarizes the ideal daily intake of food groups that can support liver health, as well as the key nutritional concepts discussed in this chapter.

Two dietary approaches, the DASH diet and the Mediterranean diet, emerged as promising strategies for managing NAFLD. Both emphasize whole foods, reduced intake of processed products, and a balanced macronutrient profile. Self-assessment tools were introduced to facilitate adherence to these dietary patterns.

Behavioral change is essential for long-term success in managing NAFLD. Setting realistic goals, identifying and overcoming barriers, and leveraging social support are crucial components of this process.

In conclusion, a comprehensive approach combining dietary modifications, physical activity, and behavioral changes is essential for managing NAFLD. By understanding the role of macronutrients, incorporating diverse food groups, and adopting suitable dietary patterns, individuals can improve liver health and overall well-being.

Acknowledgements

We would like to express our sincere gratitude to Health Canada and to Carneiro and Leloup for granting permission to use visual materials from their respective works in this chapter.

Additionally, we acknowledge the role of Perplexity AI in the preparation of this chapter. This tool was specifically utilized for translation and editing, helping to refine the content from the original language into English. We emphasize that the chapter's content was entirely developed by the authors, and Perplexity AI was employed solely to enhance language quality and ensure compliance with scientific publication standards.

Conflict of interest

The authors declare no conflict of interest.

Author details

Narges Mobasheri*, Leila Ghahremani and Mahin Nazari
Shiraz University of Medical Sciences, Shiraz, Iran

*Address all correspondence to: mobasheri.mn@gmail.com

References

[1] Liver EA for the S of the, Diabetes EA for the S of, Obesity EA for the S of. EASL-EASD-EASO clinical practice guidelines on the management of metabolic dysfunction-associated steatotic liver disease (MASLD). Obesity Facts. 2024;**17**(4):374-444. DOI: 10.1159/000443344

[2] Chalasani N, Younossi Z, Lavine JE, Charlton M, Cusi K, Rinella M, et al. The diagnosis and management of nonalcoholic fatty liver disease: Practice guidance from the American Association for the Study of Liver Diseases. Hepatology. 2018;**67**(1):328-357. DOI: 10.1002/hep.29367

[3] Leoni S, Tovoli F, Napoli L, Serio I, Ferri S, Bolondi L. Current guidelines for the management of non-alcoholic fatty liver disease: A systematic review with comparative analysis. World Journal of Gastroenterology. 2018;**24**(30):3361. DOI: 10.3748/wjg.v24.i30.3361

[4] Kwak MS, Kim D. Non-alcoholic fatty liver disease and lifestyle modifications, focusing on physical activity. The Korean Journal of Internal Medicine. 2018;**33**(1):64. DOI: 10.3904/kjim.2017.343

[5] Houttu V, Csader S, Nieuwdorp M, Holleboom AG, Schwab U. Dietary interventions in patients with non-alcoholic fatty liver disease: A systematic review and meta-analysis. Frontiers in Nutrition. 2021;**8**:716783. DOI: 10.3389/fnut.2021.716783

[6] Beygi M, Nazarpour S, Mohammadi S, Sadeghian M, Mohammadi M, Gholami F, et al. Management of metabolic-associated fatty liver disease/metabolic dysfunction-associated steatotic liver disease: From medication therapy to nutritional interventions. Nutrients. 2024;**16**(14):2220. DOI: 10.3390/nu16142220

[7] Carneiro L, Leloup C. Mens sana in corpore Sano: Does the glycemic index have a role to play? Nutrients. 2020;**12**(10):2989. DOI: 10.3390/nu12102989

[8] Gao Y, Li X, Gao Y, Zhang Y, Xu M, Zhao J. Carbohydrates deteriorate fatty liver by activating the inflammatory response. Nutrition Research Reviews. 2022;**35**(2):252-267. DOI: 10.1017/S0954422421000202

[9] Huneault HE, Lim GE, Johnson JD. The impact and burden of dietary sugars on the liver. Hepatology Communications. 2023;**7**(11):e0297. DOI: 10.1097/HC9.0000000000000297

[10] DiNicolantonio JJ, Subramonian AM, O'Keefe JH. Added fructose as a principal driver of non-alcoholic fatty liver disease: a public health crisis. Archives of Disease in Childhood. 2017;**4**(2):e000631. DOI: 10.1136/openhrt-2017-000631

[11] Zhang S, Guo X, Jin W, Ma Y, Zhang L, Ren Y, et al. Added sugar intake and its forms and sources in relation to risk of non-alcoholic fatty liver disease: Results from the Tianjin chronic low-grade systemic inflammation and health cohort study. British Journal of Nutrition. 2023;**129**(12):2094-2101. DOI: 10.1017/S000711452200277X

[12] Pathak MP, Sharma A, Sharma S, Sharma P, Kumar N, Dhiman M, et al. Therapeutic potential of bioactive phytoconstituents found in fruits in the treatment of non-alcoholic fatty liver disease: A comprehensive review. Heliyon. 2023;**9**(4):11. DOI: 10.1016/j.heliyon.2023.e15347

[13] Wang R, Zhu Y, Zhao Y, Liu X, Zhang H, Zhao Y, et al. Fruit and vegetable intake and the risk of non-alcoholic fatty liver disease: A meta-analysis of observational studies. Frontiers in Nutrition. 2024;**11**:1398184. DOI: 10.3389/fnut.2024.1398184

[14] Du LJ, Xing Q, Zhang L, Jiang Y, Jia YY, Zhao XY, et al. Inverse association of fruit and vegetable consumption with nonalcoholic fatty liver disease in Chinese patients with type 2 diabetes mellitus. Nutrients. 2022;**14**(21):4559. DOI: 10.3390/nu14214559

[15] Mishra V. Plant Metabolites and Vegetables for Gastrointestinal Disease Prevention and Treatment. In: Plant Metabolites and Vegetables as Nutraceuticals. 1st ed. Ontario, Canada: Apple Academic Press; 2024. p. 299-331

[16] Sohouli MH, Fatahi S, Sharifi-Zahabi E, Santos HO, Tripathi N, Lari A, et al. Associations between dietary total antioxidant capacity and odds of non-alcoholic fatty liver disease (NAFLD) in adults: A case–control study. Journal of Nutritional Science. 2020;**9**:e48. DOI: 10.1017/jns.2020.41

[17] Kargulewicz A, Stankowiak-Kulpa H, Grzymisławski M. Dietary recommendations for patients with nonalcoholic fatty liver disease. Gastroenterology Review/Przegląd Gastroenterologiczny. 2014;**9**(1):18-23. DOI: 10.5114/pg.2014.40845

[18] Khazaei Y, Asghari S, Izadi A, Soleimani D, Azadbakht L, Heshmati J. Association between protein intake from different animal and plant origins and the risk of non-alcoholic fatty liver disease: A case-control study. Clinical Nutrition Research. 2023;**12**(1):29. DOI: 10.7762/cnr.2023.12.1.29

[19] Chen S, Guo X, Zhang X, Yu S, Yang H, Zheng L, et al. Associations of macronutrients intake with MRI-determined hepatic fat content, hepatic fibroinflammation, and NAFLD. The Journal of Clinical Endocrinology & Metabolism. 2023;**108**(12):e1660-e1669. DOI: 10.1210/clinem/dgad346

[20] Ampong I, Watkins A, Gutierrez-Merino J, Ikwuobe J, Griffiths HR. Dietary protein insufficiency: An important consideration in fatty liver disease? British Journal of Nutrition. 2020;**123**(6):601-609. DOI: 10.1017/S0007114519003064

[21] Lang S, Farrell GC, Schattenberg JM, Lotter H, Kuhn GA, Nimphius W, et al. High protein intake is associated with histological disease activity in patients with NAFLD. Hepatology Communications. 2020;**4**(5):681-695. DOI: 10.1002/hep4.1509

[22] Riazi K, Azhari H, Charette JH, Underwood FE, King JA, Afshar EE, et al. Dietary patterns and components in nonalcoholic fatty liver disease (NAFLD): What key messages can health care providers offer? Nutrients. 2019;**11**(12):2878. DOI: 10.3390/nu11122878

[23] Dai W, Xie Y, Zhao Y, Hu F, Lu W, Fu Y, et al. Dairy product consumption was associated with a lower likelihood of non-alcoholic fatty liver disease: A systematic review and meta-analysis. Frontiers in Nutrition. 2023;**10**:1119118. DOI: 10.3389/fnut.2023.1119118

[24] Yuzbashian E, Asghari G, Mirmiran P, Amouzegar A, Azizi F. Dairy product consumption and risk of non-alcoholic fatty liver disease: A systematic review and meta-analysis of observational studies. Nutrition, Metabolism and Cardiovascular Diseases. 2023;**33**(8):1461-1471. DOI: 10.1016/j.numecd.2023.04.018

[25] Muñoz-Alvarez KY, Gutiérrez-Aguilar R, Frigolet ME. Metabolic effects of milk fatty acids: A literature review. Nutrition Bulletin. 2024;**49**(1):19-39. DOI: 10.1111/nbu.12657

[26] Li A, Deng L, Mao Y, Zhu L, Ren F. Dairy products and constituents: A review of their effects on obesity and related metabolic diseases. Critical Reviews in Food Science and Nutrition. 2024;**64**(33):12820-12840. DOI: 10.1080/10408398.2023.2257782

[27] Berg E, Baumgard L, Gabler N, Pearce S, Rhoads R, Selsby J, et al. Impacts of non-and whole-fat milk supplementation on metabolism-associated fatty liver disease (MAFLD) in C57BL/6 mice. Physiology. 2024;**39**(S1):390. DOI: 10.1152/physiol.2024.39.S1.390

[28] Montemayor S, Cuevas-Sierra A, Martínez JA, Milagro FI. Dietary patterns, foods, and nutrients to ameliorate non-alcoholic fatty liver disease: A scoping review. Nutrients. 2023;**15**(18):3987. DOI: 10.3390/nu15183987

[29] Zare Z, Salehi-Abargouei A, Shahvazi S, Nadjarzadeh A, Fallahzadeh H, Namayandeh SM, et al. The effect of the dietary approaches to stop hypertension diet on total antioxidant capacity, superoxide dismutase, catalase, and body composition in patients with non-alcoholic fatty liver disease: A randomized controlled trial. Frontiers in Nutrition. 2023;**10**:1163516. DOI: 10.3389/fnut.2023.1163516

[30] Rombach M, Cong L, Dean DL. Leave the milk for the calf and spread the word: Exploring factors determining US consumers' willingness to try plant-based milk alternatives and their word-of-mouth sharing about plant-based milk alternatives. Beverages. 2024;**10**(2):27. DOI: 10.3390/beverages10020027

[31] Grachchenkov D, Popova N, Shcherbinin A, Krasulya O, Potoroko I. Technological aspects of the production of lactose-free dairy products. In: E3S Web of Conferences. Paris, France: EDP Sciences; 2024. DOI: 10.1051/e3sconf/202453710011

[32] Rekha R, Maruthamuthu K. What factors drive consumer preference of dairy products with education as moderator? An empirical approach. International Review of Management and Marketing. 2024;**14**(4):161-168. DOI: 10.32479/irmm.16315

[33] Arias A, Hernández-Rojas M, Romero-González J, Fregoso-Aguilar T, Martínez-Castillo J. Palm oil and coconut oil saturated fats: Properties, food applications, and health. World Journal of Food Science and Technology. 2023;**7**(1):9-19. DOI: 10.11648/j.wjfst.20230701.12

[34] Fridén M, Åkesson A, Larsson SC. Substitutions of saturated fat intakes with other macronutrients and foods and risk of NAFLD cirrhosis and all-cause hepatocellular carcinoma: A prospective cohort study. The American Journal of Clinical Nutrition. 2024;**120**(1):187-195. DOI: 10.1016/j.ajcnut.2024.05.018

[35] Lawrence GD. Saturated Fats: Time to Assess Their Beneficial Role in a Healthful Diet. Dietetics. Basel, Switzerland: MDPI; 2024;**3**(4):452-462. DOI: 10.3390/dietetics3040033

[36] Vásconez EAC, Lara VEG. Nutrition, obesity and their relationship with liver diseases. Salud, Ciencia y Tecnología-Serie de Conferencias. 2024;**3**:562-562

[37] Sánchez-Torrijos Y, Bozic M, Rodríguez-Peralvarez M, Montero-Álvarez JL. Dietary approach

to NAFLD. In: Romero-Gomez M, editor. Non-Alcoholic Fatty Liver Disease. Cham: Springer; 2020. p. 271-287. DOI: 10.1007/978-3-319-95828-6_15

[38] Ahmed A, Irfan U, Saleem F, Iqbal J, Idrees J, Akhtar MF. The consequences of poor dietary patterns on the proliferation of non-alcoholic fatty liver disease. Cogent Food & Agriculture. 2024;**10**(1):2325206. DOI: 10.1080/23311932.2024.2325206

[39] Chhimwal J, Patial V, Padwad Y. Beverages and non-alcoholic fatty liver disease (NAFLD): Think before you drink. Clinical Nutrition. 2021;**40**(5):2508-2519. DOI: 10.1016/j.clnu.2021.04.011

[40] Naomi ND, Trijsburg L, Ocké MC, Sluik D, Feskens EJM, Imamura F, et al. Sugar-sweetened beverages, low/no-calorie beverages, fruit juice and non-alcoholic fatty liver disease defined by fatty liver index: The SWEET project. Nutrition & Diabetes. 2023;**13**(1):6. DOI: 10.1038/s41387-023-00237-3

[41] Tseng TS, Gu X, Li X, Jiang X, Gu J, Huang J. Sugar-sweetened beverages and artificially sweetened beverages consumption and the risk of nonalcoholic fatty liver (NAFLD) and nonalcoholic steatohepatitis (NASH). Nutrients. 2023;**15**(18):3997. DOI: 10.3390/nu15183997

[42] Mullish BH. Risk factors for liver cancer and chronic liver disease-related death: Are sugar substitutes better than the real thing? Gastroenterology. 2024;**166**(1):213-214. DOI: 10.1053/j.gastro.2023.09.032

[43] Kositamongkol C, Sanguankeo A, Upala S. Beverage consumption in patients with metabolic syndrome and its association with non-alcoholic fatty liver disease: A cross-sectional study. Frontiers in Nutrition. 2024;**11**:1257969. DOI: 10.3389/fnut.2024.1257969

[44] Liu Y, Wang Y, Lai X, Tan Y, Tao Q, Zhu Y, et al. Coffee and the risk of nonalcoholic fatty liver disease: A systematic review and meta-analysis of 11 observational studies. Research Square; 2023. DOI: 10.21203/rs.3.rs-2917946/v1.

[45] Dolati S, Nameni G, Abdollahi S, Heshmati J. Tea and coffee consumption impact on the non-alcoholic fatty liver disease: A systematic review and meta-analysis. Journal of Research in Clinical Medicine. 2024;**12**(1):5-5. DOI: 10.34172/jrcm.2024.33358

[46] Naomi N, Trijsburg L, Ocké MC, Sluik D, Feskens EJM, Imamura F, et al. Association of Sugar-Sweetened Beverages, low/No-calorie beverages and fruit juice intakes with non-alcoholic fatty liver disease: The SWEET project. Current Developments in Nutrition. 2022;**6**:934. DOI: 10.1093/cdn/nzac067.054

[47] Zhang Z, Manivannan S, Keogh JB, Clifton PM. A prospective study of fruit juice consumption and the risk of overall and cardiovascular disease mortality. Nutrients. 2022;**14**(10):2127. DOI: 10.3390/nu14102127

[48] Rooholahzadegan F, Badali T, Heshmati J, Nameni G, Gholizadeh F, Saneei P, et al. The effect of DASH diet on glycemic response, meta-inflammation and serum LPS in obese patients with NAFLD: A double-blind controlled randomized clinical trial. Nutrition & Metabolism. 2023;**20**(1):11. DOI: 10.1186/s12986-023-00733-4

[49] Park SY, Freedman ND, Haiman CA, Le Marchand L, Wilkens LR, Setiawan VW. Diet quality association with nonalcoholic fatty liver disease by

cirrhosis status: The multiethnic cohort. Current Developments in Nutrition. 2020;**4**(3):nzaa024. DOI: 10.1093/cdn/nzaa024

[50] Katsiki N, Stoian AP, Rizzo M. Dietary patterns in non-alcoholic fatty liver disease (NAFLD): Stay on the straight and narrow path! Clínica e Investigación en Arteriosclerosis (English Edition). 2022;**34**:23-30. DOI: 10.1016/j.artere.2022.07.002

[51] Badali T, Rooholahzadegan F, Heshmati J, Nameni G, Gholizadeh F, Saneei P, et al. The effect of DASH diet on atherogenic indices, pro-oxidant-antioxidant balance, and liver steatosis in obese adults with non-alcoholic fatty liver disease: A double-blind controlled randomized clinical trial. Health Promotion Perspectives. 2023;**13**(1):77. DOI: 10.34172/hpp.2023.10

[52] Haigh L, Bremner S, Houghton D, Henderson E, Avery L, Hardy T, et al. The effectiveness and acceptability of Mediterranean diet and calorie restriction in non-alcoholic fatty liver disease (NAFLD): A systematic review and meta-analysis. Clinical Nutrition. 2022;**41**(9):1913-1931. DOI: 10.1016/j.clnu.2022.06.037

[53] Anania C, Perla FM, Olivero F, Pacifico L, Chiesa C. Mediterranean diet and nonalcoholic fatty liver disease. World Journal of Gastroenterology. 2018;**24**(19):2083. DOI: 10.3748/wjg.v24.i19.2083

[54] Ryan MC, Itsiopoulos C, Thodis T, Ward G, Trost N, Hofferberth S, et al. The Mediterranean diet improves hepatic steatosis and insulin sensitivity in individuals with non-alcoholic fatty liver disease. Journal of Hepatology. 2013;**59**(1):138-143. DOI: 10.1016/j.jhep.2013.02.012

[55] Kawaguchi T, Charlton M, Kawaguchi A, Yamamura S, Nakano D, Tsutsumi T, et al. Effects of Mediterranean diet in patients with nonalcoholic fatty liver disease: A systematic review, meta-analysis, and meta-regression analysis of randomized controlled trials. Seminars in Liver Disease. 2021;**41**(3):225-234. DOI: 10.1055/s-0041-1723751

[56] Bekkouche L, Bouchenak M, Malaisse WJ, Yahia DA. The Mediterranean diet adoption improves metabolic, oxidative, and inflammatory abnormalities in Algerian metabolic syndrome patients. Hormone and Metabolic Research. 2014;**46**(4):274-282. DOI: 10.1055/s-0033-1363657

[57] Khavandegar A, Mohamadzadeh Rostami F, Mohammadi M, Hosseini B. Adherence to the Mediterranean diet can beneficially affect the gut microbiota composition: A systematic review. BMC Medical Genomics. 2024;**17**(1):91. DOI: 10.1186/s12920-024-01861-3

[58] Apovian CM, Murphy MC, Cullum-Dugan D, Lin PH, Gilbert KM, Coffman G, et al. Validation of a web-based dietary questionnaire designed for the DASH (dietary approaches to stop hypertension) diet: The DASH online questionnaire. Public Health Nutrition. 2010;**13**(5):615-622. DOI: 10.1017/S1368980009991996

[59] Warren-Findlow J, Reeve CL, Racine EF. Psychometric validation of a brief self-report measure of diet quality: The DASH-Q. Journal of Nutrition Education and Behavior. 2017;**49**(2):92-99.e1. DOI: 10.1016/j.jneb.2016.09.004

[60] Alnooh G, Almutairi F, Alajlan D, Alrehaili M, Alanazi A, Alshammari S, et al. Identification of the most suitable mobile apps to support dietary approaches to stop hypertension (DASH)

diet self-management: Systematic search of app stores and content analysis. Nutrients. 2023;**15**(15):3476. DOI: 10.3390/nu15153476

[61] Bekar C, Goktas Z. Validation of the 14-item Mediterranean diet adherence screener. Clinical Nutrition ESPEN. 2023;**53**:238-243. DOI: 10.1016/j.clnesp.2022.12.026

[62] García-Conesa MT, Philippou E, Pafilas C, Massaro M, Quarta S, Andrade V, et al. Exploring the validity of the 14-item Mediterranean diet adherence screener (Medas): A cross-national study in seven European countries around the Mediterranean region. Nutrients. 2020;**12**(10):2960. DOI: 10.3390/nu12102960

[63] Hershey MS, Sotos-Prieto M, Ruiz-Canela M, Martinez-Gonzalez MA, Cassidy A, Moffatt S, et al. The Mediterranean lifestyle and the risk of depression in middle-aged adults. The Journal of Nutrition. 2022;**152**(1):227-234. DOI: 10.1093/jn/nxab333

[64] Hutchins-Wiese HL, Bales CW, Starr KNP. Mediterranean diet scoring systems: Understanding the evolution and applications for Mediterranean and non-Mediterranean countries. British Journal of Nutrition. 2022;**128**(7):1371-1392. DOI: 10.1017/S0007114521002476

[65] Health Canada. Canada's Food Guide: Snapshot [Internet]. 2019. Reproduced with permission from the Minister of Health, 2024. Available from: https://food-guide.canada.ca/en/food-guide-snapshot/

Chapter 5

Role of Micronutrients in MAFLD

Ana-Marija Liberati Pršo and Željko Krznarić

Abstract

Metabolic dysfunction-associated fatty liver disease (MAFLD) has become recognized as a global public health issue and one of the leading causes of chronic liver disease, potentially progressing to conditions such as steatohepatitis, fibrosis, cirrhosis, and hepatocarcinoma. Diet and lifestyle changes are vital for preventing and treating MAFLD, but they can also play a role in its development. Micronutrients (vitamins and minerals) derived from the diet are essential for optimal functioning due to their antioxidant properties, influence on enzyme activities, and role in immune system regulation. However, data suggest that their intake can have both beneficial and detrimental effects on fatty liver disease, potentially leading to toxicity or exacerbating MAFLD. This chapter aims to explore the important micronutrients linked to MAFLD, with a particular focus on vitamin D, which has been largely studied and frequently prescribed in recent years.

Keywords: metabolic dysfunction-associated fatty liver disease, liver steatosis, micronutrients, vitamin deficiencies, mineral deficiencies, recommended intake

1. Introduction

Metabolic dysfunction-associated fatty liver disease (MAFLD), which is closely linked to overweight, obesity, and insulin resistance, is often viewed as the liver manifestation of "metabolic syndrome." Key mechanisms characterizing MAFLD, including oxidative stress, changes in glucose and lipid metabolism, glucotoxicity, lipotoxicity, and inflammation, are significantly influenced by both macro- and micronutrients. Accumulating results of research have shown a strong association between nutrient intake and MAFLD, stressing their roles in glucose, lipid, and protein metabolism, as well as in antioxidant effects, modulation of the immune system, and carcinogenesis. These findings highlight the importance of lifestyle modifications (e.g., calorie restriction, low-carb and low-fat diets, increased physical activity to aid weight loss, and targeted supplementation) as some of the most effective strategies for managing MAFLD [1].

Patients with MAFLD often consume diets low in micronutrients, making them susceptible to vitamin and mineral deficiencies [2]. Moreover, changes in the gut microbiome can significantly impact micronutrient absorption, which in turn contributes to existing vitamin deficiencies. In obese MAFLD patients, inflammatory adipokines released from dysfunctional adipose tissue can further aggravate these deficiencies. These complex interactions emphasize the necessity to address vitamin deficiencies in managing and improving health outcomes for MAFLD patients [3, 4]. Recent research has pinpointed the importance of specific micronutrients in key immune-inflammatory and metabolic processes related to MAFLD pathogenesis and treatment—vitamins A, D, C, B9, and E, as well as curcumin, epigallocatechin-3-gallate (EGCG), luteolin, luteolin-7-glucoside, caffeic acid, caffeine, oleuropein, quercetin, rutin, resveratrol, choline, and minerals like iron, copper, selenium, magnesium, and zinc. Some of these micronutrients (vitamins A, C, E, resveratrol, silibinin, silymarin, vanillin [apocynin], and pentoxifylline) have been extensively studied and are also the focal point of several clinical trials due to their potential benefits in MAFLD treatment [5–7].

The purpose and scope of this chapter are to resume the function of the aforementioned micronutrients, their role in MAFLD etiopathogenesis, and particular protective functions of each of them, and to discuss their protective/harmful levels and recommended intake as well.

2. Vitamins

2.1 Vitamin A

Vitamin A, a fat-soluble vitamin that must be obtained through the diet, is primarily found in the form of retinoic acid and its downstream metabolites. It is predominantly stored in hepatic stellate cells and has normal serum levels ranging from 0.30 to 0.70 mg/L for retinol and 5.00 to 20.00 mg/L for α-tocopherol [8–10]. Adequate levels of this vitamin are vital for numerous physiological functions such as cell proliferation and differentiation, glucose and lipid metabolism, vision, immune regulation, and embryogenesis [11].

Vitamin A plays a key role in liver health and the management of hepatic steatosis due to its antioxidant properties and its impact on hepatic glucose and lipid metabolism. It interacts with nuclear receptors such as peroxisome proliferator-activated receptors (PPAR) PPARα, PPARβ/γ, and PPARγ (transcription factors that regulate gene expression related to lipid metabolism), as well as Farnesoid X receptor (FXR), a bile acid-activated receptor (BAR), primarily expressed in the liver and intestine that regulates genes involved in the bile acid synthesis, transport, and reabsorption. In addition, it also participates in carbohydrate and lipid metabolism [5, 11–13]. Vitamin A contributes to MAFLD management through several mechanisms such as lipid metabolism modulation, increased insulin sensitivity, antioxidant effects, and anti-inflammatory properties [5].

Research indicates that patients with MAFLD often have a vitamin A deficiency that can exacerbate liver damage due to high levels of oxidative stress; as hepatic vitamin A levels drop, the progression of nonalcoholic fatty liver disease (NAFLD) intensifies. Low vitamin A levels are associated with a higher level of hepatic fibrosis and higher liver-related mortality [9, 14]. As MAFLD advances to more severe stages of fibrosis, disrupted vitamin A homeostasis leads to significant vitamin A deficiency in the liver, resulting in decreased serum retinol levels [9, 14, 15].

Retinoic acid treatments have shown hepatoprotective effects. They are observed *via* reduced mitochondrial reactive oxygen species, enhancing mitochondrial antioxidant enzyme superoxide dismutase 2 (SOD2), by regulating lipid metabolism (retinoid X receptors alpha [RXRsα]) and decreasing pro-inflammatory and pro-fibrogenic activities in hepatic stellate cells [7]. To maintain plasma retinol levels around 2 μmol/L, a daily intake of 700–900 μg of vitamin A and 80% hepatic storage in a healthy individual are essential [16].

Despite these findings, the clinical use of vitamin A for MAFLD treatment remains limited due to the lack of clinical trials in this domain and the narrow therapeutic range it can be used.

2.2 Vitamins B

Currently, only two water-soluble B vitamins have shown promising therapeutic approaches for MAFLD: B3 and B12.

Vitamin B3 (niacin) acts as a precursor for important coenzymes involved in lipid metabolism: nicotinamide adenine dinucleotide (NAD) and nicotinamide adenine dinucleotide phosphate (NADPH). Research has shown that B3 supplementation can lower plasma triglyceride concentrations, reduce hepatic cholesterol levels, enhance redox potential, inhibit liver weight gain, and improve liver enzyme levels in dyslipidemic patients [17, 18].

Vitamin B4 (choline) is an important nutrient that is a crucial component of phosphatidylcholine, a cell membrane phospholipid. The liver is the primary organ responsible for choline metabolism; its deficiency can lead to hepatosteatosis and hepatocyte death. In humans, choline deficiency impacts MAFLD by disrupting phospholipid synthesis, impairing lipoprotein secretion, causing oxidative damage through mitochondrial dysfunction, and inducing endoplasmic reticulum stress. This stress leads to disturbances in mitochondrial bioenergetics and fatty acid beta-oxidation [19]. Phosphatidylethanolamine N-methyltransferase (PEMT) facilitates the conversion of phosphatidylethanolamine to phosphatidylcholine. Phosphatidylcholine is necessary for the formation of very low-density lipoprotein (VLDL), which transports triacylglycerols from the liver to the bloodstream. Low phosphatidylcholine levels result in inadequate VLDL production that in turn may lead to fat accumulation in hepatocytes [20–22].

Choline requirements vary greatly among individuals, and the status of choline biomarkers can help predict the risk of NAFLD [19]. The adequate intake (AI) levels for choline are set at 550 mg/day for men and 425 mg/day for women [22].

The two forms of vitamin B12 are methylcobalamin and 5′-deoxyadenosyl-cobalamin and are predominantly stored in the liver. It is essential for deoxyribonucleic acid (DNA) synthesis, DNA replication, and adequate mitochondrial function [23]. In patients with MAFLD, the absorption of vitamin B12 is often impaired, resulting in significantly lower serum levels that can be associated with higher levels of hepatosteatosis (grade 2–3) [6, 24]. Research shows that vitamin B12 supplementation in MAFLD patients may improve serum levels of homocysteine (HCY), fasting blood glucose, and malondialdehyde (MDA)—a marker of oxidative stress derived from lipid peroxidation. In addition, studies show that daily administration of 1000 μg of cyanocobalamin for 3 months contributes to the reduction of serum homocysteine levels, decreases oxidative stress in hepatocyte endoplasmic reticulum, and may potentially slow the progression of MAFLD [24].

2.3 Vitamin C

Vitamin C (ascorbic acid) is a water-soluble vitamin and a potent antioxidant that plays a crucial role in maintaining human health. As a strong antioxidant, it participates in various oxidation-reduction reactions that are involved in liver lipid balance and regulating its circulation [25]. Research shows that vitamin C may reduce the risk of MAFLD because it helps reduce hepatic fatty acid load by promoting the expression of PPARα-dependent genes that play a key role in β-oxidation of fatty acids and by decreasing inflammation in liver cells. Additionally, vitamin C can enhance the activity of key antioxidant enzymes like manganese superoxide dismutase (SOD) and glutathione peroxidase (GPx) and reduce the formation of mitochondrial reactive oxygen species (ROS). Lastly, there has been accumulating evidence that it may also influence adiponectin regulation and is believed to lower hepatic lipid buildup, insulin resistance, and inflammation due to protective effects against MAFLD [26, 27].

Animal studies indicate that a vitamin C deficiency exacerbates dyslipidemia and liver-related issues as opposed to increased intake of vitamin C that can reduce the severity of dyslipidemia and hepatic lipid accumulation. It also lowers oxidative stress markers in the liver, decreases hepatocellular ballooning along with inflammation, and provides protective effects [28]. In patients with nonalcoholic (NASH), vitamin C supplementation has been shown to significantly improve liver fibrosis, whereas deficiency may exacerbate dyslipidemia and liver damage [29]. A daily intake of at least 146.07 mg appears to have a protective effect against liver steatosis [30].

However, despite these benefits, some contentious studies suggest that high-dose vitamin C supplementation may lead to increased body weight, fat accumulation, elevated levels of aspartate aminotransferase (AST) and alanine aminotransferase (ALT) liver enzymes after excessive consumption, and inflammation [31]. Given these mixed findings, more research is needed to fully understand vitamin C's impact on MAFLD and to establish appropriate dosing guidelines for individuals who have a metabolically unhealthy status.

2.4 Vitamin D (hormone)

Vitamin D (VD) is a vital fat-soluble vitamin and steroid prohormone essential for various biological functions. To perform its roles, vitamin D must undergo transport, hydroxylation, and binding with the vitamin D receptor (VDR) [32]. Serum 25-hydroxyvitamin D (25(OH)D), the primary circulating form of vitamin D and a key indicator of vitamin D status, is influenced by factors such as sun exposure, age, body mass index, dietary intake, and genetic variability [33].

Vitamin D's biological availability and effects can vary due to genetic differences. The VDR, a critical player in the vitamin D metabolic pathway and part of the steroid/thyroid hormone receptor family [32], activates target genes by binding to vitamin D-responsive elements in their promoter regions. The target genes regulate a range of functions in immune cells, including T helper cells (Th) Th1, Th2, Th17, T regulatory cells, and natural killer T cells [34]. Additionally, VDR influences processes related to MAFLD, such as lipid and glucose metabolism, cholesterol efflux, bile acid homeostasis, hepatic fibrogenesis, cellular differentiation, apoptosis, and immune response [35].

In addition, a range of health issues, including autoimmune and infectious diseases, cardiovascular conditions, cancer, endocrine disorders, and neurodegenerative diseases, have been linked to vitamin D deficiency [36–39].

There is a notable epidemiological overlap between NAFLD and vitamin D deficiency, as both conditions are commonly observed in obese individuals with metabolic disorders. The risk of developing MAFLD, the most prevalent chronic liver disease, has been associated with lower levels of circulating 25-hydroxyvitamin D [40].

However, the relationship between 25(OH)D levels and NAFLD can vary across different ethnic groups—vitamin D levels and NAFLD prevalence differ significantly among racial and ethnic populations. Research shows that Caucasians generally have higher serum levels of 25(OH)D compared to Hispanics and African Americans, with African Americans typically having the lowest levels. Conversely, the prevalence of NAFLD is higher in Hispanics and Caucasians compared to African Americans. Additionally, lower levels of 25(OH)D are strongly associated with NAFLD in Caucasians and Chinese American populations, while the association is less pronounced in African American and Hispanic individuals [41, 42]. There may also be gender-specific differences in the relationship between vitamin D levels and NAFLD risk [43].

Insulin resistance is a crucial factor in the development of MAFLD and is closely linked to increased oxidative stress and lipotoxicity. One of the key mediators in this process is nuclear factor κ-β (NF-κB). When activated, NF-κB triggers a pro-inflammatory response, leading to the release of cytokines such as IL-1β, IL-6, and TNF-α, which in turn activate Kupffer cells. These cytokines contribute to the histological features of NASH and are more commonly expressed in the liver of patients with NASH compared to obese individuals with normal livers [44]. The gravity of MAFLD correlates with higher levels of these cytokines. Research has shown that vitamin D supplementation can impact these inflammatory processes. For instance, Neyestani et al. [45] found that a daily intake of 1000 IU of vitamin D, either alone or in combination with calcium, reduced the secretion of pro-inflammatory cytokines IL-1β and IL-6 in type 2 diabetic patients over 12 weeks [46]. Additionally, another study demonstrated that weekly supplementation of 50,000 IU of vitamin D led to a significant reduction in triglyceride levels in NAFLD patients [47].

Liver cells have vitamin D receptors (VDR), which can help protect the liver from inflammation caused by chronic hepatitis when vitamin D is administered. Additionally, by increasing VDR expression, insulin sensitivity is enhanced. This improvement in insulin sensitivity involves the activation of Glut-4 transporters located in the muscle cells that facilitate glucose uptake into cells and subsequently lower blood glucose levels. Moreover, vitamin D treatment improves the expression of these receptors and modulates free fatty acids (FFAs), contributing to better metabolic outcomes. Vitamin D also reduces liver damage by reducing the cytokeratin 18-associated apoptotic fragment M30. This indicates its anti-fibrotic, anti-inflammatory, and anti-cirrhotic effects on many metabolic-related diseases, including obesity, hypertension, insulin resistance, type 2 diabetes, metabolic syndrome, and cardiovascular disease. Sharifi et al. [43] found that vitamin D administration significantly impacted levels of TNFα and C-reactive protein.

Studies frequently report a high incidence of NAFLD (approximately 60%) among individuals with low serum 25(OH)D levels (<20 ng/mL) [40]. Cross-sectional and case-control studies reported an inverse relationship between serum 25(OH)D and NAFLD, though not universally [48]. Research suggests that vitamin D deficiency is nonlinearly associated with increased MAFLD gravity and elevated all-cause mortality [49]. Lower levels of 25(OH)D are linked to a higher prevalence of MAFLD and liver fibrosis, whereas higher levels are associated with a reduced risk of fibrosis. Specifically, 25(OH)D levels are inversely related to the extent of liver steatosis and fibrosis. In vitamin D-deficient MAFLD patients, severity may be influenced by the activation of NF-κB and mitogen-activated protein kinase (MAPK) pathways [50, 51]. Additionally, impaired liver function in these patients can further affect 25(OH)D levels through reduced conversion of vitamin D to 25(OH)D by cytochrome CYP2R1 or through decreased levels of vitamin D binding protein and levels of albumin [52].

Vitamin D has been shown to induce autophagy (in animal models) which inhibits the p53 pathway and helps prevent hepatocyte senescence. It also mitigates inflammation through the enterohepatic axis, highlighting the importance of timely supplementation [53]. Additionally, vitamin D treatment can counteract MAFLD influenced by a high-fat diet (HFD), involving gut microbiota and metabolic regulation, and can change lipid metabolism through the PPARα signaling pathway [54]. Furthermore, vitamin D counteracts TGF-β signaling in hepatic stellate cells, thus exhibiting anti-fibrotic effects [55].

Different therapeutic dosages of vitamin D have varying impacts on MAFLD. For instance, low to medium doses of 1000 IU/day over 12 months have been found to reduce liver steatosis (measured by transient elastography indices of controlled attenuation parameter) and fibrosis (measured by liver surface nodularity) in MAFLD patients [56]. Studies have also reported that administering 50,000 IU of vitamin D3 every 14 days for 4 months led to a significant reduction in serum MDA and high-sensitivity-C-reactive protein (CRP), key indicators of overall and hepatic inflammation, in patients with NAFLD [57]. Wenclewska et al. found that daily supplementation with 2000 IU of vitamin D decreased DNA damage, particularly in patients with type 2 diabetes mellitus. This reduction in DNA damage suggests that vitamin D may help alleviate oxidative stress associated with hyperglycemia. Additionally, vitamin D supplementation was linked to reduced homeostatic model assessment for insulin resistance (HOMA-IR) and triglyceride (TG)/high-density lipoprotein (HDL) ratios and increased HDL levels that are indicative of MAFLD [58].

Overall, most trials observe the therapeutic benefits of vitamin D treatment, such as reduced hepatic inflammation and improved liver function, but there are also some studies that have not found a significant relationship between MAFLD and serum vitamin D levels [59].

These findings underscore vitamin D's potential in MAFLD treatment while also highlighting its complex and context-dependent nature. The genetics and epigenetics of MAFLD may affect how vitamin D regulates these processes, suggesting a need for further research to clarify these complex interactions.

2.5 Vitamin E

There are eight natural forms of vitamin E—four tocopherols (α, β, γ, δ) and four tocotrienols (α, β, γ, δ). Among these, α-tocopherol is the most abundant and effective at inhibiting lipid oxidation. As a potent antioxidant, its effects are seen across biochemical, cellular, genetic, and signaling range [60]. In addition to modifying inflammation response and cell proliferation, vitamin E regulates key cellular signaling enzymes (5-lipoxygenase [LOX-5], cyclooxygenase-2 [COX-2], protein kinase C [PKC], and protein phosphatase 2A [PP2A]). Also, vitamin E may offer protection against the development of MAFLD by inhibiting reactive oxygen species, and by exerting anti-apoptotic and anti-inflammatory effects [7].

Through its ability to reduce oxidative stress, vitamin E decreases *de novo* lipogenesis (DNL) and intrahepatic triglyceride (IHTG) accumulation by breaking the cycle between oxidative stress and MAFLD progression [61, 62]. In addition, meta-analyses of randomized controlled trials in adults with nonalcoholic fatty liver disease (NAFLD) have shown that vitamin E supplementation, typically in doses ranging from 400 IU (268 mg) to 800 IU (536 mg), lowers serum levels of the liver enzymes ALT and AST, as well as interleukin 6 (IL-6) levels [63].

Studies show that vitamin E lowers liver steatosis and hepatocellular ballooning, and suppressing transforming growth factor beta (TGF-β) expression helps reduce the severity of liver fibrosis [7]. Additionally, vitamin E stimulates the activation and transcription of PPARγ in adipocytes, leading to increased expression of adiponectin which plays an important role in regulating blood glucose levels and fatty acid breakdown [64].

Some research also indicates that vitamin E positively affects gut microbiota in MAFLD, shifting the composition toward a healthier pool of bacteria [65, 66].

At present, the only medication-nutrient recommended by clinical guidelines for treating metabolic dysfunction-associated steatohepatitis (MASH) is vitamin E [67]. Its daily use has been linked to significant reductions in total mortality and liver decompensation in patients with MASH-induced bridging fibrosis and cirrhosis [7, 68]. Growing evidence supports that supplementation with vitamin E improves steatosis and resolves steatohepatitis in non-diabetic adults with NASH, prompting the American Association for the Study of Liver Diseases to recommend a dose of 800 IU/day for non-diabetic, non-cirrhotic adults with NASH [68].

However, despite its anti-inflammatory, anti-apoptotic, and anti-fibrotic beneficial properties, higher doses of vitamin E could potentially lead to the development of fatty liver due to endogenous adipogenesis upregulation and cholesterol synthesis that contributes to its development [9, 69]. Additionally, there may be an increased risk of certain cancers and hemorrhagic stroke [70] with high-dose supplementation. Its efficacy and safety may vary depending on patient health status, highlighting the need for a personalized approach in its clinical use.

3. Minerals

3.1 Iron

Iron is essential for physiological processes such as heme biosynthesis, DNA synthesis, oxygen transport, and the citric acid cycle [71]. Given its central role in numerous metabolic processes, iron can both prevent and promote oxidative damage when present in excess [72].

Excess ferrous iron (the reduced form of serum ferric iron) contributes to membrane and unsaturated lipids peroxidation triggering a chain reaction that damages mitochondria and other organelles, ultimately contributing to the onset and progression of metabolic disorders [73, 74]. In the context of NAFLD, excess iron can worsen the condition by activating the redox-sensitive transcription factor NF-κB (nuclear factor kappa B) in Kupffer cells which in turn initiates inflammatory, fibrotic, and cytotoxic pathways. The production of ROS is closely linked to the liver's histopathological response to iron overload. ROS induces oxidative stress, leading to lipid peroxidation, mitochondrial dysfunction, endoplasmic reticulum (ER) stress, and inflammation that contributes to tissue necrosis and apoptosis [73, 75]. ROS not only have direct cytotoxic effects but also stimulate a key protein involved in activating inflammatory, fibrogenic, and apoptotic processes—NF-κB. Iron-induced ROS and reactive nitrogen species interact with the small G-protein p21ras, activating a series of kinases that are directly linked to the NF-κB regulation. This, in turn, leads to the production of cytokines such as TNF-α and IL-6 that play central roles in promoting hepatic inflammation and fibrosis [76].

The resulting oxidative damage to hepatocytes contributes to insulin resistance, causing compensatory hyperinsulinemia. This condition enhances hepatic *de novo* lipogenesis and cholesterol synthesis while reducing fatty acid oxidation. Several studies have established a strong link between increased iron levels and insulin resistance, with excessive iron intake also contributing to pancreatic beta cell function impairment [77].

The recommended daily intake of iron is 8–18 mg [69]. Higher intake, however, may impair hepatocyte function, as growing evidence links excessive iron consumption with an increased risk of fatty liver disease in a dose-dependent manner; iron overload can promote ferroptosis, triggering inflammation in MAFLD and causing oxidative DNA damage. This is primarily due to the worsening of hepatic insulin resistance, elevated gluconeogenesis, and lipogenesis, driven by the regulation of related mRNA [78]. Elevated ferritin levels and lower transferrin saturation (TSAT) are also associated with a higher likelihood of MAFLD and liver fibrosis. Additionally, serum ferritin may worsen MAFLD through interactions with certain bacterial families involved in iron metabolism, potentially altering the gut microbiome and transcriptomic features that contribute to liver fat accumulation [79].

The average level of iron content in patients without NAFLD is 1.4 g as opposed to patients with NAFLD which have an average body iron content of 1.6 g. Studies show that the risk of NAFLD increases by 1.73-fold with each standard deviation rise in serum iron levels [77].

Hyperferritinemia is often linked to more severe metabolic dysfunction and liver injury. In addition, it is associated with abnormal iron-induced hepcidin release, influenced by genetic variants that in turn, may further increase iron absorption [80]. Given that iron depletion has been shown to improve MAFLD, maintaining serum iron within an appropriate range may be necessary for the prevention and treatment of the disease.

3.2 Copper

Copper is an essential trace element that acts as a structural and enzymatic cofactor for various antioxidant proteins and enzymes, such as cytochrome c oxidase (COX), superoxide dismutase (SOD), and ceruloplasmin. It plays a critical role in defending against oxidative stress and supporting mitochondrial function [81]. Serum copper is primarily transported through the body by binding to ceruloplasmin which regulates copper distribution, release, and linked biological functions [81]. Research suggests that a reduction in hepatic ceruloplasmin helps restore liver copper levels, alleviating liver steatosis by modulating the copper-SOC1-AMPK (AMP-activate protein kinase) signaling pathway [82].

Studies have shown that dietary copper is closely linked to lipid metabolism and that its deficiency has been associated with hepatic steatosis and insulin resistance. Both excessive and low copper levels can result in mitochondrial dysfunction and dyslipidemia. Research has highlighted the connection between copper deficiency and liver fat accumulation with NAFLD patients showing more severe liver steatosis, inflammation, and clinical symptoms when hepatic copper levels are low [1, 82]. Individuals with NAFLD have been found to have a 50% reduction in hepatic copper levels compared to control groups and those with liver impairment unrelated to NAFLD [83].

In patients with MAFLD, both hair and liver copper levels are significantly lower and correlate with increased hepatic steatosis, the severity of MASH, and metabolic alterations [84].

Copper deficiency also contributes to NAFLD development through its interaction with iron. A lack of copper can reduce the expression of ferroportin-1 and the activity of ceruloplasmin ferroxidase, hindering iron export from the liver and leading to iron accumulation [85].

Animal studies have reported that restoring intrahepatic copper levels, achieved by down-regulating copper cyanin, promotes lipolysis through the formation of copper-loaded SCO1-LKB1-AMPK complexes, leading to improvements in MAFLD. A case-control study also found that increased copper levels significantly improved MAFLD outcomes in males, underscoring copper's protective role in treating the condition [86, 87].

However, excessive copper can also be harmful. Elevated copper levels may rise the production of ROS, impairing liver function. This excess of copper downregulates lipolysis and upregulates lipogenesis, which in turn, increases hepatic triglyceride content and raises the risk of NAFLD [88, 89].

Research has also reported a positive correlation between elevated serum copper levels and the development, progression, and recurrence of various human cancers, including hepatocellular carcinoma (HCC). Data suggest a link between high circulating copper levels and the progression of NAFLD-related cirrhosis to HCC [90]. Copper may thus serve as a potential biomarker for hepatocyte transformation with a specific threshold of 163.3 μg/dL that can be useful for identifying NAFLD-cirrhotic patients with a higher risk of developing HCC [29, 88].

Given these mixed findings, the complex relationship between copper, liver metabolism, and inflammation offers new insights and therapeutic opportunities for treating the disease due to their specific link.

3.3 Zinc

Zinc is an essential trace element with crucial antioxidant, anti-inflammatory, and anti-apoptotic functions. It enhances hepatic cell lipophagy, and reduces the accumulation of lipids and lipolysis promotion. Moreover, zinc regulates cell signaling, enzyme production, insulin biosynthesis and secretion, mRNA expression, and, lastly, antioxidant defenses [91].

In the context of MAFLD, zinc deficiency plays a crucial role. It is linked to various conditions such as insulin resistance, diabetes mellitus, obesity, dyslipidemia, hypertension, reduced zinc absorption from the gastrointestinal tract, and insufficient dietary zinc intake [92, 93].

Serum zinc levels below 70 μg/dL in adults indicate zinc deficiency [94]. This risk increases with age and is further heightened by comorbidities such as chronic inflammatory and metabolic diseases, including diabetes mellitus. Diabetes mellitus can exacerbate zinc insufficiency through dysfunction of zinc transporters. Low zinc absorption, glycosuria, and hyperglycemia may lead to increased zinc excretion in the urine. Additionally, increased oxidative stress and hyperinsulinemia can deplete intracellular zinc due to increased demand. Furthermore, phytates found in plant-based foods can inhibit zinc absorption, influencing zinc status in affected individuals [95].

Growing evidence links zinc deficiency to the development of MAFLD [92, 96, 97]. In patients with biopsy-confirmed MAFLD, a J-shaped correlation has been observed between serum zinc levels and the severity of hepatic necroinflammation. Lower zinc levels are associated with advanced hepatic fibrosis in MAFLD patients, indicating a connection between zinc deficiency and liver fibrosis severity [98, 99].

Zinc supplementation has been shown to decrease oxidative stress and inflammatory cytokines such as tumor necrosis factor-alpha [100]. It also helps reduce liver and hepatocyte lipid accumulation, mitigating NAFLD. This reduction in lipid content within hepatocytes is achieved by activating fatty acid oxidation, inhibiting lipogenesis, decreasing aerobic oxidation, and increasing glycolysis, thereby altering cellular metabolism [93, 98]. Zinc supplementation also significantly lowers serum levels of AST and ALT which are key indicators of liver injury. Additionally, zinc reduces IL-6 protein expression and MDA levels, which consequently decreases lipid peroxidation and liver damage [101, 102].

While zinc generally has a good safety profile, excessive intake can be toxic. Daily doses between 150 and 450 mg can lead to copper deficiency and other complications such as anemia, altered iron metabolism, decreased high-density lipoprotein (HDL) levels, and neurotoxicity. High zinc intake can increase intestinal metallothionein, a metal-binding protein that displaces zinc and binds dietary copper, reducing copper absorption. To avoid zinc-induced copper deficiency, it is important to monitor blood copper levels during zinc supplementation [93].

Plasma zinc levels should be evaluated in patients with NAFLD and advanced fibrosis or cirrhosis to identify and address zinc deficiency. This assessment should consider potential confounding factors such as inflammation and hypoalbuminemia which are commonly present in these patients].

Further research and validation are needed to determine specific zinc dosages and treatment protocols for managing MAFLD effectively.

3.4 Selenium

Selenium plays various roles in the human body due to its structural and enzymatic functions including antioxidant functions, maintaining redox balance, thyroid hormone metabolism, cancer prevention, and immune modulation all of which emphasize why it is an essential mineral for the body. It is also significant in a metabolic disease development context because of its protective effects against oxidative stress and inflammation [103, 104].

The relationship between selenium and MAFLD appears to be dose-dependent. Research has indicated that lower blood selenium levels (below approximately 130 μg/L) are linked to a higher prevalence of advanced liver fibrosis [105, 106]. Animal studies have shown that a selenium-deficient diet leads to reduced levels of glutathione (GSH) in the liver and an increased n-6/n-3 fatty acid ratio that can negatively impact NAFLD. Selenium deficiency also results in increased lipid peroxidation, and reduced activity of glutathione peroxidase (GPx) and thioredoxin reductase (TrxR), suggesting heightened oxidative stress and impaired antioxidant capacity, which in turn is closely associated with NAFLD development [107]. In addition, a selenium-deficient diet can cause abnormalities in hepatocyte cells (altered chromatin structure and mitochondrial swelling), severe fibrosis around the portal vein, increased metalloproteinase activity, decreased levels of tissue inhibitors of metalloproteinases type 1 and 3, all of which contributes to increased liver inflammation [107].

Studies indicate that selenium supplementation has shown beneficial effects in MAFLD mouse models such as reducing hepatic injury, alleviating oxidative stress, lowering insulin resistance, and decreasing inflammation [108]. Moreover, the combination of selenium and magnesium has been found to prevent lipid accumulation induced by a high-fat diet in rats, potentially by boosting the activity of various antioxidant enzymes. Similarly, the concurrent administration of selenium and zinc has been observed to improve lipid profiles, liver function, and liver steatosis in animal studies [7].

In patients with type 2 diabetes and MAFLD, selenium intake is negatively correlated with insulin resistance, as selenium provides antioxidant benefits and mitigates endoplasmic reticulum (ER) stress in the pancreas and blood vessels. However, this positive effect diminishes when selenium intake exceeds 112 μg/day for a 70 kg individual [109].

Conversely, some studies have found that elevated selenium levels are positively correlated with increased triglycerides and low-density lipoprotein (LDL) cholesterol, higher insulin resistance, enhanced lipogenesis, and greater oxidative stress [110]. Results of a randomized controlled trial investigating selenium supplementation for prostate cancer prevention found that it even increased the incidence of diabetes mellitus type 2 [111].

These findings suggest that excessive selenium intake may affect energy metabolism on a molecular level in skeletal muscle and visceral adipose tissue, potentially influencing the development of hepatic steatosis. The recommended intake of selenium in adults is 55 μg/day, in the United States. Intake levels exceeding 150 μg/day can pose risks, with adverse effects seen at serum selenium levels above 130 μg/L [112].

The use of selenium in the treatment of MAFLD requires careful consideration of its balance between therapeutic benefits and potential toxicity. Identifying the adequate dose of selenium is crucial and continues to be an area of active research and discussion in MAFLD treatment.

3.5 Magnesium

Magnesium plays an important role in biological systems as a cation that activates or inhibits enzymes, regulates the cell cycle and differentiation, maintains genomic stability, supports protein synthesis, and balances electrolytes. It acts as a cofactor in over 300 enzymatic reactions, particularly those involving adenosine triphosphate (ATP) or guanosine triphosphate (GTP). Magnesium forms ATP-Mg and GTP-Mg complexes that are essential for many biological processes, including lipogenesis, nucleic acid synthesis, protein synthesis, coenzyme activity, methylation, lipogenesis, and glucose stabilization [46, 113].

Magnesium and insulin are interdependent—magnesium is vital for insulin function and insulin regulates intracellular magnesium levels. Low magnesium levels can impair insulin's ability to aid glucose uptake in the body which could lead to insulin resistance [46, 114]. Magnesium supplementation has been shown to decrease lipid deposition in hepatocytes induced by free fatty acids (FFA), reduce lipid accumulation by lowering lipid synthesis, and increase lipid oxidation [46, 115].

The key characteristic of MAFLD is deficiency in magnesium which can exacerbate inflammation and oxidative stress. It may impair DNA repair mechanisms, disrupt cell proliferation and differentiation, and promote tumor growth [116]. Research has shown that there is a link between magnesium intake and inflammatory biomarkers such as tumor necrosis factor-alpha (TNF-α), C-reactive protein (CRP), and vascular cell adhesion protein 1 (VCAM-1). Magnesium supplementation may influence cellular lipid metabolism by activating the AMPK/mTOR (mammalian target-of-rapamycin) pathway that stimulates autophagy [117]. *In vitro* studies indicate that magnesium supplementation increases the production of SOD, the antioxidant enzyme, that helps neutralize oxygen free radicals and protect cells from damage [118].

Lower serum magnesium levels are typically seen in patients with NAFLD and with developed HCC in comparison with those who do not develop HCC. Conversely, NAFLD patients characterized with higher serum magnesium levels (>0.864 mmol/L) experience a 27% reduction in HCC incidence [119]. Additionally, increasing magnesium intake by 100 mg, representing a 25–33% increase over the daily recommended amount, has been associated with a 49% reduction in liver-related mortality [116].

Magnesium isoglycyrrhizinate (MGIG), derived from 18α-glycyrrhizic acid, seems to be a notable magnesium-based treatment. MGIG has shown anti-inflammatory properties and serves as a hepatoprotective agent by protecting hepatic cells from damage, improving liver function, and mitigating inflammatory responses within the liver. It helps preserve cell viability by reducing apoptosis and limiting lipid accumulation, by inhibiting the expression of metabolic enzymes involved in the synthesis of cellular triglycerides. Additionally, research shows that MGIG treatment significantly lowers levels of inflammatory biomarkers (NF-κB, IL-6, transforming growth factor beta [TGF-β], and fibroblast growth factor bFGF) in both mRNA and protein forms. MGIG effectively suppresses the unfolded protein response (UPR), reducing the production of inflammatory cytokines and protecting hepatocytes from NAFLD-induced damage [120].

4. Carotenoids

Fat-soluble pigments, carotenoids, are characterized by antioxidant properties and are primarily stored in the liver. Key carotenoids studied in relation to NAFLD include astaxanthin, lutein, β-carotene, and fucoxanthin [121].

Astaxanthin is a powerful antioxidant known for scavenging peroxyl radicals, thus protecting fatty acids and biological membranes from lipid peroxidation. This suggests it may help mitigate NAFLD-related oxidative stress. Research has shown that astaxanthin, especially when combined with vitamin E, reduces lipid accumulation in hepatocytes and diminishes inflammation and fibrosis in hepatic tissue [122].

Lutein and zeaxanthin (isomer) can amplify immune function due to strong anti-inflammatory and antioxidant properties, potentially reducing the risk of cardiovascular diseases, cancer, and oxidative stress-related conditions like MAFLD. Research on Chinese adults with NAFLD revealed an inverse relationship between lutein and zeaxanthin levels and the prevalence of the disease. In a guinea pig model, lutein decreased free hepatic cholesterol by 43% and mitigated lipid peroxidation. In addition, a study focused on zeaxanthin function that was tested independently on Mongolian gerbils showed a reduction of fibrosis and lowered lipid hydroperoxides [123].

A precursor of retinol found in various fruits and vegetables, β-carotene, is known for its potent anti-inflammatory effects. It can reduce hepatic steatosis and fibrosis. β-carotene supports both the treatment and prevention of NAFLD and enhances the efficacy of other NAFLD therapies, such as rosuvastatin which was found to be more effective in combination with β-carotene than when used alone [123, 124].

Lycopene, a β-carotene isomer, has significant potential in regulating gene expression, anti-proliferative activity, gap-junction communication, modulating hormones, and the immune system due to its highly potent dietary antioxidant characteristics. These properties make lycopene a prominent focus of research regarding MAFLD. A study conducted on animals reported that lycopene can reduce oxidative stress and liver damage induced by a high-fat diet, indicating its protective role in MAFLD development. There is also interest in exploring lycopene's potential for treating MAFLD, not just preventing it. Findings suggest that bioactive antioxidants like lycopene could complement dietary interventions to enhance recovery from high-fat diet-induced liver damage [123, 125].

Fucoxanthin, a carotenoid found in the chloroplasts of brown seaweeds, exhibits strong anti-inflammatory and cancer-preventive properties due to its antioxidant activities. Its antioxidant, anti-inflammatory, and anti-lipemic effects make it a promising carotenoid for MAFLD treatment. Lastly, fucoxanthin has been shown to reduce hepatic steatosis and fibrosis in NAFLD patients and studies show that it can attenuate inflammation and adipogenesis associated with NAFLD [126].

5. Conclusions

Micronutrient deficiencies are commonly observed in patients with liver diseases, particularly those associated with metabolic dysfunction like MAFLD, and these deficiencies can impair metabolic processes and exacerbate the progression of fatty liver conditions, leading to steatohepatitis, fibrosis, and cirrhosis.

Achieving optimal levels of essential nutrients can significantly enhance insulin sensitivity, reduce lipotoxicity, lower inflammatory mediators and regulate gut microbiota. Collectively, these improvements help slow the progression from MAFLD to more severe conditions such as metabolic-associated steatohepatitis, fibrosis, and potentially hepatocellular carcinoma.

Due to its high (according to numerous authors—even therapeutical) potential in various inflammatory processes, due to its metabolism-regulating and anti-fibrotic potential, vitamin D has been extensively evaluated and studied as a specific micronutrient, important in the pathogenesis of MAFLD and its therapeutic approach as well.

Aging is associated with decreased nutrient absorption and a gradual decline in physiological integrity. Notably, aging is linked to an annual reduction in hepatic clearance by 0.80% starting from age 40, indicating a diminished liver capacity to metabolize vitamins and minerals as micronutrients.

To achieve therapeutic goals, it may be necessary to start supplementing with these nutrients well before the onset of MAFLD to maximize their reparative effects.

Conflict of interest

The authors declare no conflict of interest.

Author details

Ana-Marija Liberati Peršo[1,2]* and Željko Krznarić[3,4]

1 Clinical Hospital Sveti Duh, Zagreb, Croatia

2 Faculty of Medicine of University of Rijeka, Croatia

3 Clinical Hospital Centre Zagreb, Zagreb, Croatia

4 Faculty of Medicine of University of Zagreb, Croatia

*Address all correspondence to: anamarijaliberati@gmail.com

References

[1] Hou JZ, Wu QW, Zhang L. Association between micronutrients intake and metabolic-associated fatty liver disease: A cross-sectional study based on the National Health and nutrition examination survey. Journal of Nutritional Science. 2023;**12**:e117

[2] Kim CH, Kallman JB, Bai C, et al. Nutritional assessments of patients with non-alcoholic fatty liver disease. Obesity Surgery. 2010;**20**:154-160

[3] Thomas-Valdés S, Tostes M, Anunciação PC, et al. Association between vitamin deficiency and metabolic disorders related to obesity. Critical Reviews in Food Science and Nutrition. 2017;**57**:3332-3343

[4] De Filippis F, Pellegrini N, Vannini L, et al. High-level adherence to a Mediterranean diet beneficially impacts the gut microbiota and associated metabolome. Gut. 2016;**65**:1812-1821

[5] Liu Y, Qin X, Chen T, et al. Exploring the interactions between metabolic dysfunction-associated fatty liver disease and micronutrients: From molecular mechanisms to clinical applications. Frontiers in Nutrition. 2024;**11**:1344924

[6] Pickett-Blakely O, Young K, Carr RM. Micronutrients in nonalcoholic fatty liver disease pathogenesis. Cellular and Molecular Gastroenterology and Hepatology. 2018;**6**:451-462

[7] Munteanu C, Schwartz B. The effect of bioactive aliment compounds and micronutrients on non-alcoholic fatty liver disease. Antioxidants. 2023;**12**(4):903

[8] Fortuna VA, Martucci RB, Trugo LC, Borojevic R. Hepatic stellate cells uptake of retinol associated with retinol-binding protein or with bovine serum albumin. The Journal of Cellular Biochemistry. 2003;**90**:792-805

[9] Jeon D, Son M, Shim J. Dynamics of serum retinol and alpha-tocopherol levels according to non-alcoholic fatty liver disease status. Nutrients. 2021;**13**(5):1720

[10] Blaner WS. Vitamin A signaling and homeostasis in obesity, diabetes, and metabolic disorders. Pharmacology & Therapeutics. 2019;**197**:153-178

[11] Carazo A, Macáková K, Matoušová K, et al. Vitamin A update: Forms, sources, kinetics, detection, function, deficiency, therapeutic use and toxicity. Nutrients. 2021;**13**(5):1703

[12] Chen G. The interactions of insulin and vitamin A signaling systems for the regulation of hepatic glucose and lipid metabolism. Cells. 2021;**10**(8):2160

[13] Saeed A, Dullaart RPF, Schreuder TCMA, et al. Disturbed vitamin A metabolism in non-alcoholic fatty liver disease (NAFLD). Nutrients. 2017;**2017**(10):29

[14] Saeed A, Bartuzi P, Heegsma J, et al. Impaired hepatic vitamin A metabolism in NAFLD mice leading to vitamin A accumulation in hepatocytes. Cellular and Molecular Gastroenterology and Hepatology. 2021;**11**:309-325.e3

[15] Kamada Y, Takahashi H, Ogawa Y, et al. Characterization of nutrient intake in biopsy-confirmed NAFLD patients. Nutrients. 2022;**14**(17):3453

[16] Koprivica M, Bjelanović J. The importance of vitamin A in the nutrition. Medicinski Časopis. 2021;**55**(3):99-103

[17] Raza S, Tewari A, Rajak S, Sinha RA. Vitamins and non-alcoholic fatty liver disease: A molecular insight. Liver Research. 2021;**5**(2):62-71

[18] Pan J, Zhou Y, Pang N, Yang L. Dietary niacin intake and mortality among individuals with nonalcoholic fatty liver disease. JAMA Network Open. 2024;7(2):e2354277-e2354277

[19] Corbin KD, Zeisel SH. Choline metabolism provides novel insights into nonalcoholic fatty liver disease and its progression. Current Opinion in Gastroenterology. 2012;**28**(2):159-165

[20] DiStefano JK. The role of choline, soy isoflavones, and probiotics as adjuvant treatments in the prevention and management of NAFLD in postmenopausal women. Nutrients. 2023;**15**(12):2670

[21] Lu Y, Feng T, Zhao J, et al. Polyene phosphatidylcholine ameliorates high fat diet-induced non-alcoholic fatty liver disease via Remodeling metabolism and inflammation. Frontiers in Physiology. 2022;**13**:810143

[22] Piras IS, Raju A, Don J, et al. Hepatic PEMT expression decreases with increasing NAFLD severity. International Journal of Molecular Sciences. 2022;**23**(16):9296

[23] Stabler SP. Vitamin B12. In: Present Knowledge in Nutrition. Vol. 2020. Academic Press; 2020. pp. 257-227. eBook ISBN:9780128198421

[24] Zelber-Sagi S, Ivancovsky-Wajcman D, Fliss-Isakov N. Serum malondialdehyde is associated with non-alcoholic fatty liver and related liver damage differentially in men and women. Antioxidants. 2020;**9**:578

[25] Njus D, Kelley PM, Tu YJ, Schlegel HB. Ascorbic acid: The chemistry underlying its antioxidant properties. Free Radical Biology and Medicine. 2020;**159**:37-43

[26] Wei J, Lei G-H, Fu L, et al. Association between dietary vitamin C intake and non-alcoholic fatty liver disease: A cross-sectional study among middle-aged and older adults. PLoS One. 2016;**11**:e0147985

[27] Lee SW, Baek SM, Kang KK, et al. Vitamin C deficiency inhibits nonalcoholic fatty liver disease progression through impaired de novo lipogenesis. The American Journal of Pathology. 2021;**191**(9):1550-1563

[28] Park SH, Han AL, Kim NH, Shin SR. Liver histological improvement after administration of high-dose vitamin C in Guinea pig with nonalcoholic steatohepatitis. International Journal for Vitamin and Nutrition Research. 2019;**88**:263-269

[29] Tyczyńska M, Hunek G, Szczasny M, et al. Supplementation of micro- and macronutrients—A role of nutritional status in non-alcoholic fatty liver disease. International Journal of Molecular Sciences. 2024;**25**(9):4916

[30] Ezhilarasan D, Lakshmi T. A molecular insight into the role of antioxidants in nonalcoholic fatty liver diseases. Oxidative Medicine and Cellular Longevity. 2022;**2022**(1):9233650

[31] Zeng Q, Zhao L, Meng C, et al. Prophylactic and therapeutic effects of different doses of vitamin C on high-fat-diet-induced non-alcoholic fatty liver disease in mice. Biomedicine & Pharmacotherapy. 2020;**131**:110792

[32] Gallagher JC, Rosen CJ. Vitamin D: 100 years of discoveries, yet controversy continues. The Lancet Diabetes & Endocrinology. 2023;**11**(5):362-374

[33] El-Hajj Fuleihan G, Bouillon R, Clarke B, et al. Serum 25-hydroxyvitamin D levels: Variability, knowledge gaps, and the concept of a desirable range. Journal of Bone and Mineral Research. 2015;**30**(7):1119-1133

[34] Carlberg C. Vitamin D and its target genes. Nutrients. 2022;**14**(7):1354

[35] Barchetta I, Cimini FA, Cavallo MG. Vitamin D and metabolic dysfunction-associated fatty liver disease (MAFLD): An update. Nutrients. 2020;**12**(11):3302

[36] Szymczak-Pajor I, Miazek K, Selmi A, et al. The action of vitamin D in adipose tissue: Is there the link between vitamin D deficiency and adipose tissue-related metabolic disorders? International Journal of Molecular Sciences. 2022;**23**(2):956

[37] Charoenngam N, Holick MF. Immunologic effects of vitamin D on human health and disease. Nutrients. 2020;**12**(7):2097

[38] de la Guía-Galipienso F, Martínez-Ferran M, Vallecillo N, et al. Vitamin D and cardiovascular health. Clinical Nutrition. 2021;**40**(5):2946-2957

[39] Ismailova A, White JH. Vitamin D, infections and immunity. Reviews in Endocrine and Metabolic Disorders. Apr 2022;**23**(2):265-277

[40] Zhang R, Wang M, Wang M, et al. Vitamin D level and vitamin D receptor genetic variation were involved in the risk of non-alcoholic fatty liver disease: A case-control study. Frontiers in Endocrinology. 2021;**12**:648844

[41] Jiang X, O'Reilly PF, Aschard H, et al. Genome-wide association study in 79,366 European-ancestry individuals informs the genetic architecture of 25-hydroxyvitamin D levels. Nature Communications. 2018;**9**(1):260

[42] El Khoudary SR, Samargandy S, Zeb I, et al. Serum 25-hydroxyvitamin-D and nonalcoholic fatty liver disease: Does race/ethnicity matter? Findings from the MESA cohort. Nutrition, Metabolism and Cardiovascular Diseases. 2020;**30**(1):114-122

[43] Sharifi N, Amani R. Vitamin D supplementation and non-alcoholic fatty liver disease: A critical and systematic review of clinical trials. Critical Reviews in Food Science and Nutrition. 2019;**59**(4):693-703

[44] Sakurai Y, Kubota N, Yamauchi T, Kadowaki T. Role of insulin resistance in MAFLD. International Journal of Molecular Sciences. 2021;**22**(8):4156

[45] Neyestani TR, Nikooyeh B, Alavi-Majd H, et al. Improvement of vitamin D status via daily intake of fortified yogurt drink either with or without extra calcium ameliorates systemic inflammatory biomarkers, including adipokines, in the subjects with type 2 diabetes. The Journal of Clinical Endocrinology & Metabolism. 2012;**97**(6):2005-2011

[46] Barbagallo M, Veronese N, Dominguez LJ. Magnesium in aging, health and diseases. Nutrients. 2021;**13**(2):463

[47] Foroughi M, Maghsoudi Z, Ghiasvand R, et al. Effect of vitamin D supplementation on C-reactive protein in patients with nonalcoholic fatty liver. International Journal of Preventive Medicine. 2014;**5**(8):969

[48] Liu T, Xu L, Chen FH, Zhou YB. Association of serum vitamin D level and nonalcoholic fatty liver disease: A meta-analysis. European Journal

of Gastroenterology & Hepatology. 2020;**32**(2):140-147

[49] Zhang JJ, Yu HC, Li Y, et al. Association between serum 25-hydroxy vitamin D concentrations and mortality among individuals with metabolic dysfunction–associated fatty liver disease: A prospective cohort study. The American Journal of Clinical Nutrition. 2022;**116**(5):1409-1417

[50] Ciardullo S, Muraca E, Cannistraci R, et al. Low 25 (OH) vitamin D levels are associated with increased prevalence of nonalcoholic fatty liver disease and significant liver fibrosis. Diabetes/Metabolism Research and Reviews. 2023;**39**(5):e3628

[51] Kim HS, Rotundo L, Kothari N, et al. Vitamin D is associated with severity and mortality of non-alcoholic fatty liver disease: A US population-based study. Journal of Clinical and Translational Hepatology. 2017;**5**(3):185

[52] Bikle Daniel D. Vitamin D: Production, Metabolism and Mechanisms of Action. 2021 Dec 31. Endotext [Internet]. South Darthmouth, MA: MDText.com, Inc,; 2000

[53] Liu Y, Wang M, Xu W, et al. Active vitamin D supplementation alleviates initiation and progression of nonalcoholic fatty liver disease by repressing the p53 pathway. Life Sciences. 2020;**241**:117086

[54] Zhang XL, Chen L, Yang J, et al. Vitamin D alleviates non-alcoholic fatty liver disease via restoring gut microbiota and metabolism. Frontiers in Microbiology. 2023;**14**:1117644

[55] Beilfuss A, Sowa JP, Sydor S, et al. Vitamin D counteracts fibrogenic TGF-β signalling in human hepatic stellate cells both receptor-dependently and independently. Gut. 2015;**64**(5): 791-799

[56] Lukenda Zanko V, Domislovic V, Trkulja V, et al. Vitamin D for treatment of non-alcoholic fatty liver disease detected by transient elastography: A randomized, double-blind, placebo-controlled trial. Diabetes, Obesity and Metabolism. 2020;**22**(11):2097-2106

[57] Sharifi N, Amani R, Hajiani E, Cheraghian B. Does vitamin D improve liver enzymes, oxidative stress, and inflammatory biomarkers in adults with non-alcoholic fatty liver disease? A randomized clinical trial. Endocrine. 2014;**47**:70-80

[58] Wenclewska S, Szymczak-Pajor I, Drzewoski J, et al. Vitamin D supplementation reduces both oxidative DNA damage and insulin resistance in the elderly with metabolic disorders. International Journal of Molecular Sciences. 2019;**20**(12):2891

[59] Lee HK, Shin SR, Han AL. Metabolic dysfunction associated fatty liver disease (MAFLD) and serum vitamin D concentration in South Korea. Asia Pacific Journal of Clinical Nutrition. 2022;**31**(2):201-207

[60] Szymańska R, Nowicka B, Trela A, Kruk J. Vitamin E: Structure and forms. In: Molecular nutrition. Academic Press; 2020. pp. 67-90. eBook ISBN: 9780128119075

[61] Poonyam P, Kritsanaviparkporn C, Chommaitree P, Soodcharoen A. The effects of combined vitamin E and C for treatment of non-alcoholic fatty liver disease (NAFLD): A systematic review and meta-analysis of randomized controlled trials. Asian Pacific Journal of Cancer Prevention. 2022;**23**:2891-2899

[62] Sato K, Gosho M, Yamamoto T, et al. Vitamin E has a beneficial effect on nonalcoholic fatty liver disease: A meta-analysis of randomized controlled trials. Nutrition. 2015;**31**:923-930

[63] Fouda A, Abdelaziz AE, Hussien M, et al. A randomized controlled trial comparing the effects of vitamin E, Ursodeoxycholic acid and Pentoxifylline on Egyptian non-alcoholic steatohepatitis patients. European Review for Medical & Pharmacological Sciences. 2021;**25**(23):7449-7459

[64] Ciarcià G, Bianchi S, Tomasello B, et al. Vitamin E and non-communicable diseases: A review. Biomedicine. 2022;**10**(10):2473

[65] Choi Y, Lee S, Kim S, et al. Vitamin E (α-tocopherol) consumption influences gut microbiota composition. International Journal of Food Sciences and Nutrition. 2020;**71**(2):221-225

[66] Jennison E, Byrne CD. The role of the gut microbiome and diet in the pathogenesis of non-alcoholic fatty liver disease. Clinical and Molecular Hepatology. 2021;**27**(1):22

[67] Cusi K, Isaacs S, Barb D, et al. American Association of Clinical Endocrinology Clinical Practice Guideline for the diagnosis and Management of Nonalcoholic Fatty Liver Disease in primary care and endocrinology clinical settings: co-sponsored by the American Association for the Study of Liver Diseases (AASLD). Endocrine Practice. 2022;**28**:528-562

[68] Vilar-Gomez E, Vuppalanchi R, Gawrieh S, et al. Vitamin E improves transplant-free survival and hepatic decompensation among patients with nonalcoholic steatohepatitis and advanced fibrosis. Hepatology. 2020;**71**:495-509

[69] Niu Z, Liu J, Peng H, Wu X, et al. Dietary composition and its association with metabolic dysfunction-associated fatty liver disease among Chinese adults: A cross-sectional study. Arab Journal of Gastroenterology. 2024;**25**(2):205-213

[70] Montemayor S, García S, Monserrat-Mesquida M, et al. Dietary patterns, foods, and nutrients to ameliorate non-alcoholic fatty liver disease: A scoping review. Nutrients. 2023;**15**(18):3987

[71] Richardson DR, Lane DJ, Becker EM, et al. Mitochondrial iron trafficking and the integration of iron metabolism between the mitochondrion and cytosol. Proceedings of the National Academy of Sciences. 2010;**107**(24):10775-10782

[72] Simcox JA, McClain DA. Iron and diabetes risk. Cell Metabolism. 2013;**17**:329-341

[73] Zhang L, Dai X, Wang L, et al. Iron overload accelerated lipid metabolism disorder and liver injury in rats with non-alcoholic fatty liver disease. Frontiers in Nutrition. 2022;**9**:961892

[74] Murotomi K, Tawara H, Sutoh M, Yasunaga M. Iron-accumulating splenocytes may exacerbate non-alcoholic steatohepatitis through the production of proinflammatory cytokines and reactive oxygen species. Experimental Biology and Medicine. 2022;**247**(10):848-855

[75] Xu GX, Wei S, Yu C, et al. Activation of Kupffer cells in NAFLD and NASH: Mechanisms and therapeutic interventions. Frontiers in Cell and Developmental Biology. 2023;**11**:1199519

[76] de Oliveira J, Denadai MB, Costa DL. Crosstalk between Heme Oxygenase-1 and iron metabolism in macrophages: Implications for the modulation of inflammation and immunity. Antioxidants. 2022;**11**(5):861

[77] Wang JW, Jin CH, Ke JF, et al. Serum iron is closely associated with metabolic dysfunction-associated fatty liver disease in type 2 diabetes: A real-world study. Frontiers in Endocrinology. 2022;**13**:942412

[78] Altamura S, Müdder K, Schlotterer A, et al. Iron aggravates hepatic insulin resistance in the absence of inflammation in a novel db/db mouse model with iron overload. Molecular Metabolism. 2021;**51**:101235

[79] Wang Q, Zhu M, Li H, et al. Hyperferritinemia correlates to metabolic dysregulation and steatosis in Chinese biopsy-proven nonalcoholic fatty liver disease patients. Diabetes, Metabolic Syndrome and Obesity. 2022;**15**:1543-1552

[80] Tsurusaki S, Tsuchiya Y, Koumura T, et al. Hepatic ferroptosis plays an important role as the trigger for initiating inflammation in nonalcoholic steatohepatitis. Cell Death & Disease. 2019;**10**(6):449

[81] Tsang T, Davis CI, Brady DC. Copper biology. Current Biology. 2021;**31**(9):R421-R427

[82] Chen Y, Wu C, Li G, et al. Comparison of copper concentration between non-alcoholic fatty liver disease patients and normal individuals: A meta-analysis. Frontiers in Public Health. 2023;**11**:1095916

[83] Aigner E, Strasser M, Haufe H, et al. A role for low hepatic copper concentrations in nonalcoholic fatty liver disease. American Journal of Gastroenterology. 2010;**105**(9):1978-1985

[84] Lee SH, Kim MJ, Kim YS, et al. Low hair copper concentration is related to a high risk of nonalcoholic fatty liver disease in adults. Journal of Trace Elements in Medicine and Biology. 2018;**50**:28-33

[85] Ma C, Han L, Zhu Z, et al. Mineral metabolism and ferroptosis in non-alcoholic fatty liver diseases. Biochemical Pharmacology. 2022;**205**:115242

[86] Blades B, Ayton S, Hung YH, et al. Copper and lipid metabolism: A reciprocal relationship. Biochimica et Biophysica Acta (BBA)-General Subjects. 2021;**1865**(11):129979

[87] Lan Y, Wu S, Wang Y, et al. Association between blood copper and nonalcoholic fatty liver disease according to sex. Clinical Nutrition. 2021;**40**(4):2045-2052

[88] Zhong CC, Zhao T, Hogstrand C, et al. Copper (Cu) induced changes of lipid metabolism through oxidative stress-mediated autophagy and Nrf2/PPARγ pathways. The Journal of Nutritional Biochemistry. 2022;**100**:108883

[89] Chen C, Zhou Q, Yang R, et al. Copper exposure association with prevalence of non-alcoholic fatty liver disease and insulin resistance among US adults (NHANES 2011-2014). Ecotoxicology and Environmental Safety. 2021;**218**:112295

[90] Himoto T, Masaki T. Current trends on the involvement of zinc, copper, and selenium in the process of Hepatocarcinogenesis. Nutrients. 2024;**16**(4):472

[91] Chasapis CT, Ntoupa PSA, Spiliopoulou CA, Stefanidou ME. Recent aspects of the effects of zinc on human health. Archives of Toxicology. 2020;**94**:1443-1460

[92] Akdas S, Yazihan N. Serum zinc level and dietary zinc intake status in

non-alcoholic fatty liver disease: A meta-analysis and systematic review. In: Hepatology Forum Vol. 1(2). Turkish Association for the Study of the Liver; May 2020. p. 59

[93] Barbara M, Mindikoglu AL. The role of zinc in the prevention and treatment of nonalcoholic fatty liver disease. Metabolism Open. 2021;**11**:100105

[94] Hess SY. National risk of zinc deficiency as estimated by national surveys. Food and Nutrition Bulletin. 2017;**38**(1):3-17

[95] Stiles LI, Ferrao K, Mehta KJ. Role of zinc in health and disease. Clinical and Experimental Medicine. 2024;**24**(1):38

[96] Abdallah AAM, Abdelrahman MM, Attia HMAAS, et al. Decreased serum zinc, selenium, and vitamin E as possible risk factors of hepatic fibrosis in non-alcoholic fatty liver disease. Nutrition and Health. May 2022;**22**:2601060221103032

[97] Kim MC, Lee JI, Kim JH, et al. Serum zinc level and hepatic fibrosis in patients with nonalcoholic fatty liver disease. PLoS One. 2020;**15**(10):e0240195

[98] Kosari F, Jamali R, Ramim T, Abad EMJ. The correlation between serum zinc level and liver histology in non-alcoholic steatohepatitis. Iranian Journal of Pathology. 2019;**14**(1):17

[99] Chen SD, Zhang H, Rios RS, et al. J-shaped relationship between serum zinc levels and the severity of hepatic necro-inflammation in patients with MAFLD. Nutrition, Metabolism and Cardiovascular Diseases. 2022;**32**(5):1259-1265

[100] Prasad AS. Lessons learned from experimental human model of zinc deficiency. Journal of Immunology Research. 2020;**1**:9207279

[101] Hosseini R, Ferns GA, Sahebkar A, et al. Zinc supplementation is associated with a reduction in serum markers of inflammation and oxidative stress in adults: A systematic review and meta-analysis of randomized controlled trials. Cytokine. 2021;**138**:155396

[102] Fathi M, Alavinejad P, Haidari Z, Amani R. The effect of zinc supplementation on steatosis severity and liver function enzymes in overweight/obese patients with mild to moderate non-alcoholic fatty liver following calorie-restricted diet: A double-blind, randomized placebo-controlled trial. Biological Trace Element Research. 2020;**197**:394-404

[103] Hariharan S, Dharmaraj S. Selenium and selenoproteins: It's role in regulation of inflammation. Inflammopharmacology. 2020;**28**:667-695

[104] Barchielli G, Capperucci A, Tanini D. The role of selenium in pathologies: An updated review. Antioxidants. 2022;**11**(2):251

[105] Wang X, Seo YA, Park SK. Serum selenium and Non-alcoholic Fatty Liver Disease (NAFLD) in US adults: National Health and Nutrition Examination Survey (NHANES) 2011-2016. Environmental Research. 2021;**197**:111190

[106] Wu J, Zeng C, Yang Z, et al. Association between dietary selenium intake and the prevalence of nonalcoholic fatty liver disease: A cross-sectional study. Journal of the American College of Nutrition. 2020;**39**(2):103-111

[107] Han J, Liang H, Yi J, et al. Long-term selenium-deficient diet induces

liver damage by altering hepatocyte ultrastructure and MMP1/3 and TIMP1/3 expression in growing rats. Biological Trace Element Research. 2017;**175**:396-404

[108] Zhu M, Niu Q, Zhang J, et al. Amorphous selenium nanodots alleviate non-alcoholic fatty liver disease via activating VEGF receptor 1 to further inhibit phosphorylation of JNK/p38 MAPK pathways. European Journal of Pharmacology. 2022;**932**:175235

[109] Steinbrenner H, Duntas LH, Rayman MP. The role of selenium in type-2 diabetes mellitus and its metabolic comorbidities. Redox Biology. 2022;**50**:102236

[110] Wang X, Zhang W, Chen H, et al. High selenium impairs hepatic insulin sensitivity through opposite regulation of ROS. Toxicology Letters. 2014;**224**(1):16-23

[111] Stanisławska IJ, Figat R, Kiss AK, Bobrowska-Korczak B. Essential elements and isoflavonoids in the prevention of prostate cancer. Nutrients. 2022;**14**(6):1225

[112] Levander OA, Burk RF. Update of human dietary standards for selenium. In: Selenium: Its Molecular Biology and Role in Human Health. Boston, MA: Springer US; 2006. pp. 399-410

[113] Fiorentini D, Cappadone C, Farruggia G, Prata C. Magnesium: Biochemistry, nutrition, detection, and social impact of diseases linked to its deficiency. Nutrients. 2021;**13**(4):1136

[114] Kostov K. Effects of magnesium deficiency on mechanisms of insulin resistance in type 2 diabetes: Focusing on the processes of insulin secretion and signaling. International Journal of Molecular Sciences. 2019;**20**(6):1351

[115] Găman MA, Dobrică EC, Cozma MA, et al. Crosstalk of magnesium and serum lipids in dyslipidemia and associated disorders: A systematic review. Nutrients. 2021;**13**(5):1411

[116] Simón J, Delgado TC, Martinez-Cruz LA, Martínez-Chantar ML. Magnesium, little known but possibly relevant: A link between NASH and related comorbidities. Biomedicine. 2021;**9**(2):125

[117] Nielsen FH. Magnesium deficiency and increased inflammation: Current perspectives. Journal of Inflammation Research. 2018;**11**:25-34

[118] Liu M, Dudley SC Jr. Magnesium, oxidative stress, inflammation, and cardiovascular disease. Antioxidants. 2020;**9**(10):907

[119] Yu YC, Paragomi P, Wang R, et al. High serum magnesium is associated with lower risk of hepatocellular carcinoma among patients with nonalcoholic fatty liver disease. Cancer. 2023;**129**(15):2341-2347

[120] Jiang W, Xu S, Guo H, et al. Magnesium isoglycyrrhizinate prevents the nonalcoholic hepatic steatosis via regulating energy homeostasis. Journal of Cellular and Molecular Medicine. 2020;**24**(13):7201-7213

[121] Maoka T. Carotenoids as natural functional pigments. Journal of Natural Medicines. 2020;**74**(1):1-16

[122] Wu L, Mo W, Feng J, et al. Astaxanthin attenuates hepatic damage and mitochondrial dysfunction in non-alcoholic fatty liver disease by up-regulating the FGF21/PGC-1α pathway. British Journal of Pharmacology. 2020;**177**(16):3760-3777

[123] Clugston RD. Carotenoids and fatty liver disease: Current knowledge and research gaps. Biochimica et Biophysica Acta (BBA)-Molecular and Cell Biology of Lipids. 2020;**1865**(11):158597

[124] Yao P, Liu Y. Terpenoids: Natural compounds for non-alcoholic fatty liver disease (NAFLD) therapy. Molecules. 2022;**28**(1):272

[125] Ibrahim IM, Althagafy HS, Abd-Alhameed EK, et al. Promising hepatoprotective effects of lycopene in different liver diseases. Life Sciences. 2022;**310**:121131

[126] Yang S, Li J, Yan L, et al. Molecular mechanisms of fucoxanthin in alleviating lipid deposition in metabolic associated fatty liver disease. Journal of Agricultural and Food Chemistry. 2024;**72**(18):10391-10405

Chapter 6

Lifestyle Intervention of Metabolic Dysfunction-Associated Steatotic Liver Disease

Xinyi Lu, Zhengyang Bao, Yu Chen and Daozhen Chen

Abstract

Metabolic dysfunction-associated fatty liver disease (MASLD) remains a major underlying cause of persistent liver disease worldwide. Lifestyle treatments, especially those involving regular exercise and balanced diet plans, are considered the cornerstone techniques for managing MASLD. The purpose of this chapter is to guide readers in a comprehensive assessment of the translation and treatment status of lifestyle interventions in managing MASLD through a wealth of clinical and preclinical data. Specifically, the importance of diet types and the impact of various dietary components on the occurrence and severity of MASLD are discussed. Managing the timing of energy intake has certain positive effects on MASLD, regardless of caloric restriction. In addition, exercise, regardless of type and intensity, is equally important as dietary intervention, with the gut microbiota seemingly playing an essential role. By leveraging personalized metabolic and lifestyle treatments, a viable non-pharmacological treatment path is provided for MASLD patients.

Keywords: lifestyle treatment, dietary, intermittent fasting, caloric restriction, exercise, MASLD, probiotics

1. Introduction

In today's contemporary culture, with substantial adjustments in way of life and dietary behaviors, MASLD, commonly known as Non-Alcoholic Fatty Liver Disease (NAFLD), has become one of the most common types of chronic liver disease worldwide. It not just impacts the health of millions but is also associated with various metabolic disorders, such as obesity, diabetes, and cardiovascular diseases. The development of MASLD generally starts with the accumulation of excess fat, largely triglycerides in liver cells. This fat buildup is an outcome of metabolic disorders, such as insulin resistance, metabolic syndrome, and obesity. Ultimately, the fatty liver can bring about inflammation, which might progress to liver fibrosis and cirrhosis. Oxidative stress, mitochondrial dysfunction, and inflammatory responses also play significant functions in this procedure.

At present, drug therapy mainly focuses on its pathogenic factors, pathogenesis, and related metabolic disorders as targets, including hypoglycemic drugs (such as pioglitazone, glucagon-like peptide-1 (GLP-1) receptor agonists, and sodium-glucose cotransporter-2 (SGLT-2) inhibitors), antioxidants (such as vitamin E), statins or other lipid-lowering drugs, bile and non-bile acid Farnesoid X receptor (FXR) agonists, etc. However, there is still a lack of specific drugs. The European Association for the Study of the Liver (EASL), the European Association for the Study of Diabetes (EASD), and the European Association for the Study of Obesity (EASO) practice guidelines recommend lifestyle intervention as the primary treatment for patients with MASLD. Therefore, optimizing lifestyle through reasonable diet and exercise intervention is undoubtedly the important link in the treatment of MASLD.

Dietary intervention is the foundation of MASLD treatment. The Mediterranean diet (MD) is particularly recommended, emphasizing the intake of high fiber, low sugar, moderate protein, and healthy fats. Reducing the intake of saturated fats and easily digestible carbohydrates, as well as avoiding high-fructose foods and beverages, is especially important for improving liver health. In addition, dietary behaviors, such as eating speed and frequency, are also related to the development of MASLD. Exercise therapy, such as aerobic exercise and resistance training, can also be part of MASLD treatment, helping to increase muscle mass, improve insulin sensitivity, and having a positive impact on hepatic steatosis. There is also evidence to suggest that combined dietary and exercise intervention is more effective than individual interventions. Nevertheless, when carrying out these interventions, it is important to make customized treatment strategies tailored to the specific needs and conditions of MASLD individuals. Such individualized approaches are more probable to lead to boosted adherence, greater efficacy, and continual health benefits over the long term, thus offering much better and a lot more durable end results for those affected by MASLD (**Figure 1**).

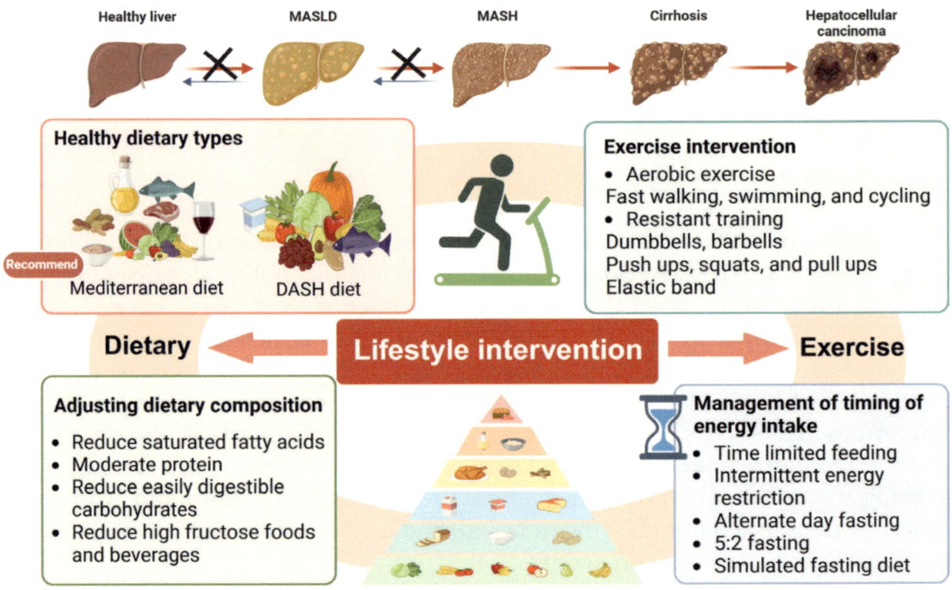

Figure 1.
Lifestyle interventions in the management of MASLD.

DOI: http://dx.doi.org/10.5772/intechopen.1007122

2. Dietary intervention

MASLD is the liver indication of metabolic syndrome. Unhealthy dietary practices, consisting of extreme intake of saturated fatty acids, fructose, and soft drinks, insufficient consumption of omega (ω)-3 fatty acids and dietary fiber, in addition to constant and irregular consuming patterns, not only aggravate the event and development of MASLD, yet also boost the risk of establishing metabolic dysfunction-associated steatohepatitis (MASH). Experimental and scientific evidence recommends that the possible devices underlying the occurrence and development of MASLD include boosted hepatic neolipogenesis, inhibition of lipid oxidation, increased insulin resistance, interruption of circadian rhythms, and dysbiosis of the digestive tract microbiota. In response to these variables, dietary interventions should be the primary focus in handling MASLD among healthy and balanced way of living interventions. Adjusting dietary framework, lowering calorie intake, recurring eating patterns, and so on may offer an ideal, long-lasting dietary intake pattern, therefore improving metabolism.

2.1 Types of diet

2.1.1 Mediterranean diet

MD is a healthful eating pattern that emphasizes a plant-based foundation, with an abundance of fruits, vegetables, whole grains, legumes, and nuts. It primarily uses olive oil as the chief source of fat and includes moderate consumption of fish and poultry, while limiting red meat and processed foods. Moderate consumption of red wine is encouraged, and herbs and spices are used, instead of salt, to season dishes. MD is a high-fat diet, with fat accounting for 35–45% of total energy intake, carbohydrates accounting for 35–40%, and protein accounting for 15–20%, which has been proven to promote cardiovascular health and improve metabolic parameters.

In a 6-week randomized cross diet intervention study on non-diabetic subjects (6 females/6 males) with biopsy-proven MASLD, compared with the low-fat high-carbohydrate diet, liver steatosis in MD was relatively reduced and insulin sensitivity was improved [1]. Similarly, in another double-blind, parallel design, randomized controlled trial (RCT), Asian MASLD patients received MD with (n = 31) or without (n = 28) pentadecanoic acid (C15:0) supplementation and control (habitual diet without C15:0 supplementation) (n = 29). Compared to the control, body weight (BW), proton density fat fraction (PDFF) of the liver, total cholesterol, γ-glutamyl transferase (GGT), and triglyceride (TG) concentrations were significantly reduced. In addition, supplementing C15:0 can further reduce low-density lipoprotein (LDL)-cholesterol and increase the abundance of *Bifidobacterium adolescentis* [2]. In addition, in an MD intervention for non-diabetic white patients with biopsy-confirmed MASLD and elevated transaminase (n = 20), the average weight, average waist circumference, and average transaminase levels, including alanine aminotransferase (ALT) and aspartate aminotransferase (AST), were significantly reduced, but no significant changes in intestinal permeability were observed after the trial [3]. Therefore, more research is needed on the relationship between MD and changes in intestinal permeability.

Interestingly, MD seems to be one of the more suitable diets for children and adolescents with MASLD. A study conducted on children aged 9–17 years diagnosed with MASLD showed that those with MD experienced significant reductions in liver steatosis and insulin resistance, and notable improvements in liver enzymes, without a significant decrease in energy intake required for growth [4]. Another study on adolescents aged 11–18 years with MASLD similarly demonstrated that, in addition to improvements in the aforementioned indicators, the MD group exhibited increased serum total antioxidant capacity, paraoxonase-1, and glutathione peroxidase (GPx) levels, along with decreased C-reactive protein (CRP) levels, suggesting a positive impact on inflammation and oxidative stress [5].

2.1.2 DASH diet

The Dietary Approaches to Stop Hypertension (DASH) is a dietary plan specifically designed to help lower high blood pressure and has also been considered to improve MASLD in recent years. However, there is a lack of related research compared to MD. DASH diet emphasizes the consumption of plenty of fruits, vegetables, whole grains, and low-fat dairy products, while limiting the intake of saturated fats, cholesterol, and total fats. It also encourages moderate consumption of fish, poultry, and nuts, and reduces the intake of red meat, sugar, sugary drinks, and foods with added salt. By increasing the intake of minerals like potassium, calcium, and magnesium while reducing sodium intake, the DASH diet not only aids in blood pressure management but also promotes cardiovascular health.

In a 12-week randomized controlled trial of MASLD patients (n = 70), the DASH diet had a significant effect on improving liver fibrosis and hepatic steatosis and reducing ALT levels compared to a healthy diet (both containing 50–55% carbohydrates, 15–20% protein, and 30% total fat) [6]. In another 8-week randomized controlled clinical trial of overweight and obese MASLD patients (n = 60), the DASH diet significantly reduced body weight, body mass index (BMI), ALT, alkaline phosphatase (ALP), and improved the markers of insulin metabolism. Moreover, the DASH diet is beneficial for the level of malondialdehyde (MDA), glutathione (GSH), and inflammatory markers, such as serum high-sensitivity C-reactive protein [7]. A systematic review suggests that the DASH diet, like MD, can reduce the risk of MASLD [8]. However, limited evidence suggests that currently further research is needed, including equal calorie diet patterns, longer intervention times, and measurement of inflammatory markers, to obtain more informative results.

2.2 Adjusting dietary composition

Adjusting dietary composition is taken into consideration as a vital approach for handling and boosting MASLD.

2.2.1 Selection of high-quality fats

Excessive consumption of saturated and trans fats in the diet regimen can cause fat buildup in the liver and liver dysfunction. Saturated fats are largely located in red meat, full-fat milk items, and specific deep-fried foods, while trans fats are common in readily baked items, fast food, and partially hydrogenated vegetable oils. These fats not only boost the threat of heart diseases but are also likewise directly connected with liver steatosis. A study compared the hazards of saturated fat (SAT) and unsaturated fat (UNSAT) on liver metabolism by administering an additional 1000 calories of saturated or unsaturated fats or monosaccharides per day to overweight subjects (n = 38) for 3 weeks. Overfeeding SAT increased intrahepatic triglycerides by about 40% compared with UNSAT. In addition, SAT induced insulin resistance and endotoxemia, and significantly increased various plasma ceramides, indicating that reducing SAT intake may help reduce the risk of increased intrahepatic triglyceride and related diabetes [9].

Changing harmful fats with healthy and balanced fats is valuable for the healing of MASLD individuals. Polyunsaturated fats, such as omega-3 fatty acids located in fish, flaxseeds, and walnuts, help reduce swelling and liver fat accumulation. Monounsaturated fatty acids, such as those in olive oil and avocados, can improve lipid profiles and insulin sensitivity, thus playing a role in reducing liver fat. Several studies have shown that the use of high-quality fat source sesame oil with a hypocaloric diet significantly reduces the weight, body mass index, waist circumference, and fatty liver grading of MASLD patients. In addition, serum levels of AST and ALT were significantly reduced [10, 11]. Sesame oil contains lipophilic unsaponifiable substance—sesame lignan. Sesamin can inhibit lipid accumulation by regulating key factors involved in lipogenesis and lipolysis, such as fatty acid synthase (FASN), sterol regulatory element-binding protein 1c (SREBP-1c), forkhead box protein O-1 (FOXO1), and adipose triglyceride lipase (ATGL). Sesamin attenuates palmitate-induced lipotoxicity and regulates hepatic lipid metabolism in HepG2 cells by activating the estrogen receptor alpha/Ca^{2+}/calmodulin-dependent protein kinase kinase β/AMP-activated protein kinase (ERα/CaMKKβ/AMPK) signaling pathway [12], making it a promising candidate for the treatment of hepatic steatosis.

2.2.2 Controlling carbohydrate intake

Refined carbohydrates like white bread, white rice, sweets, and sugary drinks can quickly raise blood glucose and insulin levels, promoting fat synthesis. Dietary fructose, sucrose, or high-fructose corn syrup has been shown to have a special tendency to induce fatty liver and inflammation in experimental animals [13]. The administration of fructose can also induce other characteristics of metabolic syndrome, including elevated blood pressure, elevated serum triglycerides, and insulin resistance. If the diet has a high sugar content (40%), even a calorie-restricted diet can induce fatty liver, accompanied by upregulation of fructose-dependent transporter glucose transporter 5 (Glut5) and fructokinase [14].

In addition, the endogenous production of fructose by the liver can cause systemic metabolic changes [15]. Aldehyde reductase can metabolize glucose into sorbitol, which is then converted into fructose by sorbitol dehydrogenase. Therefore, if aldose reductase is highly expressed or activated in the liver, some of the absorbed glucose may be converted into fructose. Mice with aldose reductase deficiency can prevent glucose-induced fatty liver.

Consumption of sugary-sweetened beverages is also closely linked to the development of MASLD in humans. Clinical studies have confirmed the role of fructose in MASLD. For instance, compared to aspartame-sweetened drinks, consuming sucrose-sweetened soft drinks can increase ectopic fat accumulation and lipid levels, as well as the risk of cardiovascular and metabolic diseases [16]. Conversely, a fructose-restricted diet can reduce liver fat, visceral fat, and *de novo* lipogenesis in obese children, while also improving insulin kinetics and glucose tolerance [17, 18].

Complex carbohydrates, such as whole grains, legumes, and fiber-rich vegetables, are recommended, which provide stable energy sources and promote gut health and metabolic balance. The low glycemic index of these food aids in their slow digestion and absorption, helping to maintain stable blood glucose levels. Studies report that compared with the traditional diet for diabetes, moderate carbohydrate restriction can moderately improve blood sugar control in a short period, and reduce circulating and hepatic triacylglycerol levels in individuals with type 2 diabetes, which is beyond the influence of weight loss itself.

2.2.3 Moderate protein intake

There is relatively little research done on the quality, quantity, and composition of protein in MASLD dietary management. Moderate protein intake prolongs satiety and reduces the risk of overeating. This satiety and the boost to basal metabolic rate assist in weight loss and improvement of metabolic syndrome symptoms, thus positively affecting MASLD management. Researchers have found that while low-protein very-low-carbohydrate diets can reduce BW in MASLD rats, they may also lead to metabolic disorders and changes in the gut microbiome composition. However, diets with high-protein content and very low carbohydrates can partially mitigate these limitations. Specifically, in low-protein rats, there is an increase in very-low-density lipoprotein receptor expression and elevated liver oxidative stress, which subsequently activate the expression of nuclear factor erythroid 2-related factor 2 (Nrf2). This activation causes inflammation through TLR4/TRIF/NLRP3 (Toll-like receptor 4/TIR-domain-containing adaptor-inducing interferon-β/NOD-, LRR-, and pyrin domain-containing protein 3) and TLR4/MyD88/NF-κB (Toll-like receptor 4/myeloid differentiation primary response 88/nuclear factor kappa B) pathways, leading to hepatic lipid accumulation. In contrast, rats with higher protein content in their diet can partially prevent changes in very-low-density lipoprotein receptor (VLDLR) and the TLR4-inflammasome pathway [19].

However, the safety of high-protein diets still needs to be evaluated. First, a high intake of protein can increase the burden on the kidneys. The kidneys are responsible for excreting nitrogenous waste products, particularly urea, during protein metabolism. When protein intake is too high, the kidneys must work harder to eliminate these metabolic byproducts, which may accelerate renal function decline, especially in individuals already at risk for kidney dysfunction. Moreover, excessive dietary protein may disrupt nitrogen balance in the body and could potentially lead to liver dysfunction. For individuals with existing MASLD, the liver already bears an extra burden, and a high-protein diet might further exacerbate metabolic stress on the liver. Although protein is essential for liver repair and regeneration, overconsumption could result in the accumulation of protein metabolism byproducts in liver cells, thereby exacerbating liver damage. Therefore, MASLD patients should focus on obtaining high-quality protein from lean fish, poultry, legumes, and tofu, which provide essential amino acids without adding extra liver burden, aiding muscle repair and immune function.

In summary, moderate protein intake has shown positive effects and may provide useful references for the treatment of MASLD in humans. However, further research and clinical trials are needed to determine the applicability and best practices of these effects in humans.

2.3 Management of timing of energy intake

The timing of energy intake is a risk factor for MASLD and metabolic dysfunction. Intermittent fasting (IF) is a non-pharmacological dietary method for managing obesity and metabolic syndrome, which includes regular complete or near-complete abstinence from food and energy containing fluids. IF protocols mainly include time-restricted feeding (TRF), intermittent energy restriction (IER), alternate-day fasting (ADF), 5:2 fasting, and simulated fasting diet (fasting-mimicking diet (FMD)) (**Table 1**). Recently, IF has gained great popularity in mainstream culture as an intervention that may mitigate the metabolic dysfunction underlying MASLD and MASH. The beneficial effects of IF on weight loss, insulin sensitivity, and oxidative stress have been well documented in both preclinical and clinical studies [20], making it a promising approach for treating MASLD and MASH.

2.3.1 Preclinical studies on IF in MASLD and MASH

The effects of different intermittent fasting methods in MASLD animal models have been extensively studied. While positive results have been obtained, the conclusions are not consistent. In high-fat diet-induced obese rats, both ADF and TRF were able to reduce body weight and body mass index. The TRF group showed an increase in total white blood cell (WBC) count, lymphocytes, and monocytes, while the ADF group showed an increase in platelet count. However, the blood lipid profile and liver stress markers were not altered by IF [21]. Some researchers additionally reported that the muscular tissue glucose transporter 4 (Glut4) protein material and blood glucose degrees in the high-fat with ADF group were substantially lower compared to the common diet group [22]. In examining the effects of three types of recurring fasting in high-fat diet-induced obese computer mice, ADF and TRF significantly led to weight loss, while TRF and the 5:2 diet plan minimized visceral fat [23]. As a result, further evaluation and synthesis of these conclusions are important for reviewing the pros and cons of periodic fasting.

Additionally, comparative researches have checked out the effects of IF versus continuous calorie restriction (CCR) in rodent models of MASLD. While both treatments have actually been revealed to minimize liver fat and boost metabolic wellness, IF appears to offer one-of-a-kind benefits in preserving lean body mass and metabolic adaptability. In particular, IF has actually been connected with better enhancements in insulin sensitivity and reductions in hepatic swelling contrasted to CCR, recommending that the regular fasting durations may provide extra metabolic benefits past straightforward calorie reduction [24]. In addition, the capability of IF to improve

Type of intermittent fasting	Definition
Time-restricted feeding	Food intake is confined to a specific number of hours each day, typically ranging from 4 to 12 hours, without necessarily altering the actual caloric consumption
Intermittent energy restriction	Calorie restriction occurs on several non-consecutive days, interspersed with regular calorie intake.
Alternate-day fasting	Involves fasting every other day, alternating between fasting days with little to no calorie intake and non-fasting days with normal eating.
5:2 fasting	Entails eating normally for five days a week and reducing calorie intake to 500–600 calories on the other two days.
Simulated fasting diet	Typically lasts for a period of about 5 days, during which specific foods are consumed to maintain low calorie and protein intake while providing essential nutrients to support basic bodily functions.

Table 1.
Types and definitions of IF.

metabolic versatility—the capability to switch in between fat and sugar metabolic process—may make it a more sustainable and efficient long-lasting intervention for clients.

2.3.2 IF and gut-liver axis

IF has actually been shown to influence the structure of the gut microbiome, benefiting the development of helpful bacteria and decreasing populations of hazardous bacteria [25]. Preclinical research studies have actually demonstrated that IF can bring back digestive tract barrier feature, lowering the translocation of endotoxins to the liver and consequently undermining liver inflammation. For example, in rodent designs of MASLD, IF was associated with increased levels of *Akkermansia muciniphila*, an intestinal bacterium known for its anti-inflammatory properties, and reduced levels of pro-inflammatory species, such as *Escherichia coli* [26].

Gut microbiota also plays an important role in activating adipose tissue browning and treating metabolic diseases. IF can selectively stimulate the development of beige fat within white adipose tissue and significantly improve obesity, insulin resistance, and hepatic steatosis. Specifically, IF treatment leads to changes in the composition of the gut microbiota, resulting in an increase in fermentation products such as acetate and lactate, and a selective upregulation of monocarboxylate transporter 1 (MCT1) expression in beige cells. However, mice depleted of gut microbiota exhibit resistance to IF-induced beige [27].

Moreover, the regulation of gut microbiota by IF may also affect metabolites. For example, the process of bile acid metabolism is related to lipid metabolism rate and liver health. Digestive tract bacteria change primary bile acids into secondary bile acids, influencing lipid food digestion and metabolic signaling. IF can alter bile acid structure, which impacts metabolic paths with activation of receptors like Farnesoid X receptor and G-protein-coupled bile acid receptor (TGR5). These pathways are vital for keeping energy equilibrium and insulin sensitivity [28]. In addition, short-chain fatty acids (SCFAs), including acetate, propionate, and butyrate, are key bacterial metabolites that play significant roles in gut health and metabolism. IF has been shown to increase the production of SCFAs, which act as energy sources for colonocytes, regulators of glucose and lipid metabolism, and anti-inflammatory agents. Higher levels of fecal acetate and propionate are associated with lower resting regulatory T cells (rTregs) ($CD4^+CD45RA^+CD25^+$) and higher peripheral blood T helper 17 cells (Th17)/rTregs ratios, which can serve as immunological features of MASH patients [29].

Importantly, fasting periods can help align the gut microbiota activity with host circadian rhythms, optimizing metabolic processes. The synchronization of feeding-fasting cycles with microbiome shifts supports efficient nutrient utilization and metabolic homeostasis. These findings underscore the importance of the gut-liver axis in mediating the benefits of IF in liver disease.

2.3.3 Effectiveness and challenges of IF in a patient of MASLD

Based on animal experiments, recent clinical trials have also adopted various IF protocols, such as ADF and TRF, to evaluate their impact on liver health in MASLD patients. These studies typically involve carefully monitoring fasting regimens over several weeks or months, providing insights into the short-term and potential long-term effects of IF.

Trials frequently observe weight loss among participants following IF regimens, along with reductions in visceral fat and improved muscle-to-fat ratios. The liver enzymes such as ALT and AST, biomarkers of liver injury, of IF participants decreased. Additionally, markers of systemic inflammation often diminish, suggesting reduced hepatic inflammation and potentially slowing MASLD progression. Moreover, numerous researches report decreases in fasting glucose degrees and decreases in triglycerides, which are critical in reducing the dangers connected with MASLD. Luckily, with the help of imaging strategies, such as magnetic resonance imaging (MRI) and ultrasound (US), adjustments in liver steatosis can now be quantified. Several experiments have additionally shown that IF can considerably minimize liver fat material.

The favorable outcomes related to IF in MASLD patients may originate from a number of mechanisms. Metabolic switching: fasting promotes a button from glucose to fat metabolic process, improving lipolysis and minimizing hepatic fat buildup. Improved lipid metabolic rate: IF may alter lipid profiles, minimizing triglyceride degrees and improving cholesterol proportions. Gut microbiota inflection: modifications in gut microbiota makeup observed in IF studies suggest prospective interactions with the gut-liver axis, supporting liver health.

While the findings are encouraging, numerous factors to consider stay for applying IF in scientific method. To start with, conformity and sustainability. For some clients, ensuring long-lasting adherence to the IF regimen may be difficult and call for assistance and personalized approaches. Second, there are considerable differences in between people. The feedback to IF might vary due to individual elements, such as genetics, standard metabolic status, and way of living, and these variables must be thought about when developing therapy strategies. Additional research study is required to check out the long-lasting influences and security of continual IF, specifically in diverse client populations. Lastly, integration with various other intervention measures needs to be taken into consideration. Integrating IF with various other lifestyle changes, such as exercise and dietary adjustments, can enhance its efficacy and ensure general management of MASLD.

2.4 Reduction of caloric intake

Caloric restriction (CR) refers to the practice of reducing food intake while ensuring adequate nutrition, thereby lowering the total daily energy intake. This dietary approach is believed to extend the lifespan of organisms, improve metabolic health, and potentially combat certain age-related diseases [30]. In experimental research, long-term adherence to moderate caloric restriction has shown positive health benefits across various biological models, although its long-term effects and feasibility in humans are still under investigation.

The liver is critical in managing energy equilibrium. In the context of MASLD, extreme caloric intake is a substantial vehicle driver of fat buildup in the liver. This occurs because excess calories, particularly from carbohydrates and fats, can be converted into triglycerides within the liver, resulting in hepatic steatosis. Over time, this leads to the development and progression of MASLD. Hence, managing caloric intake is vital to mitigating liver fat accumulation and improving overall liver health.

2.4.1 The potential of CR in preclinical and clinical trials

Studies have shown that CR interventions have positive effects on ALT, liver steatosis, and liver stiffness, and there is a dose-response relationship between the degree of CR and the beneficial impacts on liver function and weight loss [31]. Despite its effectiveness, weight loss is often not sustained in most people, partly due to physiological adaptations that suppress energy expenditure, a process known as adaptive thermogenesis [32]. In high-fat-fed mouse models, recombinant Growth Differentiation Factor 15 (GDF15) was found to reduce obesity and improve glycemic control by inhibiting food intake through a Glial cell line-derived neurotrophic factor family receptor alpha-like (GFRAL)-dependent mechanism. In addition to suppressing appetite, GDF15 counteracts the compensatory reduction in energy expenditure, leading to greater weight loss and reduction in MASLD compared to CR alone. The role of GDF15 in maintaining energy expenditure during CR requires a GFRAL-β-adrenergic signaling axis, which increases fatty acid oxidation and calcium futile cycling in mouse skeletal muscle. Thus, therapeutic targeting of the GDF15-GFRAL pathway may help sustain skeletal muscle energy expenditure during CR [33].

In addition, mice models have shown that CR plays an important role in reversing the MASH-like pathology and effectively delaying the development of hepatocellular carcinoma (HCC). The gene expression profile revealed radiation-related activation of the peroxisome proliferator-activated receptor gamma (PPAR-γ)/CD 36 (cluster of differentiation 36) pathway for transmembrane fatty acid translocation before the development of MASH-like state, but CR can inhibit this process, making the CR-related pathway a promising strategy for preventing HCC caused by radiation or other DNA damaging agents [34].

Interestingly, another study shows that compared with the widely used diabetes drug semaglutide, CR is better at improving body weight and liver steatosis, although it is inferior to semaglutide in improving glucose tolerance. Both are effective for hypertriglyceridemia [35], supporting that CR is also a promising method for improving metabolic diseases in addition to medication.

Based on animal models, CR in MASLD management also exhibits several beneficial biological effects. Moderate CR can lead to temporal changes in liver and skeletal muscle metabolism. Short-term CR can affect triglyceride levels, liver insulin sensitivity, and glucose production, while moderate weight loss can affect muscles, including insulin-mediated glucose uptake and insulin signaling [36]. However, considering the long-term maintenance of initial weight loss and metabolic outcomes under similar net energy intake, there is currently a lack of research to evaluate the sustainability and practicality of different CR methods, such as intermittent CR and CCR [37].

Due to the limited improvement achieved by single CR, recent studies have explored the effects of adjusting dietary structures, such as low-carbon diets in combination with CR on MASLD. The extremely low-calorie ketogenic diet achieved excellent weight loss and significantly reduced liver fat fraction compared to the standard low calorie diet, demonstrating that rapid mobilization of liver fat may be an effective alternative to treating MASLD [38]. Interestingly, the use of CR combined with molecular target agonists such as peroxisome proliferator-activated receptor alpha (PPARα) also showed better improvement effects. The oleoylethanolamine (OEA) group showed lower levels of NF-κB and interleukin 6 (IL-6), and approximately twice as high levels of interleukin 10 (IL-10). In addition, OEA supplements led to a significant increase in fat-free mass, but had no significant effect on MASLD fibrosis score, suggesting a role in improving inflammation levels and body composition [39].

Therefore, understanding the mechanisms and practical effects through these experiments enables scientists to better design human clinical trials and personalized dietary interventions to promote health management and disease improvement in MASLD patients.

2.4.2 Considerations and challenges

When implementing a calorie decrease technique, while this method may profit several people with MASLD, there are prospective threat elements and factors to consider to be aware of.

1. Nutritional deficiency. Excessive calorie decrease can lead to dietary shortages, particularly if there is inadequate interest to diet's high quality. It's essential to make certain the diet consists of all vital nutrients to stop deficiency-related problems.

2. Muscle mass loss. Significant calorie decrease, or not enough healthy protein intake, can cause muscular tissue loss. Preserving sufficient healthy protein consumption and taking part in ideal strength training can aid preserve lean body mass.

3. Lowered metabolic rate. Long-term low-calorie diet plans may bring about a reduction in the body's basic metabolic price. This happens as the body adapts by minimizing power expenditure in response to inadequate calorie intake, possibly making additional weight management more difficult.

4. Mental impact. Strict calorie reduction can lead to troublesome eating habits, including binge eating and disordered consuming. Mental variables such as stress and anxiety might also raise, specifically during weight loss plateaus or when objectives are hard to attain.

3. Exercise

Exercise intervention refers to the organized execution of exercise programs targeted at boosting health and wellness conditions or dealing with particular disease. In the monitoring of MASLD, exercise intervention plays an important role. The primary objectives are to improve liver health and overall metabolic status by increasing energy expenditure, reducing liver fat, enhancing insulin sensitivity, and decreasing inflammation and oxidative stress. Common forms of exercise intervention include aerobic exercise and resistance training. These exercise modalities help in weight reduction, improve cardiovascular health, and effectively lower the risk of MASLD progression. Through personalized and gradually progressive exercise plans, exercise intervention serves as a safe and effective lifestyle modification strategy for MASLD patients.

3.1 Types of exercise

The choice of exercise mode has a crucial impact on the effectiveness of intervention, and patients should choose a more suitable way for themselves. A systematic review summarized the effects of aerobic exercise and resistance exercise on MASLD. Both aerobic and resistance exercises are effective at reducing hepatic steatosis in individuals with MASLD when performed with similar frequency, duration, and period (40–45 minutes per session, three times a week for 12 weeks). Despite these similarities in reducing liver fat, the two exercise types have distinct characteristics [40]. A large number of clinical trials have further evaluated the effects of aerobic exercise, resistance exercise, or combined exercise on metabolic syndrome, obesity, and cardiovascular risk factors (**Table 2**). In short, the energy consumption of resistance exercise is significantly lower than that of aerobic exercise. Although aerobic exercise or a combination of aerobic exercise and resistance exercise may seem more effective for cardiovascular disease, resistance exercise may be more feasible than

Study	Experimental subjects	Study design	Results
Villareal et al. [41]	Obese older adults	Aerobic training (n = 40), resistance training (n = 40), or combined aerobic and resistance training (n = 40) or control group (n = 40)	The physical function test scores of the combination group increased more than those of the aerobic and resistance groups. The peak oxygen consumption of the combination and aerobic groups increased more than that of the resistance group. The strength increase of the combination group and resistance group is higher than that of the aerobic group. Compared with the aerobic group, the combination group and resistance group showed less weight loss.
Dieli-Conwright et al. [42]	Patients with sedentary, overweight, or obese breast cancer	Aerobic and resistance exercise (n = 50) or usual care (n = 50)	Combined resistance and aerobic exercise effectively attenuated metabolic syndrome, sarcopenic obesity, and relevant biomarkers including insulin, IGF-1, leptin, and adiponectin.
Lee et al. [43]	Adults with overweight or obesity and elevated blood pressure.	Resistance (n = 102), aerobic (n = 101), combined resistance plus aerobic exercise (n = 101), or no-exercise control (n = 102)	The cardiovascular disease risk status improved in the aerobic and combination groups, but not in the resistance group, and there was no difference between the aerobic and combination groups. There was no significant improvement in the four individual cardiovascular disease risk factors: body fat, systolic blood pressure, LDL-cholesterol, and fasting blood glucose.
Rezende et al. [44]	Sedentary postmenopausal women with biopsy-proven MASLD	Aerobic physical activity (n = 19) or control group (n = 21)	The exercise group showed a decrease in waist circumference, an increase in high-density lipoprotein cholesterol levels, and an improvement in cardiovascular and pulmonary function, but there was no significant difference in inflammatory factors between the two groups.
Harris et al. [45]	Patients with MASLD	Moderate-intensity aerobic exercise training (n = 15) or standard clinical care (n = 8	The serum biomarkers of liver fibrosis inflammation induced by exercise training were improved, including [1] ALT improvement ≥17 IU/L (mean reduction 24% vs. 10%, respectively) [2] improvement in CK18 (−61 vs. +71 ng/mL).

Table 2.
The effects of different exercise modes on MASLD, metabolic syndrome, obesity, and cardiovascular risk factors.

aerobic exercise for MASLD patients with poor cardiovascular health or those who cannot tolerate or participate in aerobic exercise.

3.2 Intensity of exercise

Exercise intervention not only emphasizes the intensity of exercise, but also the duration of exercise. Only by combining the two can ideal exercise effects be achieved. Several studies have compared the effects of different exercise intensities on the intervention of MASLD. In the MASLD mice model fed a high-fat, high-carbohydrate diet, both high-intensity interval training (HIIT) and moderate-intensity continuous training (MIT) inhibited weight gain, improved systemic metabolic parameters, and ameliorated the progression of MASH. However, HIIT was superior to MIT in reducing obesity, enhancing systemic glucose tolerance, and improving hepatic steatosis, inflammation, and fibrosis, without any change in body weight [46].

Similar to the results in animal experiments, HIIT showed more weight loss than MIT for overweight or obese individuals [47]. In addition, exercise of different intensities seems to be equally effective in reducing hepatic triglyceride levels and improving insulin sensitivity [48, 49]. Interestingly, exercise-induced improvements in cardiovascular health are related to intensity [50]. A high-intensity or a combination of high-intensity and low-intensity exercise programs can significantly reduce cardiac metabolic markers in obese adolescents [51]. Moreover, it is worth noting that studies suggest HIIT has not reported any adverse events in the management of MASLD, and HIIT is feasible globally [52]. These results fully demonstrate the potential of exercise intensity in MASLD intervention.

3.3 Combining exercise and diet

Combining diet with exercise has significant advantages in health management and disease prevention. Compared to monotherapy, its synergistic effects can bring more comprehensive and lasting health benefits [53]. For example, studies evaluated the effects of a low glycemic index Mediterranean diet (LGIMD), aerobic exercise, or a combination of both on MASLD. The results showed that all treatments were effective in reducing MASLD scores, but LGIMD combined with aerobic exercise was the most effective [54], which may be partially attributed to the synergistic effect of these two lifestyle interventions on the gut microbiota composition of MASLD patients [55]. When conducting association tests on aerobic exercise programs, MD, and combinations of these programs for gut microbiota, it was found that nine genera had statistical significance. Specifically, *Ruminococcus*, *Lachnospiraceae*, *GCA-900066575*, *Clostridia vadin BB60 group*, *Enterorhabdus*, *Coprobacter*, *UCG002* (*Oscillospiraceae*), *Intestimonas*, and *Ruminococcaceae_g_UBA1819* were elevated in the combination therapy group [56]. *Ruminococcus* is believed to promote liver protection in MASLD by improving the integrity of the gastrointestinal barrier and regulating the gut microbiome. Another study evaluated the effects of probiotic supplementation combined with exercise on patients with MASLD. The combination of probiotics and exercise resulted in greater reductions in AST, γ-glutamyl transferase, low-density lipoprotein, total cholesterol, and homeostatic model assessment of insulin resistance compared to exercise alone [57]. These results emphasize the role of gut microbiota in exercise and dietary interventions for the treatment of MASLD.

In addition, a study showed that when ADF was combined with aerobic exercise treatment, body weight and hepatic triglyceride levels decreased compared to the single exercise group and the control group, but there was no significant difference compared to the ADF group [58]. However, CR or aerobic exercise can increase peak VO2 in obese elderly patients with heart failure, and this effect may be additive [59]. Therefore, more research is needed to evaluate the effects of different dietary interventions combined with exercise therapy on MASLD.

3.4 Precautions and personalized guidance

Individualized guidance and reasonable planning are essential in the process of creating exercise strategies. It is required to take into consideration the client's standard health and wellness status, degree of cardio and lung feature, along with the existence of other comorbidities such as cardio or joint diseases.

Wellness assessment and initial consultation. Prior to executing any type of new exercise plan, especially for people who have been inactive for a long time or have chronic health problems, a thorough health and wellness assessment is critical, including analyzing cardio features, metabolic standing, liver function, and the extent of liver disease. Speak with doctors, exercise physiologists, or signed up dietitians when creating exercise plans to get expert guidance and suggestions.

Principle of gradual progression. Dressmaker exercise intends according to the individual's wellness condition, fitness degree, and way of life to take full advantage of the advantages and sustainability of the exercise. For newbies or those resuming exercise, it is advisable to follow a concept of gradual development to avoid injury or tiredness from overtraining. Beginning with low-intensity, cardio exercises, progressively increase exercise period and strength every week. The exercise plan needs to be integrated into day-to-day live, thinking about work, family, and social life.

Monitoring and feedback. Regularly evaluate the effectiveness of activity to ensure goals are being met and adjust as needed. Monitor indicators, such as weight, waist circumference, blood pressure, blood sugar, and the impact of exercise on liver function. Make adjustments based on the body's response to the exercise plan and consult professionals immediately if discomfort is felt.

Social support and motivation maintenance. Studies have shown that joining exercise groups or receiving family support significantly improves adherence to an exercise plan. Gain support from family, friends, or peers to enhance engagement and a sense of commitment. Set small, incremental goals to achieve progressively to boost confidence and motivation.

4. Conclusion

A healthy lifestyle, characterized by a nutritious diet and regular physical activity, stands as the sole evidence-based intervention for treating MASLD. Despite the potential for future pharmacological treatments, current strategies rely heavily on metabolic or lifestyle intervention.

Incorporating polyunsaturated fatty acids from fish and flaxseeds, reducing the intake of refined carbohydrates like fructose and soft drinks, increasing the consumption of complex carbohydrates containing dietary fiber, and maintaining an adequate protein intake are key to achieving a healthier dietary structure. Additionally, reducing calorie intake is a straightforward method, but combining it with intermittent fasting can enhance patient adherence and minimize other bodily impacts.

While exercise is vital to a healthy lifestyle, many MASLD patients lead sedentary lives and find it challenging to stick to exercise routines. Establishing reasonable exercise durations and intensities based on individual age, physical fitness, and exercise habits, along with appropriate dietary adjustments, can greatly benefit overall metabolic improvement and slow disease progression.

Lastly, there is a call for more research into synergistic interventions for MASLD, such as regulating and improving gut microbiota homeostasis and gut barrier health. More comprehensive and reliable recommendations are necessary.

Acknowledgements

This study was supported by National Natural Science Foundation of China (82473350), Qinghai Province Key Research and Development and Transformation Plan Specific fund of Science and Technology Assistance to Qinghai (No. 2022-QY-216), and Jiangsu Province Graduate Research and Practice Innovation Plan Project (KYCX23_1938).

Conflict of interest

The authors declare no conflict of interest.

Author details

Xinyi Lu[1,2], Zhengyang Bao[2], Yu Chen[2*] and Daozhen Chen[1,2*]

1 The Affiliated Wuxi Maternity and Child Health Care Hospital of Nanjing Medical University, Jiangsu, China

2 Affiliated Women's Hospital of Jiangnan University, Jiangnan University, Jiangsu, China

*Address all correspondence to: cy-78@hotmail.com and chendaozhen@163.com

References

[1] Ryan MC, Itsiopoulos C, Thodis T, Ward G, Trost N, Hofferberth S, et al. The Mediterranean diet improves hepatic steatosis and insulin sensitivity in individuals with non-alcoholic fatty liver disease. Journal of Hepatology. 2013;**59**(1):138-143

[2] Chooi YC, Zhang QA, Magkos F, Ng M, Michael N, Wu X, et al. Effect of an Asian-adapted Mediterranean diet and pentadecanoic acid on fatty liver disease: The TANGO randomized controlled trial. The American Journal of Clinical Nutrition. 2024;**119**(3):788-799

[3] Biolato M, Manca F, Marrone G, Cefalo C, Racco S, Miggiano GA, et al. Intestinal permeability after Mediterranean diet and low-fat diet in non-alcoholic fatty liver disease. World Journal of Gastroenterology. 2019;**25**(4):509-520

[4] Akbulut UE, Isik IA, Atalay A, Eraslan A, Durmus E, Turkmen S, et al. The effect of a Mediterranean diet vs. a low-fat diet on non-alcoholic fatty liver disease in children: A randomized trial. International Journal of Food Sciences and Nutrition. 2021;**73**(3):357-366

[5] Yurtdaş G, Akbulut G, Baran M, Yılmaz C. The effects of Mediterranean diet on hepatic steatosis, oxidative stress, and inflammation in adolescents with non-alcoholic fatty liver disease: A randomized controlled trial. Pediatric Obesity. 2021;**17**(4):e12872

[6] Sangouni AA, Nadjarzadeh A, Rohani FS, Sharuni F, Zare Z, Rahimpour S, et al. Dietary approaches to stop hypertension (DASH) diet improves hepatic fibrosis, steatosis and liver enzymes in patients with non-alcoholic fatty liver disease: A randomized controlled trial. European Journal of Nutrition. 2023;**63**(1):95-105

[7] Razavi Zade M, Telkabadi MH, Bahmani F, Salehi B, Farshbaf S, Asemi Z. The effects of DASH diet on weight loss and metabolic status in adults with non-alcoholic fatty liver disease: A randomized clinical trial. Liver International. 2015;**36**(4):563-571

[8] Zheng J, Zhao L, Dong J, Chen H, Li D, Zhang X, et al. The role of dietary factors in nonalcoholic fatty liver disease to hepatocellular carcinoma progression: A systematic review. Clinical Nutrition. 2022;**41**(10):2295-2307

[9] Luukkonen PK, Sädevirta S, Zhou Y, Kayser B, Ali A, Ahonen L, et al. Saturated fat is more metabolically harmful for the human liver than unsaturated fat or simple sugars. Diabetes Care. 2018;**41**(8):1732-1739

[10] Atefi M, Entezari MH, Vahedi H, Hassanzadeh A, Laranjo M. Sesame oil ameliorates alanine aminotransferase, aspartate aminotransferase, and fatty liver grade in women with nonalcoholic fatty liver disease undergoing low-calorie diet: A randomized double-blind controlled trial. International Journal of Clinical Practice. 2022;**2022**:1-11

[11] Vahedi H, Atefi M, Entezari MH, Hassanzadeh A. The effect of sesame oil consumption compared to sunflower oil on lipid profile, blood pressure, and anthropometric indices in women with non-alcoholic fatty liver disease: A randomized double-blind controlled trial. Trials. 2022;**23**(1):551

[12] Pham TH, Lee GH, Jin SW, Lee SY, Han EH, Kim ND, et al. Sesamin ameliorates lipotoxicity and lipid

accumulation through the activation of the estrogen receptor alpha signaling pathway. Biochemical Pharmacology. 2023;**216**:115768

[13] Al-Nagdy S, Miller DS, Yudkin J. Changes in body composition and metabolism induced by sucrose in the rat. Nutrition and Metabolism. 1970;**12**(4):193-219

[14] Roncal-Jimenez CA, Lanaspa MA, Rivard CJ, Nakagawa T, Sanchez-Lozada LG, Jalal D, et al. Sucrose induces fatty liver and pancreatic inflammation in male breeder rats independent of excess energy intake. Metabolism. 2011;**60**(9):1259-1270

[15] Lanaspa MA, Ishimoto T, Li N, Cicerchi C, Orlicky DJ, Ruzycki P, et al. Endogenous fructose production and metabolism in the liver contributes to the development of metabolic syndrome. Nature Communications. 2013;**4**(1):2434

[16] Maersk M, Belza A, Stødkilde-Jørgensen H, Ringgaard S, Chabanova E, Thomsen H, et al. Sucrose-sweetened beverages increase fat storage in the liver, muscle, and visceral fat depot: A 6-mo randomized intervention study. The American Journal of Clinical Nutrition. 2012;**95**(2):283-289

[17] Schwarz J-M, Noworolski SM, Erkin-Cakmak A, Korn NJ, Wen MJ, Tai VW, et al. Effects of dietary fructose restriction on liver fat, De novo lipogenesis, and insulin kinetics in children with obesity. Gastroenterology. 2017;**153**(3):743-752

[18] Lustig RH, Mulligan K, Noworolski SM, Tai VW, Wen MJ, Erkin-Cakmak A, et al. Isocaloric fructose restriction and metabolic improvement in children with obesity and metabolic syndrome. Obesity. 2015;**24**(2):453-460

[19] Wu IT, Yeh W-J, Huang W-C, Yang H-Y. Very low-carbohydrate diet with higher protein ratio improves lipid metabolism and inflammation in rats with diet-induced nonalcoholic fatty liver disease. The Journal of Nutritional Biochemistry. 2024;**126**:109583

[20] de Cabo R, Longo DL, Mattson MP. Effects of intermittent fasting on health, aging, and disease. New England Journal of Medicine. 2019;**381**(26):2541-2551

[21] Bilibio BLE, dos Reis WR, Compagnon L, de Batista DG, Sulzbacher LM, Pinheiro JF, et al. Effects of alternate-day fasting and time-restricted feeding in obese middle-aged female rats. Nutrition. 2023;**116**:112198

[22] Higashida K, Fujimoto E, Higuchi M, Terada S. Effects of alternate-day fasting on high-fat diet-induced insulin resistance in rat skeletal muscle. Life Sciences. 2013;**93**(5-6):208-213

[23] Habiby M, Ezati P, Soltanian D, Rahehagh R, Hosseini F. Comparison of three methods of intermittent fasting in high-fat-diet-induced obese mice. Heliyon. 2024;**10**(4):e25708

[24] Zhang Q, Zhang C, Wang H, Ma Z, Liu D, Guan X, et al. Intermittent fasting versus continuous calorie restriction: Which is better for weight loss? Nutrients. 2022;**14**(9):1781

[25] Teker HT, Ceylani T. Intermittent fasting supports the balance of the gut microbiota composition. International Microbiology. 2022;**26**(1):51-57

[26] Rong B, Wu Q, Saeed M, Sun C. Gut microbiota—A positive contributor in the process of intermittent fasting-mediated obesity control. Animal Nutrition. 2021;7(4):1283-1295

[27] Li G, Xie C, Lu S, Nichols RG, Tian Y, Li L, et al. Intermittent fasting promotes

white adipose browning and decreases obesity by shaping the gut microbiota. Cell Metabolism. 2017;**26**(4):672-85.e4

[28] Chiang JYL, Ferrell JM. Bile acid receptors FXR and TGR5 signaling in fatty liver diseases and therapy. American Journal of Physiology. Gastrointestinal and Liver Physiology. 2020;**318**(3):G554-GG73

[29] Rau M, Rehman A, Dittrich M, Groen AK, Hermanns HM, Seyfried F, et al. Fecal SCFAs and SCFA-producing bacteria in gut microbiome of human NAFLD as a putative link to systemic T-cell activation and advanced disease. United European Gastroenterology Journal. 2018;**6**(10):1496-1507

[30] Acosta-Rodríguez V, Rijo-Ferreira F, Izumo M, Xu P, Wight-Carter M, Green CB, et al. Circadian alignment of early onset caloric restriction promotes longevity in male C57BL/6J mice. Science. 2022;**376**(6598):1192-1202

[31] Haigh L, Kirk C, El Gendy K, Gallacher J, Errington L, Mathers JC, et al. The effectiveness and acceptability of Mediterranean diet and calorie restriction in non-alcoholic fatty liver disease (NAFLD): A systematic review and meta-analysis. Clinical Nutrition. 2022;**41**(9):1913-1931

[32] Müller MJ, Enderle J, Bosy-Westphal A. Changes in energy expenditure with weight gain and weight loss in humans. Current Obesity Reports. 2016;**5**(4):413-423

[33] Wang D, Townsend LK, DesOrmeaux GJ, Frangos SM, Batchuluun B, Dumont L, et al. GDF15 promotes weight loss by enhancing energy expenditure in muscle. Nature. 2023;**619**(7968):143-150

[34] Shang Y, Morioka T, Daino K, Nakayama T, Nishimura M, Kakinuma S. Ionizing radiation promotes, whereas calorie restriction suppresses, NASH and hepatocellular carcinoma in mice. International Journal of Cancer. 2023;**153**(8):1529-1542

[35] Chen S-Y, Beretta M, Olzomer EM, Alexopoulos SJ, Shah DP, Byrne FL, et al. Head-to-head comparison of BAM15, semaglutide, rosiglitazone, NEN, and calorie restriction on metabolic physiology in female db/db mice. Biochimica et Biophysica Acta (BBA)—Molecular Basis of Disease. 2024;**1870**(1):166908

[36] Kirk E, Reeds DN, Finck BN, Mayurranjan MS, Patterson BW, Klein S. Dietary fat and carbohydrates differentially alter insulin sensitivity during caloric restriction. Gastroenterology. 2009;**136**(5):1552-1560

[37] Lee HA, Moon H, Kim Y, Lee HA, Kim HY. Effect of 12-week intermittent calorie restriction compared to standard of care in patients with nonalcoholic fatty liver disease: A randomized controlled trial. Trials. 2023;**24**(1):490

[38] Cunha GM, Guzman G, Correa De Mello LL, Trein B, Spina L, Bussade I, et al. Efficacy of a 2-month very low-calorie ketogenic diet (VLCKD) compared to a standard low-calorie diet in reducing visceral and liver fat accumulation in patients with obesity. Frontiers in Endocrinology. 2020;**11**:607

[39] Tutunchi H, Ostadrahimi A, Saghafi-Asl M, Roshanravan N, Shakeri-Bavil A, Asghari-Jafarabadi M, et al. Expression of NF-κB, IL-6, and IL-10 genes, body composition, and hepatic fibrosis in obese patients with NAFLD—Combined effects of oleoylethanolamide supplementation and calorie restriction: A triple-blind randomized controlled clinical trial. Journal of Cellular Physiology. 2020;**236**(1):417-426

[40] Hashida R, Kawaguchi T, Bekki M, Omoto M, Matsuse H, Nago T, et al. Aerobic vs. resistance exercise in non-alcoholic fatty liver disease: A systematic review. Journal of Hepatology. 2017;**66**(1):142-152

[41] Villareal DT, Aguirre L, Gurney AB, Waters DL, Sinacore DR, Colombo E, et al. Aerobic or resistance exercise, or both, in dieting obese older adults. New England Journal of Medicine. 2017;**376**(20):1943-1955

[42] Dieli-Conwright CM, Courneya KS, Demark-Wahnefried W, Sami N, Lee K, Buchanan TA, et al. Effects of aerobic and resistance exercise on metabolic syndrome, sarcopenic obesity, and circulating biomarkers in overweight or obese survivors of breast cancer a randomized controlled trial. Journal of Clinical Oncology. 2018;**36**(9):875-883

[43] Lee D-c, Brellenthin AG, Lanningham-Foster LM, Kohut ML, Li Y. Aerobic, resistance, or combined exercise training and cardiovascular risk profile in overweight or obese adults: The CardioRACE trial. European Heart Journal. 2024;**45**(13):1127-1142

[44] Rezende REF, Duarte SMB, Stefano JT, Roschel H, Gualano B, de Sá Pinto AL, et al. Randomized clinical trial: Benefits of aerobic physical activity for 24 weeks in postmenopausal women with nonalcoholic fatty liver disease. Menopause. 2016;**23**(8):876-883

[45] Harris SJ, Smith N, Hummer B, Schreibman IR, Faust AJ, Geyer NR, et al. Exercise training improves serum biomarkers of liver fibroinflammation in patients with metabolic dysfunction-associated steatohepatitis. Liver International. 2023;**44**(2):532-540

[46] Fredrickson G, Barrow F, Dietsche K, Parthiban P, Khan S, Robert S, et al. Exercise of high intensity ameliorates hepatic inflammation and the progression of NASH. Molecular Metabolism. 2021;**53**:101270

[47] Berge J, Hjelmesæth J, Hertel JK, Gjevestad E, Småstuen MC, Johnson LK, et al. Effect of aerobic exercise intensity on energy expenditure and weight loss in severe obesity—A randomized controlled trial. Obesity. 2021;**29**(2):359-369

[48] Zhang H-J, He J, Pan L-L, Ma Z-M, Han C-K, Chen C-S, et al. Effects of moderate and vigorous exercise on nonalcoholic fatty liver disease. JAMA Internal Medicine. 2016;**176**(8):1074-1082

[49] Ryan BJ, Schleh MW, Ahn C, Ludzki AC, Gillen JB, Varshney P, et al. Moderate-intensity exercise and high-intensity interval training affect insulin sensitivity similarly in obese adults. The Journal of Clinical Endocrinology & Metabolism. 2020;**105**(8):e2941-e2e59

[50] Gorostegi-Anduaga I, Corres P, MartinezAguirre-Betolaza A, Pérez-Asenjo J, Aispuru GR, Fryer SM, et al. Effects of different aerobic exercise programmes with nutritional intervention in sedentary adults with overweight/obesity and hypertension: EXERDIET-HTA study. European Journal of Preventive Cardiology. 2018;**25**(4):343-353

[51] González-Ruíz K, Correa-Bautista JE, Izquierdo M, García-Hermoso A, Martínez-Vizcaíno V, Lobelo F, et al. Exercise dose on hepatic fat and cardiovascular health in adolescents with excess of adiposity. Pediatric Obesity. 2021;**17**(4):e12869

[52] Keating SE, Croci I, Wallen MP, Cox ER, Thuzar M, Pham U, et al. High-intensity interval training is safe, feasible and efficacious in nonalcoholic

steatohepatitis: A randomized controlled trial. Digestive Diseases and Sciences. 2022;**68**(5):2123-2139

[53] Mucinski JM, Salvador AF, Moore MP, Fordham TM, Anderson JM, Shryack G, et al. Histological improvements following energy restriction and exercise: The role of insulin resistance in resolution of MASH. Journal of Hepatology. 2024;**S0168-8278**(24):02323-7

[54] Franco I, Bianco A, Mirizzi A, Campanella A, Bonfiglio C, Sorino P, et al. Physical activity and low glycemic index Mediterranean diet: Main and modification effects on NAFLD score. Results from a randomized clinical trial. Nutrients. 2020;**13**(1):66

[55] Cheng R, Wang L, Le S, Yang Y, Zhao C, Zhang X, et al. A randomized controlled trial for response of microbiome network to exercise and diet intervention in patients with nonalcoholic fatty liver disease. Nature. Communications. 2022;**13**(1):2555

[56] Calabrese F, Disciglio V, Franco I, Sorino P, Bonfiglio C, Bianco A, et al. A low glycemic index Mediterranean diet combined with aerobic physical activity rearranges the gut microbiota signature in NAFLD patients. Nutrients. 2022;**14**(9):1773

[57] Kazeminasab F, Miraghajani M, Mokhtari K, Karimi B, Rosenkranz SK, Santos HO. The effects of probiotic supplementation and exercise training on liver enzymes and cardiometabolic markers in patients with non-alcoholic fatty liver disease: A systematic review and meta-analysis of randomized clinical trials. Nutrition & Metabolism. 2024;**21**(1):59

[58] Ezpeleta M, Gabel K, Cienfuegos S, Kalam F, Lin S, Pavlou V, et al. Effect of alternate day fasting combined with aerobic exercise on non-alcoholic fatty liver disease: A randomized controlled trial. Cell Metabolism. 2023;**35**(1): 56-70.e3

[59] Kitzman DW, Brubaker P, Morgan T, Haykowsky M, Hundley G, Kraus WE, et al. Effect of caloric restriction or aerobic exercise training on peak oxygen consumption and quality of life in obese older patients with heart failure with preserved ejection fraction. Journal of the American Medical Association. 2016;**315**(1):36-46

Chapter 7

Pregnancy and Metabolic Dysfunction-Associated Steatotic Liver Disease (MASLD): Relationship with Obesity, Clinical Outcomes, and Diagnosis

María del Rosario Herrero Macedo, Alejandra Díaz García, Cristian Alexis Oviedo Garza and Scherezada Maria Isabel Mejia Loza

Abstract

During pregnancy, elevated levels of transaminases, bilirubin, and the international normalized ratio require a thorough evaluation, in which the gastroenterologist plays a key role in the diagnosis. Metabolic dysfunction-associated steatotic liver disease (MASLD) results from the excess accumulation of fat in hepatocytes. The prevalence of MASLD has been increasing in recent years and has a close association with overweight and obesity. In pregnancy, weight gain is expected due to changes in body composition and metabolism; however, prepregnancy obesity and excessive weight gain are associated with adverse outcomes, including a higher risk of developing cardiometabolic diseases and negative fetal-neonatal outcomes. The pathogenesis of MASLD is multifactorial; during pregnancy, hormonal and metabolic changes promote adipose tissue deposition, reduce insulin sensitivity, and lead to hyperlipidemia. Choosing a diagnostic method during pregnancy is challenging, but noninvasive approaches that combine biomarkers and imaging techniques are appropriate.

Keywords: MASLD, MASH, steatosis, obesity, pregnancy, fetal, neonatal, metabolic syndrome

1. Introduction

During pregnancy, there are important anatomical, physiological, and biochemical changes, with an impact on almost all organs and systems to support the normal development and growth of the fetus through complex hormonal and metabolic pathways. Weight gain is characteristic of this process; however, excessive weight gain or obesity throughout pregnancy has an impact on the natural history of metabolic dysfunction-associated steatotic liver disease (MASLD) [1–3].

The prevalence of MASLD in pregnancy has almost tripled in the last decade. MASLD is defined as the presence of excess triglyceride storage in the liver in the presence of at least one cardiometabolic risk factor. The metabolic risk factors in the definition of MASLD are overweight or obesity, dysglycemia or type 2 diabetes, dyslipidemia, and hypertension [3–5].

Type 2 diabetes and obesity are the metabolic diseases with the strongest impact on the natural history of MASLD and determinants of the risk of cirrhosis and hepatocellular carcinoma. The duration and severity of obesity are associated with an increased risk of progression [2, 3].

The obesity epidemic has affected reproductive-aged women, with obesity present in over 30% of U.S. women ages 20–39 years. Pregnancy is considered a relative state of obesity. In a retrospective study using the United States 2007–2016 National Inpatient Sample (NIS) database, obesity was present in nearly 40% of pregnancies with MASLD (vs 6–7% in other groups) [4].

It has recently been observed that MASLD may impact maternal and offspring outcomes, including gestational diabetes mellitus (GDM), gestational hypertension, cesarean delivery, preterm birth, preeclampsia, and abnormal fetal growth.

2. Epidemiology

MASLD is considered one of the most common causes of chronic liver disease and global health problem, which has shown an increase in prevalence in recent years. It has a close relationship with type 2 diabetes mellitus, obesity, and other metabolic risk factors [3].

It is estimated that the worldwide prevalence of MASLD in the general population currently is more than 30% and the prevalence in pregnant women has nearly tripled in the last decade. Data from the United States National Inpatient Sample from 2007 to 2015 reports that 10.5 to 28.9 per 100,000 pregnancies have MASLD and is independently associated with a higher incidence of hypertensive complications, postpartum hemorrhage, preeclampsia, HELLP syndrome, and preterm birth [2, 3, 6, 7].

Likewise, obesity has risen in adults in the United States, with a significant increase from 30.5% in 1999–2000 to 42.4% in 2017–2018, as reported by the National Health and Nutrition Examination Survey (NHANES). The global prevalence of MASLD parallels obesity rates, affecting up to 80–90% of adults with obesity, and the increasing prevalence of obesity among women of reproductive age represents a public health problem. US natality data also showed that prepregnancy obesity among women aged 20–39, varying from 22.6% to 37.6% by state, increased significantly between 2016 and 2019, with an average increase of 11% [2–8].

For pregnant women, the prevalence of MASLD was around 14–18% across the studies using ultrasonography and/or fatty liver index for the MASLD diagnosis. The increasing prevalence of MASLD is alarming as it is associated with an increase in cardiovascular risk and cardiovascular diseases (CVDs) [8, 9].

3. Physiology of pregnancy and metabolic changes

The pathogenesis of MASLD is multifactorial including genetic factors and lifestyle. However, other factors also described are the gut microbiota dysbiosis and altered intestinal permeability. These may overlap with pregnancy, while it should be noted that the dynamic hormonal and metabolic changes during pregnancy itself may contribute to hepatic changes across the pregnancy trimesters [2].

To better understand the underlying pathophysiology of MASLD in the context of pregnancy, it is important to highlight key physiologic adaptations of the maternal metabolism [2].

We describe the physiological changes that occur during pregnancy. Initially, pregnancy is an "anabolic phase" with the aim of creating a reservoir of energy, primarily in lipids, to meet the demands of the developing fetus and breastfeeding. During the first trimester, maternal glucose homeostasis is regulated by insulin, estrogen, and cortisol, prolonging blood glucose clearance, promoting adipose tissue deposition, and suppressing energy expenditure. Gradually, pregnancy transitions into a "catabolic phase," or "fetal anabolic phase," using stored energy to allow the fetal growth. This metabolic shift is characterized by reduced insulin sensitivity, allowing glucose and free fatty acids to cross the placenta [2, 7].

In the third trimester, maternal basal metabolic rate increases by 20% compared to nonpregnant women. Of note, Abeysekera et al. reported that women accumulate lean mass during pregnancy despite increased total energy expenditure and no significant changes in energy intake. This suggests more efficient energy storage [1].

A percentage of the weight gain during pregnancy is secondary to uterine and breast growth and the expansion of circulating volume. And a small fraction is secondary to the effect of metabolic alterations that favor the accumulation of intracellular water, fat, and protein, which are called maternal reserves. On average, a pregnant woman gains approximately 12.5 kg and an increase greater than this is seen to be related to numerous pregnancy complications as well as long-term morbidity and mortality. Also, obesity interacts with hereditary factors to create insulin resistance [1].

Further potential pathophysiologic mechanisms include the development of a persistent, low-grade inflammation that can follow excess adipose tissue accumulation centrally and in the liver. As such, increased circulating levels of pro-inflammatory adipokines, chemokines, and cytokines (e.g., tumor necrosis factor-α and interleukin-6) from the adipose tissue and the liver are associated with the development and the severity of insulin resistance, MASLD and GDM [2].

Leptin, the prototype adipokine, plays an important role in linking obesity and MASLD by regulating appetite and energy balance. Elevated leptin levels characterize obesity and contribute to hepatic steatosis and inflammation [2].

The pathophysiology of MASLD is closely related to adipose tissue dynamics, with the expansion of white adipose tissue depots in obesity leading to adipocyte dysfunction and insulin resistance, which further trigger lipolysis [2, 10].

First the adipocyte dysfunction is characterized by redistribution of nonesterified fatty acids and subsequent imbalance of the release of anti- and pro-inflammatory cytokines. This favors hepatic lipid storage and leads to hepatic insulin resistance with reduced postprandial glycogen storage and increased glucose production, resulting in higher circulating fatty acid levels, which, together with the aforementioned dysregulated adipokines, favor pro-steatogenic effects and intrahepatic fat accumulation. Furthermore, a high intake of dietary fat and carbohydrates further amplifies *de novo* lipogenesis and fat accumulation in the liver [2, 3, 8].

Although the pathophysiological relationship that exists between maternal obesity, subsequent hyperglycemia, and MASLD is not fully understood, insulin resistance appears to be a cornerstone in both hepatic steatosis and central obesity, which subsequently impacts on glucose metabolism during pregnancy and even postpartum [2].

Insulin resistance is defined as impaired insulin action in its target tissues, resulting from genetic risk and acquired factors, mainly hypercaloric nutrition, gut dysbiosis, and specifically adipose tissue dysfunction. It is characterized by altered glucose metabolism and predisposition to type 2 diabetes, and it also causes several subclinical abnormalities that predispose to cardiovascular disease and accelerate its onset [1, 3].

The mechanisms causing this decrease in insulin sensitivity include numerous endocrine and inflammatory factors. Particularly pregnancy-related hormones such as progesterone, placenta-derived growth hormone, prolactin, and cortisol; cytokines such as tumor necrosis factor; and hormones derived from central fat, especially leptin and its interaction with prolactin, are all involved in insulin resistance during pregnancy [1].

Also, a 50–60% reduction in insulin sensitivity occurs with advancing gestation in women with normal glucose tolerance and those with GDM [2].

Moreover, pregnancy induces significant physiologic changes in the maternal lipid metabolism, including adipose tissue accumulation and hyperlipidemia. Plasma concentrations of lipids, lipoproteins, and apolipoproteins increase significantly during pregnancy. Elevated estrogen, progesterone, and insulin levels promote lipid deposition in early and midpregnancy, with increased fatty acid synthesis and lipoprotein lipase expression. Consequently, circulating levels of fatty acids, triglycerides, cholesterol, and phospholipids rise throughout pregnancy, peaking in the third trimester [1, 2].

This increased lipid synthesis and excessive food intake contribute to maternal fat accumulation during the first two trimesters. Maternal hyperlipidemia is one of the most consistent changes in lipid metabolism during advanced stages of pregnancy. Triacylglycerol and cholesterol concentrations increase during the third trimester compared with those in nonpregnant women [1].

4. Maternal and fetal outcomes

It has been widely described that MASLD is associated with an increased risk of CVDs, chronic kidney disease, hepatic and extrahepatic malignancies, and liver-related outcomes, including liver failure and hepatocellular carcinoma (HCC) [2].

Women who are overweight or obese have higher rates of adverse outcomes complicating pregnancy. Extreme obesity defined as prepregnancy BMI ≥ 50 kg/m^2 has heightened risks of gestational hypertension, GDM, cesarean section, prolonged hospital stays, and adverse neonatal outcomes such as macrosomia as well as higher rates of preterm and small or large for gestational age birth (**Figure 1**) [10].

The above findings suggest maternal insulin resistance that promotes placental growth, negatively affects placental efficiency, and may contribute to lower fetal birth weight [8].

These complications increase with the presence of MASLD, which further impairs metabolic regulation and liver function [1, 2].

Fetal outcomes are reflected in increased perinatal mortality and short-term morbidity and, in childhood, increased risk of features of the metabolic syndrome and doubling in the risk of obesity. Babies of overweight or obese mothers are less able to initiate and maintain breastfeeding. In an autopsy study of 81 stillbirths, GDM was associated with a four times higher risk of presenting fetal hepatic steatosis. Also patients with excessive gestational weight gain and GDM were more likely to have children with the rising-high-BMI trajectory [10–12].

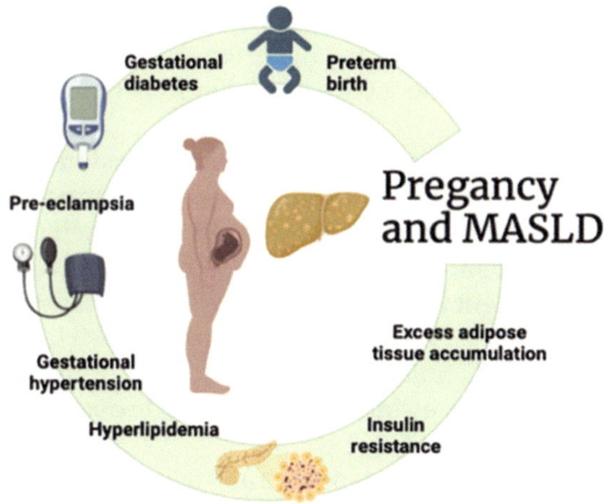

Figure 1.
Pathophysiology of MASLD during pregnancy and fetal outcome. MASLD metabolic dysfunction-associated steatotic liver disease.

In a retrospective study, pregnant patients with MASLD exhibited an increased risk of preterm birth compared to those without the condition (AOR 2.05, 95% CI 1.81–2.33). Moreover, the MASLD group presented higher occurrences of fetal growth restriction (AOR 1.32, 95% CI 1.06–1.64) and low birth weight (<2500 g), but not for being born small for gestational age (SGA) [9–13].

Maternal prepregnancy obesity, rapid weight gain during pregnancy, lack of physical activity, unhealthy diet consumption, GDM, and maternal MASLD have all been linked to pediatric steatotic liver disease (**Figure 2**) [10].

The aforementioned physiological changes during pregnancy, such as increases in circulatory volume and insulin resistance, as well as pro-inflammatory responses and dyslipidemia, can predispose to the development of cardiovascular complications beyond hypertensive disorders of pregnancy (HDP) [2].

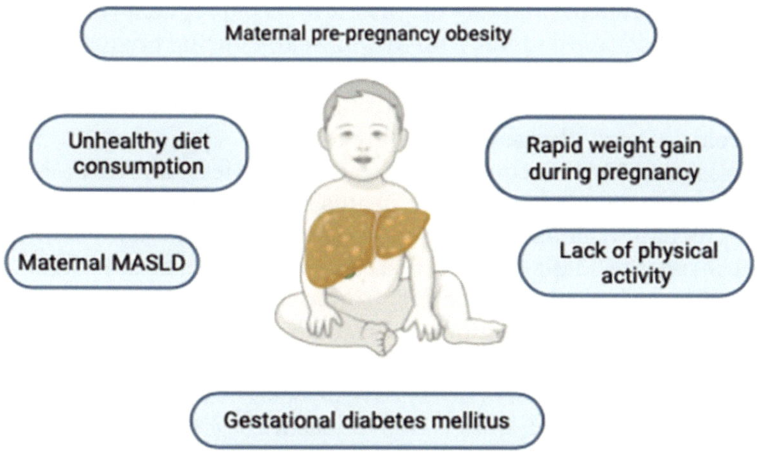

Figure 2.
Maternal and gestational risk factors for the development, severity, and natural history of pediatric MASLD.

One study found that during delivery hospitalization, the risk of heart failure was more than 3 times higher, gestational hypertensive complications were 3.3 times higher, and cardiac arrhythmia was 2.6 times higher in patients with MASLD compared to those without [9].

Particularly notable are the very high rates of hypertension and GDM. As discussed above, obesity and metabolic syndrome are characterized by insulin resistance, which results in low-grade inflammation, endothelial activation, and increased sodium reabsorption. These latter effects play a central role in preeclampsia. Increasing maternal weight is linked to a higher risk of late-onset preeclampsia with severe features. A cross-sectional study in Sri Lanka by Herath et al. showed that pregnant women with MASLD hold a twofold higher risk of developing gestational hypertension and preeclampsia, even after controlling for variables such as BMI, age, and hyperglycemia in pregnancy [1, 2, 14].

In a prospective study of 476 pregnancies, first-trimester ultrasound evidence of maternal MASLD was strongly associated with gestational diabetes, affecting at least 5% of pregnancies worldwide. Furthermore, there is a greater incidence of postpartum hemorrhage compared to those without (6% vs. 3–5%, respectively) [1, 2, 15].

Nevertheless, there is not enough information about the risk of new-onset MASLD in postpartum women who experience adverse pregnancy outcomes (APOs) during pregnancy. However, women with a history of APOs had a 58% higher risk of new-onset MASLD after delivery than those without. Patients at highest risk of developing new-onset MASLD after delivery are those who presented with HDP or GDM. By contrast, the risk of new-onset MASLD did not significantly increase in women with other APOs such as preterm birth, neonatal low birth weight, and placental abruption [11].

Exploring this topic may provide new insights into the pathogenic mechanisms by which APOs increase the susceptibility of women to subsequent metabolic diseases, including MASLD.

5. Diagnostic of MASLD during pregnancy

The aforementioned incidence of MASLD in pregnancy highlights the need for early detection with reliable and safe diagnostic tools in pregnant women. First, the need to identify at-risk individuals with MASLD early during pregnancy with the aim of impacting on the course of the disease, and then it is important to identify affected women for stratification and early therapeutic management, which includes nonpharmacological and pharmacological treatment [1, 2].

The diagnosis of MASLD requires the presence of at least one cardiometabolic risk factor in an individual with documented steatosis [3].

Through pregnancy, global liver function is modified by hemodynamic and biochemical changes to adapt to the increased metabolic demand. Primary systemic vasodilation may occur as early as the first trimester, inducing an increase in plasma volume and hyperdynamic circulatory status, with a 30–50% increase in cardiac output. All these changes affect liver function [1].

Abnormal liver function tests (LFTs) have low diagnostic value for MASLD since these are not MASLD-specific; in fact, individuals with MASLD and normal aminotransferase levels can still have steatohepatitis, fibrosis, or cirrhosis. The normal levels of LFTs depend on the pregnancy trimester. Aspartate transaminase (AST), alanine transaminase (ALT), γ-glutamyl transpeptidase (GGT), and bilirubin levels are slightly lower compared with values in nonpregnant women, while alkaline phosphatase has higher values due to its physiological increase produced by the placenta. Conversely, serum albumin concentrations decrease during pregnancy. By the end of pregnancy, albumin concentrations may approach 3 g/100 mL compared with 4.3 g/100 mL in nonpregnant women [1–3, 7, 16].

Therefore, elevated levels of AST, ALT, total bilirubin, and international normalized ratio INR (results from a calculation in which an individual patient PT test value is divided by the laboratory's pooled normal plasma standard PT) in pregnancy require evaluation for de novo or previously unrecognized liver disease [17].

Pregnancy is associated with physiologic changes that may simulate liver disease. For example, the hyperestrogenic state may result in spider angioma and palmar erythema, which has typically been associated with cirrhosis, and hemodynamic changes associated with pregnancy (increased plasma volume and cardiac output, decreased systemic and splanchnic vascular resistance, and activation of the renin-angiotensin-aldosterone system) can present or exacerbate manifestations of portal hypertension [17].

Other changes that we have to keep in mind for the diagnosis is that hepatic arterial and portal venous blood flows are substantially increased and liver stiffness increases from the second to the third trimester and returns to baseline levels during the postpartum period. On color Doppler ultrasonography (CDUS), portal blood flow increases, while hepatic arterial resistance decreases in the third trimester [1, 7].

Currently, liver biopsy is the gold standard for diagnosing liver diseases including MASLD; however, its invasive procedure associated with some risks makes it neither feasible nor ethical in pregnant women [18, 19].

Based on the above, noninvasive diagnostic methods have been developed and these can be used during pregnancy. Despite advances in biomarker development, these noninvasive methods have limitations in sensitivity and specificity, particularly for detecting early and moderate fibrosis. Therefore, imaging methods are often employed to complement biomarker data. However, there is no consensus on the optimal timing for assessing MASLD during pregnancy. This lack of standardized guidelines highlights the need for further research to determine the most appropriate periods for screening and diagnosis [19, 20].

The European Association for the Study of the Liver have recommended clinical care pathway with an emphasis on the use of noninvasive tests (NITs). It has been shown that a combination of values from blood test and anthropometric data enables a better prediction of fibrosis. The following scores have been described for their predictive power for fibrosis: FIB-4, APRI, and NFS (NAFLD fibrosis score). FIB-4 is the most widely established and available tool and should be acceptable to most individuals even in pregnant women [2, 3].

Liver imaging is important for the diagnosis and follow-up of liver conditions and during pregnancy helps to guide the differential diagnoses and identifies parenchymal or vascular complications [7].

Ultrasound is the study of first choice in pregnancy, followed by transient liver elastography and noninvasive scores, depending on availability. Fibrosis leads to modify mechanical properties of the liver, which can be assessed by special ultrasound devices wich elastography, such as Acoustic Radiation Force Impulse (ARFI), Shear Wave and vibration-controlled transient elastography (VCTE), liver stiffness measurement (LSM) and controlled attenuation parameter (CAP) values are determined which allow for a estimation of the degree of fibrosis and steatosis, respectively, are utilized for risk stratification and diagnosis [2, 3].

While computed tomography or magnetic resonance imaging is largely used in research to quantify hepatic fat, a practical advantage of using ultrasound in early pregnancy is that it can be performed safely at the time of routine first-trimester ultrasound measurement. In addition, sonographic evidence of hepatic fat in early pregnancy, especially the presence of hepatorenal contrast, was found to predict dysglycemia and GDM in midpregnancy. However, the limitation of liver ultrasound is interobserver variance may affect the results [21, 22].

Overall, selecting an accurate and safe diagnostic approach for early MASLD diagnosis in pregnant women is challenging.

6. Treatment

The management in pregnancy involves early diagnosis in addition to nutritional measures and physical activity mainly focused on liver-related outcomes with impact on metabolic syndrome. Liver-related outcomes usually refer to cirrhosis decompensation, decline in liver function, occurrence of HCC, and liver transplantation [3, 7, 23].

It has been demonstrated in clinical trials that weight reduction achieved by caloric restriction, either with or without increased physical activity, leads to improvements in MASLD biomarkers, including liver enzymes, steatosis, MASH, and fibrosis (**Figure 3**) [3].

In patients with MASLD, dietary and behavioral therapy-induced weight loss should be recommended to improve liver injury, aiming at a sustained reduction of >5% to reduce liver fat, 7–10% to improve liver inflammation, and >10% to improve fibrosis. Improving diet quality similar to the Mediterranean dietary pattern, limiting the consumption of ultraprocessed foods rich in sugars and saturated fat, and avoiding sugar-sweetened beverages should be recommended [3].

In a prospective cohort conducted in the United States, it was found that those with higher intake of red meat, including both processed and unprocessed red meat, contributed to a significant, dose-dependent increased risk of developing incident MASLD, and this association was largely mediated by obesity. Therefore, patients should moderate their consumption and continue with a varied diet [24].

Gestational weight gain recommendations aim to optimize outcomes for the woman and the infant. The Institute of Medicine (IOM) guidelines recommend a total weight gain of 6.8–11.3 kg (15–25 lb) for overweight women (BMI of 25–29.9; BMI is calculated as weight in kilograms divided by height in meters squared). IOM recommendation seems to be adequate for underweight and normal-weight pregnant women but not for obese ones, so there is an urgent need to obtain a consensus on the correct and reasonable gestational weight gain during pregnancy [6, 25].

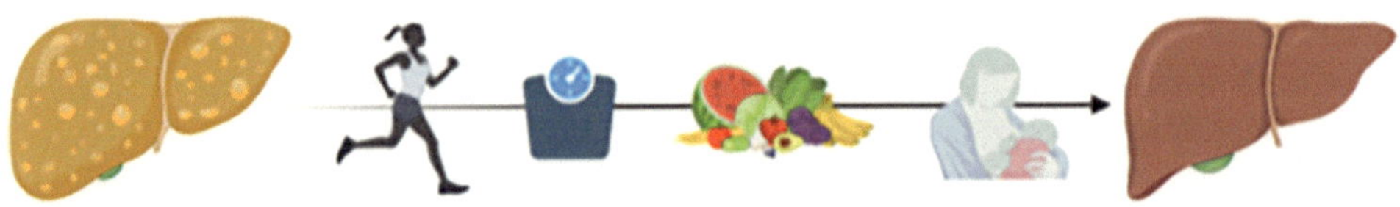

Figure 3.
Treatment of MASLD includes physical activity and exercise, weight loss, and nutritional measures. Breastfeeding may offer protection against postpartum obesity and MASLD. MASLD metabolic dysfunction-associated steatotic liver disease.

Breastfeeding may offer protection against postpartum obesity and MASLD. It is encouraged in patients because lactation decreases maternal lipid, glucose, and insulin levels while improving insulin sensitivity. Duration of lactation for a longer time has been associated with a lower rate of future MASLD among offspring and a lower incidence of maternal metabolic complications including increased postpartum weight loss and a reduction in heart disease and diabetes [6, 26].

Lower prevalence of MASLD was seen among children who were exclusively breastfed for 6 months, compared to those who received mixed feeding and those who never breastfed, but the confidence interval included the null (19.3% vs. 20.0% vs. 24.0% respectively; OR 0.78 [0.56–1.09]; $p = 0.14$) [27].

Beyond reducing steatosis, physical activity and exercise enhance insulin sensitivity, independently of weight loss, and modulate regulatory T cells, reducing the risk of gestational weight gain, GDM, gestational hypertensive disorders, cesarean birth, preterm birth, lower birth weight, and postpartum recovery time [8].

Benefits and minimal maternal-fetal risk have been documented with physical activity and exercise during pregnancy. It must be tailored to the individual's preference and ability, preferably >150 minutes/week of moderate or 75 minutes/week of vigorous-intensity physical activity [3, 28].

Additionally, some meta-analyses have used low-dose aspirin previously described for its effect on reducing preeclampsia incidence and cardiovascular benefits; therefore, it may also attenuate MASLD progression by moderating inflammatory processes by inhibiting TNF-α production and enhancing antioxidant mechanisms. Considering the heightened cardiovascular risk observed in pregnant patients with MASLD, the use of aspirin into therapeutic protocols merits consideration [9].

While evidence from nonpregnant populations indicates improvements in liver function and histological markers, the safety and efficacy of vitamin E in pregnant women with MASLD remain understudied. Further research is essential to ascertain its impact on maternal and fetal outcomes [9].

Because there is no currently approved pharmacotherapy for MASLD management in pregnancy, the treatment is still based on lifestyle interventions [23, 29].

7. Conclusion

MASLD during pregnancy is a major health problem due to its increasing incidence and complex pathophysiology, which may further exacerbate insulin resistance, dyslipidemia, and chronic low-grade inflammation.

MASLD is a condition that affects a large number of pregnant women, especially those with obesity and gestational diabetes. MASLD can have serious consequences for maternal and fetal health, including an increased risk of cardiovascular disease, diabetes, and liver disease. Early and accurate diagnosis using noninvasive testing and treatment measures that include lifestyle changes such as a healthy diet and regular exercise, as well as consideration of breastfeeding, are essential. Further research is needed to determine the most effective and safe treatment for pregnant women with MASLD.

Screening for MASLD in pregnant women is currently insufficient so early identification may potentially improve morbidity outcomes. Hence, we highlight the importance of considering metabolic health in pregnant women, particularly during prenatal care visits or preconception counseling.

Author details

María del Rosario Herrero Macedo*, Alejandra Díaz García, Cristian Alexis Oviedo Garza and Scherezada Maria Isabel Mejia Loza
Hospital Juárez de México, Mexico

*Address all correspondence to: charoherrero@gmail.com

References

[1] Cunningham FG, Leveno KJ, Dashe JS, Hoffman BL, Spong CY, Casey BM. Williams Obstetrics 26th ed. New York: McGraw-Hill Education/Medical; 2022

[2] Leca BM, Lagojda L, Kite C, Karteris E, Kassi E, Randeva HS, et al. Maternal obesity and metabolic (dysfunction) associated fatty liver disease in pregnancy: A comprehensive narrative review. Expert Review of Endocrinology and Metabolism. 2024;**19**(4):335-348. DOI: 10.1080/17446651.2024.236579

[3] European Association for the Study of the Liver (EASL), European Association for the Study of Diabetes (EASD), European Association for the Study of Obesity (EASO), Tacke F, Horn P, Wai-Sun Wong V, et al. EASL-EASD-EASO clinical practice guidelines on the management of metabolic dysfunction-associated steatotic liver disease (MASLD). Obesity Facts. 2024;**17**(4):374-444. DOI: 10.1159/000539371

[4] Sarkar M, Grab J, Dodge JL, Gunderson EP, Rubin J, Irani RA, et al. Non-alcoholic fatty liver disease in pregnancy is associated with adverse maternal and perinatal outcomes. Journal of Hepatology. 2020;**73**(3):516-522. DOI: 10.1016/j.jhep.2020.03.049

[5] Rinella ME, Lazarus JV, Ratziu V, Francque SM, Sanyal AJ, Kanwal F, et al. Multisociety Delphi consensus statement on new fatty liver disease nomenclature. Journal of Hepatology. 2023;**79**(6):1542-1556. DOI: 10.1016/j.jhep.2023.06.003

[6] Dalfra' MG, Burlina S, Lapolla A. Weight gain during pregnancy: A narrative review on the recent evidences. Diabetes Research and Clinical Practice. 2022;**188**:109913. DOI: 10.1016/j.diabres.2022.109913

[7] Porrello G, Cannella R, Bernuau J, Agman A, Brancatelli G, Dioguardi Burgio M, et al. Liver imaging and pregnancy: What to expect when your patient is expecting. Insights Into Imaging. 2024;**15**(1):66. DOI: 10.1186/s13244-024-01622-x

[8] Karachaliou GS, Suzuki A. Metabolic dysfunction-associated steatotic liver disease: Emerging risk factors for adverse pregnancy outcomes. Clinical Liver Disease (Hoboken). 2024;**23**(1):e0121. DOI: 10.1097/CLD.0000000000000121

[9] Niu C, Zhang J, Khalid N, Zhu K, Syed T, Liu H, et al. Cardiovascular complications during delivery hospitalizations in patients with nonalcoholic fatty liver disease in pregnancy. European Journal of Gastroenterology & Hepatology. 2024;**36**(9):1141-1148. DOI: 10.1097/MEG.0000000000002802

[10] Mouzaki M, Woo JG, Divanovic S. Gestational and developmental contributors of pediatric MASLD. Seminars in Liver Disease. 2024;**44**(1):43-53. DOI: 10.1055/s-0044-1782210

[11] Jung YM, Lee SM, Wi W, Oh M-J, Park JS, Cho GJ, et al. Adverse pregnancy outcomes as a risk factor for new-onset metabolic dysfunction-associated steatotic liver disease in postpartum women: A nationwide study. JHEP Reports. 2024;**6**(4):101033. DOI: 10.1016/j.jhepr.2024.101033

[12] Hu Z, Tylavsky FA, Han JC, Kocak M, Fowke JH, Davis RL, et al. Maternal metabolic factors during

pregnancy predict early childhood growth trajectories and obesity risk: The CANDLE Study. International Journal of Obesity. 2019;**43**(10):1914-1922

[13] Hagström H, Höijer J, Ludvigsson JF, Bottai M, Ekbom A, Hultcrantz R, et al. Adverse outcomes of pregnancy in women with non-alcoholic fatty liver disease. Liver International. 2016;**36**(2):268-274. DOI: 10.1111/liv.12902

[14] Modi N, Murgasova D, Ruager-Martin R, Thomas EL, Hyde MJ, Gale C, et al. The influence of maternal body mass index on infant adiposity and hepatic lipid content. Pediatric Research. 2011;**70**(3):287-291. DOI: 10.1203/PDR.0b013e318225f9b1

[15] Milionis C, Ilias I, Koukkou E. Gestational diabetes mellitus may predispose to metabolic dysfunction-associated steatotic liver disease. World Journal of Hepatology. 2024;**16**(5):860-862. DOI: 10.4254/wjh.v16.i5.860

[16] Herath RP, Siriwardana SR, Ekanayake CD, Abeysekara V, Kodithuwakku SUA, Herath HP. Non-alcoholic fatty liver disease and pregnancy complications among Sri Lankan women: A cross sectional analytical study. PLoS ONE. 2019;**14**(4):e0215326. DOI: 10.1371/journal.pone.0215326

[17] Lao TT. Implications of abnormal liver function in pregnancy and non-alcoholic fatty liver disease. Best Practice & Research. Clinical Obstetrics & Gynaecology. 2020;**68**:2-11. DOI: 10.1016/j.bpobgyn.2020.02.011

[18] Terrault NA, Williamson C. Pregnancy-associated liver diseases. Gastroenterology. 2022;**163**(1):97-117.e1. DOI: 10.1053/j.gastro.2022.01.060

[19] Lee SM, Jung YM, Choi ES, Kwak SH, Koo JN, Oh IH, et al. Metabolic dysfunction-associated fatty liver disease and subsequent development of adverse pregnancy outcomes. Clinical Gastroenterology and Hepatology. 2022;**20**(11):2542-2550.e8

[20] Yin X, Guo X, Liu Z, Wang J. Advances in the diagnosis and treatment of non-alcoholic fatty liver disease. International Journal of Molecular Sciences. 2023;**24**(3):2844. DOI: 10.3390/ijms24032844

[21] De Souza LR, Berger H, Retnakaran R, Vlachou PA, Maguire JL, Nathens AB, et al. Non-alcoholic fatty liver disease in early pregnancy predicts dysglycemia in mid-pregnancy: Prospective study. The American Journal of Gastroenterology. 2016;**111**(5):665-670. DOI: 10.1038/ajg.2016.43

[22] Jung YM, Lee SM, Hong S, Koo JN, Oh IH, Kim BJ, et al. The risk of pregnancy-associated hypertension in women with nonalcoholic fatty liver disease. Liver International. 2020;**40**(10):2417-2426. DOI: 10.1111/LIV.14563

[23] Mandato C, Panera N, Alisi A. Pregnancy and metabolic-associated fatty liver disease. Endocrinology and Metabolism Clinics of North America. 2023;**52**(3):521-531. DOI: 10.1016/j.ecl.2023.02.005

[24] Kim MN, Lo C-H, Corey KE, Luo X, Long L, Zhang X, et al. Red meat consumption, obesity, and the risk of nonalcoholic fatty liver disease among women: Evidence from mediation analysis. Clinical Nutrition. 2022;**41**(2):356-364. DOI: 10.1016/j.clnu.2021.12.01

[25] American College of Obstetricians and Gynecologists. Committee

Opinion No. 548: Weight gain during pregnancy. Obstetrics & Gynecology. Jan 2013;**121**(1):210-212

[26] Karim G, Giri D, Kushner T, Reau N, et al. Evaluation of liver disease in pregnancy. Clinics in Liver Disease. 2023;**27**(1):133-155. DOI: 10.1016/j.cld.2022.08.009

[27] Abeysekera KWM, Orr JG, Madley-Dowd P, Fernandes GS, Zuccolo L, Gordon FH, et al. Association of maternal pre-pregnancy BMI and breastfeeding with NAFLD in young adults: A parental negative control study. The Lancet Regional Health - Europe. 2021;**10**:100206. DOI: 10.1016/j.lanepe.2021.100206

[28] American College of Obstetricians and Gynecologists. Physical activity and exercise during pregnancy and the postpartum period. Committee Opinion No. 804. Obstetrics & Gynecology. 2020;**135**(4):e178-e183

[29] Kwo PY, Cohen SM, Lim JK. ACG clinical guideline: Evaluation of abnormal liver chemistries. The American Journal of Gastroenterology. 2017;**112**(1):18-35. DOI: 10.1038/ajg.2016.517

Chapter 8

Gene-Environment Interactions in Non-alcoholic Fatty Liver Disease: Insights from Mexican American Populations

Eron G. Manusov, Vincent P. Diego, Marcio Almeida, Jacob A. Galan, Auwal A. Bala, Marco A. Arriaga, Natasha S. Garcia-Rodriguez, Renee Hernandez, Satish Kumar, John Blangero and Sarah Williams-Blangero

Abstract

Nonalcoholic Fatty Liver Disease (NAFLD) is a prevalent and complex condition influenced by both genetic and environmental factors. This chapter explores the genotype-by-environment interactions that contribute to the development and progression of NAFLD in the Mexican American population. Using advanced genetic epidemiology and bioinformatics approaches, we investigated how specific genetic variants interact with environmental factors such as depression, acculturation stress, and social determinants of health, to influence NAFLD risk and severity. Our findings reveal significant genotype-by-environment interactions for key NAFLD-related traits, including HbA1c, AST/ALT ratio, and steatosis-controlled attenuation parameter (CAP). We also discuss the application of cutting-edge proteomic and transcriptomic techniques in identifying novel biomarkers and potential therapeutic targets for NAFLD. This comprehensive analysis provides insights into the molecular mechanisms of NAFLD in Mexican Americans and provides support for developing targeted prevention strategies and personalized healthcare.

Keywords: NAFLD, Mexican Americans, gene-environment interactions, genetic epidemiology, bioinformatics, proteomics, liver fibrosis, extracellular vesicles

1. Introduction

Although there have been considerable advances in the diagnosis and management of Non-Alcoholic Fatty Liver Disease (NAFLD) and Non-Alcoholic Steatohepatitis (NASH), the exact etiology of this complex dysmetabolic process has yet to be delineated. Research and management are complex because the mechanisms underlying

NAFLD/NASH are unknown. Current thought includes a "multiple hit" hypothesis that includes diet, obesity, inflammation, mitochondrial dysfunction, increased oxidative stress, intestinal dysbiosis, and lipotoxicity [1, 2].

The heritability of NAFLD is approximately 60% in the Hispanic population in south Texas, where there is an epidemic prevalence of overweight and obesity (60%) and diabetes (32%) [3]. The heritability of hepatic steatosis was estimated at 0.52 (95% confidence interval, 0.31–0.73; $p < 1.1 \times 10^{-11}$) and the heritability of hepatic fibrosis was 0.5 (95% confidence interval, 0.28–0.72; $p < 6.1 \times 10^{-11}$) [4]. Twin and family studies re-enforce that both fatty content and transaminase serum levels are heritable [4].

This chapter focuses on the complex interplay between genetic predisposition and environmental factors in the development and progression of NAFLD among Mexican Americans. We aim to elucidate the gene-environment interactions that contribute to NAFLD risk and severity in this population, with a focus on how genetic factors interact with depression, acculturation/marginalization stress, and social determinants of health [5, 6].

We will explore:

1. The genetic and molecular basis of NAFLD, with emphasis on variants prevalent in Mexican Americans

2. Advanced statistical genetic methods for investigating gene-environment interactions

3. The application of cutting-edge proteomic and transcriptomic techniques in NAFLD research

4. The role of extracellular vesicles in NAFLD pathogenesis and their potential as diagnostic and therapeutic tools

5. Specific gene-environment interactions identified in our studies and their implications for NAFLD management in Mexican American populations.

We aim to provide a comprehensive review of how genetic and environmental factors interact to influence NAFLD risk and progression in Mexican Americans. This knowledge will provide information to develop and support prevention strategies and personalized treatment approaches, ultimately improving health outcomes in this high-risk population.

2. Genetic and molecular basis of NAFLD in Mexican Americans

The identification of genetic variants through Genome-Wide Associations Studies (GWAS) and Whole Genome-Association Study (WGAS) techniques is subject to sample size, cohort diversity, and study design choices. The collection of larger sample sizes improves representation of the population under study. However, realistically, all scientific studies are limited by budget and population participation [7, 8]. Most genetic studies employ either random sampling or case-control study designs. The advantages of these approaches include scalability, meta-analysis compatibility, statistical power, generalizability, and efficiency. These features make random sampling and case-control designs valuable in genetic research, allowing for robust, expandable, and comparable studies across different populations and research groups. When analyzing large sample sizes, these approaches allow the detection of common genetic variants with modest effects on traits of interest. For example, a study by Fujita et al. explored the role of variations with modest effects–previously identified by a large-scale meta-analysis in European populations–in the genetic background of type 2 diabetes and diabetes-related traits in a Japanese population [9]. The most common genetic variants associated with NAFLD as detected by genome-wide association studies (GWAS) can explain only a minor proportion of the trait's heritability estimate, a phenomenon known as the "heritability paradox" or "missing heritability." This limitation has been observed in studies of complex traits, including NAFLD [10].

Rare genetic variants with a minor allele frequency below one percent are the most promising candidates for explaining the heritability paradox. Studying rare genetic variants is challenging and requires the use of extended human pedigrees and whole-genome sequencing approaches to identify all genetic variants present in a sample. Multigenerational extended pedigrees are the best design for identifying multiple copies of rare genetic variants. Each family can be interpreted as a biological experiment where the parents' genetic information has been combined and transmitted to their progeny. The same process is repeated for every generation, and when combined with whole genome sequencing, extended pedigrees provide an ideal framework for estimating a trait's heritability.

Early G × E studies tested the direct or indirect effects of an individual marker or marker set genotyped in the laboratory after environmental exposure. The DNA markers were selected based on specific genes. This method focuses on inferred genetic liability and includes inherited risk. Candidate genes are selected and then tested [11]. Advanced technology and statistical genetic tools leverage empirical kinship estimates constructed from extended human pedigrees combined with whole genome sequencing approaches using dense genotyping data from single-nucleotide polymorphism arrays or next-generation sequencing.

2.1 Statistical genetic methods for liver disease

Most complex phenotypic variation involves variation at many different means and multiple environmental effects. We utilize statistical models to make inferences about the presence, importance, genomic locations, identities, and biological effect sizes of the underlying sources of genetic variation. When there is sequence variation at many genes that influence a trait, the inheritance pattern is called polygenic. Given that GWA studies have clearly shown that many different genes are involved in complex disease risk, the polygenic model of disease now dominates genetic inference. In the canonical polygenic model, a phenotype, denoted by P, is fully determined by the sum of an additive genetic component, denoted by G, and an environmental component, denoted by E (P = G + E). Assuming that the genetic and environmental effects are uncorrelated, the polygenic inheritance leads to a simple relationship among the underlying components that determine phenotypic variation: $\sigma_p^2 = \sigma_g^2 + \sigma_e^2$, where both the phenotypic variance, denoted by σ_p^2, and the additive genetic variance, denoted by σ_g^2, can, in principle, be estimated, while the residual environmental variance, denoted by σ_e^2, is computed as the difference between σ_p^2 and σ_g^2, hence the term "residual". The standard way to make inferences about the polygenic variance is to utilize the observed correlations between phenotypic correlation among different classes of relatives (with the caveat that all humans are related to some extent). These expected correlations are a direct function of genetic relatedness (i.e., the amount of the variable genome that is shared by two people). From this model based on phenotypic similarities between pairs of individuals, we can efficiently estimate the heritability, denoted by h^2, which is defined as the ratio of the additive genetic variance to the phenotypic variance, $h^2 = \sigma_g^2 / \sigma_p^2$. Heritability gives a general measure of the relative importance of genetic factors in relation to the observed total phenotypic variation of a trait.

One of the obvious simplifying assumptions of this standard model is that the additive genetic and residual environmental variance components are homogeneous (or constant) across the environments that a person experiences. For example, consider environments that only have two possible states (e.g., sex [male/female], or affection status [e.g., diabetes: yes or no], or exposure [e.g., smoking: yes or no]) or, more generally, across the spectrum of a given continuous environment [e.g., alcohol consumed, or quantitative aflatoxin exposure levels]. The basic polygenic model assumes that the amount of genetic variance is unchanging regardless of the environment(s) experienced. But this assumption is often unlikely to be true and the violation of this assumption is evidence for the important contribution of genotype-by-environment interactions. This assumption can be relaxed by introducing environment-specific genetic variance components in the dichotomous environment case or genetic variance functions in the continuous environment case. Using these more complex models, we have discovered evidence for genotype-by-environment interaction influences on liver disease-related phenotypes that is discussed below.

2.2 Epigenetic factors in NAFLD development

Genes are short functional units whose expression is regulated by specialized proteins known as transcription factors. Transcription factors are highly conserved proteins that coevolve with DNA and can detect and bind to short DNA motifs in a gene's promoter region [12]. These short DNA motifs are called transcription factor binding sites and generally have less than 10 base pairs with a highly conserved core [13]. Transcription factors receive signaling of metabolic or environmental changes and bind to their respective Transcription Factor Binding Sites (TFBS) to allow the transcription machinery to assemble and, consequently, the expression of a target gene. Transcription factors act like functional hubs controlling the expression of multiple genes in a gene pathway, allowing for the delicate orchestration of genes' expression [14]. Scientific studies focused on gene expression alterations were successful in identifying candidate genes associated with phenotypes of interest for conditions such as cancer, hypertension, and type-2 diabetes [15–17]. A differently expressed gene denotes the existence of a molecular response that may have large metabolic implications.

For many years, genetic research focused on studying the expression of individual genes, which hindered our ability to comprehend the broad transcriptional changes associated with specific phenotypes of interest [18]. The possibility of studying the global gene expression using microarray, RNA-Seq, and, more recently, single-cell RNA-Seq experiments paved the way for cost-effective scientific experiments to shed light on many relevant biological conditions [19]. RNA-Seq uses cDNA sequencing platforms to estimate gene expression abundance. The short-length sequence reads are aligned to a reference genome and quantified considering known genes of a genome. Recently, Darci Maher et al. used omics techniques such as RNAseq to identify biomarkers associated with obesity and NAFLD in approximately 300 adults [20]. Xu L. et al. recently combined RNA-seq, high-throughput chromosomal capture, and Nanopore sequencing to study chromatin structure alterations associated with NAFLD [21].

3. Bioinformatics and proteomics approaches in NAFLD

Advances in translational, precision, and personalized medicine have transformed clinical diagnostics, large epidemiological-scale surveillance, and therapeutic care. Due to new technologies, cost reductions, and high throughput capabilities, standard sequencing approaches have become commonplace in laboratories. Nucleotide detection (i.e., RNA, DNA, cDNA) has significantly contributed to multiple areas, including disease detection, surveillance classification, and treatment [22–24]. These advancements in sequencing have greatly improved disease detection; however, the analysis of nucleic acids analysis is not sufficient to provide a thorough and comprehensive depiction of complex disease phenotypes and their resulting pathophysiology [22–24]. Comparing genes and proteins to known pathways helps identify hub genes, gene interactions, and alternate pathways involved in illness. This process and the results are fundamental to "personalized or precision medicine," and are used for further research, interventions, and understanding disease pathophysiology [22–24]. The following sections will review effective peptide detection, quantify phosphoprotein profiling, discuss extracellular vesicles, and explore the use of induced pluripotent stem cells (iPSCs) in liver research.

3.1 Proteomic/phosphoproteomic characterization of NAFLD

Blood plasma is crucial to maintaining and facilitating several biological processes. With advancements in bioinformatics and proteomics, it is becoming increasingly feasible to monitor disease states and therapeutic responses through plasma samples, driving significant progress in biomarker discovery. Following centrifugation with anticoagulants like EDTA or heparin, blood and its components—lipids, proteins, metabolites, and other small molecules—can be analyzed to characterize metabolic diseases, cancer, and neurodegenerative diseases [25]. Proteins, peptides, cleaved fragments, and their proteoforms (including spliced variants, isoforms, and post-translationally modified) enter the bloodstream via active secretion or cellular leakage, providing insights into the current state of human health. Utilizing plasma as a biofluid to study NAFLD offers a non-invasive alternative to liver imaging and is highly desirable due to its higher protein concentration, allowing for the detection of proteins, metal ions, metabolites, lipids, and proteins.

Protein phosphorylation represents one of the most ubiquitous post-translational modifications and regulates most biological processes in eukaryotes [26]. Adding a phosphate group to the side-chain hydroxyl group (O.H.) of serine, threonine, and tyrosine--- catalyzed by a regulatory kinase using ATP as a substrate is a fundamental enzymatic reaction for all life processes. Protein phosphorylation in signal transduction allows for the activation and deactivation of signaling cascades that allow for the basic functions of the cells, such as cell growth, proliferation, transcription, apoptosis, autophagy, and more. Moreover, in eukaryotes, there are over 100,000 phosphorylation events, and as a result of mutations, genetic variation, DNA methylation, gene expression, and molecular interaction can lead to altered cell signaling function resulting in but not limited to cancer, diabetes, Alzheimer's, and Parkinson's [25] Phosphorylation is a dynamic process, and elucidating signaling networks requires quantifying these phosphorylation events. Identifying a complete list of substrates using proteomics will be critical to understanding how altered signaling can modulate cellular kinases and their role in chronic disease.

3.2 Advances in systems biology/mass spectrometry-based approaches for biomarker discovery

Biological markers are measurable genetic, protein, and metabolite targets from biofluids or tissues that relate to physiological states, disease, injury, or environmental exposure. They provide epidemiologists and clinicians with the data they need to make informed decisions regarding a disease state's detection, epidemiology, diagnosis, and prognosis [27–30]. Mass spectrometry has been the most sensitive and widely used method. It is a leading development of "omics" technology, enabling global identification and quantification of large protein/peptide data sets [31–35]. The large-scale study of proteins, called proteomics, generates large datasets, and studying these data requires processing information efficiently and identifying regulated proteins. Fortunately, many bioinformatic tools are freely available and relatively user-friendly.

3.3 Novel tools for understanding NAFLD pathogenesis

NAFLD encompasses several conditions associated with hepatocyte lipid deposits. Despite recent progress in identifying over 300 genomic variants statistically associated with NAFLD risk [36], our understanding of the overall risk for NAFLD remains limited. Additionally, while GWAS has identified complex disease loci, connecting the functional effects of these variants to disease pathogenesis remains challenging [37, 38]. The risk of NAFLD is likely due to a complex interplay of genetic and environmental factors. As with most major complex diseases, NAFLD is the consequence of intermediate phenotypes that are tissue and cell-specific and are closer to genes that are causally related to or involved in NAFLD pathogenesis [39].

In our recent work aimed at discovering novel biological insights into NAFLD risk, we have focused on identifying measurable intermediate phenotypes/biomarkers that are genetically correlated with lipid deposits in hepatocytes. We have achieved this through large-scale epidemiological use of induced pluripotent stem cell (iPSC) technology to generate hard-to-obtain hepatic cells. iPSCs reprogrammed from easily accessible somatic cells, including blood-derived cells stored worldwide in various large-scale genetic studies, allow the generation of hepatic cells from any individual in the context of their own genetic identity for modeling NAFLD pathophysiology (**Figure 1**) [40–43].

We have focused on identifying measurable intermediate phenotypes/biomarkers that are genetically correlated with lipid deposits in hepatocytes by epidemiological-scale use of induced pluripotent stem cell (iPSC) technology for the generation of hard-to-obtain hepatic cells (**Figure 1a**). iPSCs reprogrammed from easily accessible somatic cells, including blood-derived cells stored worldwide in various large-scale genetic studies, allow the generation of hepatic cells from any individual in the context of their own genetic identity for modeling NAFLD pathophysiology [36, 37, 44, 45]. The iPSC-generated hepatocytes show morphology like primary hepatocytes expressing hepatocyte-specific markers and are functionally active,

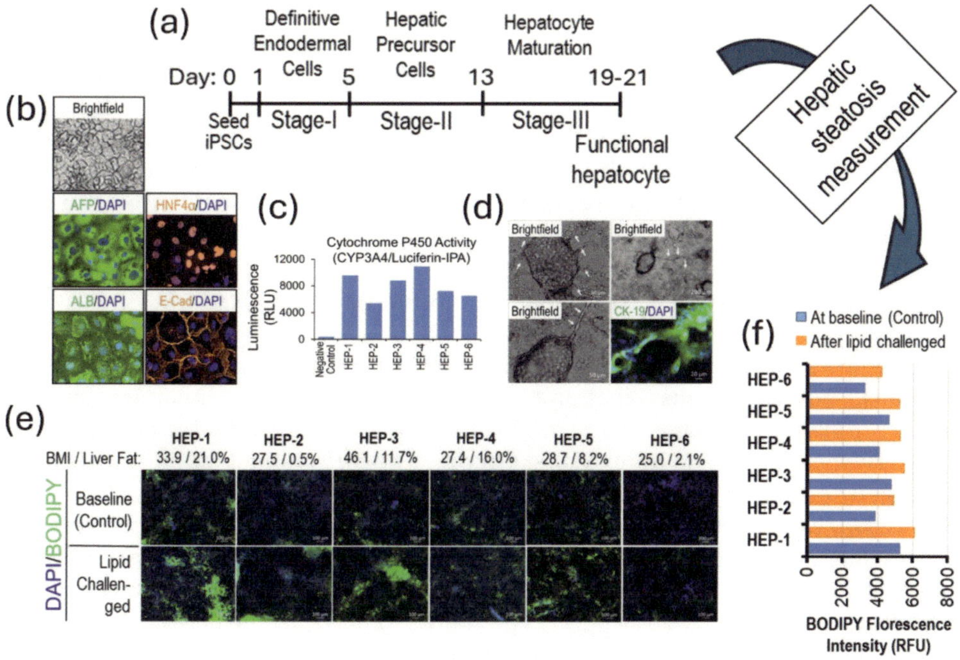

Figure 1.
In-vitro *modeling of NAFLD in iPSC-derived hepatocytes (HEPs). (a) A schematic outline of the HEP differentiation. (b) Brightfield and ICC analysis of HEPs morphology and hepatic markers (AFB, ALB, HNFα, and E-cad) expression. (c) Cytochrome P450 activity in six HEP cultures, measured by CYP3A4/Luciferin-IPA assay. (d) Bile canaliculi and CK-19 positive cholangiocytic cysts and duct-like structures (white arrows) in iPSC-derived HEP cultures. (e) Representative image panel showing BODIPY (lipid probe) fluorescence quantification at baseline and post-lipid challenge in six HEP lines. (f) Average BODIPY fluorescence intensity measured in three randomly chosen visual fields per HEP lines.*

including the cytochrome p450 activity, without any stimulation (**Figure 1b**, **d**). While most cells (~90–95%) in the iPSC-generated hepatic cultures are hepatocytes, other structures such as bile canaliculi and a few biliary/cholangiocytic cysts and duct-like structures also develop (**Figure 1d**). In the late-fetal and perinatal liver, some fetal hepatic progenitors near the portal veins commit to the cholangiocytic lineage and form mature bile ductal structures [38]. Development of these biliary structures in the iPSC-derived hepatic cultures suggests they recapitulate the developmental and functional characteristics of the liver.

In a pilot study, we examined the transcriptome-wide characteristics and NAFLD modeling potential of the iPSC-derived hepatocytes from six participants of our longitudinal Mexican American Family Study (MAFS) whose body mass index (BMI) and MRI-derived hepatic protein density fat fraction (MRI-PDFF) measures were known. A total of 6764 genes were significantly differentially expressed between iPSCs and generated hemocytes, and 3392 genes were significantly upregulated in hepatocytes. The functional annotation of the hepatocyte's upregulated genes showed significant enrichment in liver function-related pathways such as FXR/RXR activation (52.4% overlap, $p = 3.56\times10^{-21}$), LXR/RXR activation (48.8% overlap, $p = 3.77\times10^{-17}$) and hepatic fibrosis/hepatic stellate cell activation (37.6% overlap, $p = 6.32\times10^{-13}$). To validate the NAFLD modeling potential of the generated hepatocytes, we performed intracellular lipid quantification both at baseline and after a lipid challenge. The quantitative measures of cellular lipids, both at baseline and post-lipid challenge, showed a high correlation ($r^2 \geq 75\%$ and $r^2 \geq 85\%$, respectively) with individuals MRI measured liver fat, which strongly suggests that the iPSC-generated hepatocytes recapitulate their donor's bodily phenotype and are relevant cell model to investigate NAFLD etiology and pathogenesis (**Figure 1e**, **f**). These methodologies, coupled with genome-wide bulk and single-cell transcriptomics, are currently being employed in our laboratory in an epidemiological scale study to identify biomarkers of NAFLD risk.

3.4 Use of bioinformatics: Essential tools for understanding NAFLD

Proteomics is the comprehensive study of proteins—including their structures, functions, and interactions—that provides critical insights into cellular processes and disease mechanisms. In the context of NAFLD, proteomics enables the identification of disease-specific protein biomarkers, offering a deeper understanding of the protein expression and post-translational modifications associated with disease risk and progression. By identifying disease-specific protein biomarkers, proteomics resources can facilitate early diagnosis, monitor disease progression, and evaluate the efficacy of treatments. Proteomic databases and bioinformatic software help process and interpret proteomic data, offering a deeper understanding of the molecular mechanisms driving NAFLD, which aids in the development of targeted therapies [46–49]. Additionally, integrating proteomic data and clinical information can help personalize treatment plans, ultimately improving patient outcomes and reducing healthcare costs associated with chronic liver diseases.

Advanced techniques such as mass spectrometry and bioinformatics are employed to identify and quantify proteins as well as understand their modifications and interactions. Mass spectrometry, the primary technique in proteomics, identifies and quantifies proteins by measuring the mass-to-charge ratio of their ions. Two-dimensional gel electrophoresis (2-DE) is another pivotal technique that separates proteins based on their isoelectric point and molecular weight. The resolved proteins on the gel can be excised, in-gel digested with trypsin and analyzed by mass spectrometry. For example, four apolipoproteins and CD5 antigen-like protein (CD5L) have been identified by 2-DE in patients with NAFLD [39]. CD5L reflected the severity of hepatic fibrosis in NAFLD, with increased serum levels in cases of severe fibrosis. This suggests that CD5L may serve as a diagnostic marker for NASH [40].

Other techniques, such as liquid chromatography coupled with mass spectrometry (LC-MS), are commonly employed to enhance protein separation and identification. Bioinformatic tools are essential for processing and interpreting the large amounts of data generated, enabling the mapping of protein networks and pathways. Protein microarrays and X-ray crystallography also provide detailed information on protein interactions and structures. Together, these technologies offer comprehensive insights into the proteome, driving advances in drug discovery, diagnostics, and personalized medicine.

3.5 Proteomics databases in liver pathology research

Annotated databases provide compiled collections of biological data, including gene and protein sequences, functions, and interactions, along with relevant literature and experimental findings. These databases are essential research resources, enabling efficient access to high-quality, standardized information for bioinformatics analyses and experimental validation. Relevant annotated databases for proteomic analysis include general protein and disease-specific databases. Protein databases, such as UniProt [41], provide comprehensive information on protein sequences, functions, and interactions and serve as fundamental resources for identifying and characterizing proteins. The Swiss-Prot [42] database, a highly curated component of the UniProt database, focuses on providing detailed, accurate, and manually annotated protein sequence information. It includes extensive data on protein functions, structures, interactions, post-translational modifications, and relevant literature references. Swiss-Prot is known for its high-quality annotations and consistent terminology, making it an invaluable resource for researchers seeking to understand protein functions and relationships. It is regularly updated to incorporate new findings, ensuring the information remains current and reliable. Protein Data Bank (PDB) [43] offers detailed 3D structures of proteins, aiding in understanding their functions and interactions at the molecular level. Additionally, databases such as Pfam [50] and InterPro [46] provide information on protein families, domains, and functional sites, facilitating studying evolutionary relationships and functional annotations.

Disease-specific databases, such as Liver Cell Atlas [47], focus on proteins and biomarkers associated with obesity, while the Hepatocellular Carcinoma Database [48] offers targeted information to research disease mechanisms, diagnostics, and therapeutic development. These specialized resources enable researchers to correlate specific proteins with disease states, improving our understanding of pathophysiology and supporting the development of precision medicine approaches. The Gene Ontology (G.O.) [49] database provides a structured vocabulary for describing gene and protein functions across various organisms. G.O. classifies genes and proteins into categories related to biological processes, cellular components, and molecular functions, allowing researchers to consistently and systematically annotate to annotate and analyze gene products. The Kyoto Encyclopedia of Genes and Genomes (KEGG) [51] integrates information on genomes, biological pathways, diseases, and chemical substances. It provides detailed maps of metabolic and signaling pathways, helping researchers to understand complex biological systems and the roles of specific proteins within these pathways. The PIR-NREF database, part of the Protein Information Resource (PIR) [52], is a comprehensive, non-redundant protein sequence database. It integrates sequences from various sources, including GenBank, RefSeq, and UniProt, to provide a single resource for protein sequence information. In a study including 41 patients with hepatocellular carcinoma (HCC) and 51 patients with hepatitis C cirrhosis, the PIR-NREF database was crucial for proteomic profiling and tumor identification. It enabled the accurate identification and annotation of protein biomarkers detected by surface-enhanced laser desorption/ionization-time of flight mass spectrometry (SELDI-TOFMS), thus enhancing the sensitivity and specificity of hepatocellular cancer detection compared to traditional biomarkers like AFP, AFP-L3, and PIVKA-II [53]. Integrating annotated databases in proteomic research facilitates data mining and analysis by providing a centralized repository of high-quality, curated information on proteins and their functions. This enables researchers to efficiently identify patterns, predict protein interactions, and generate hypotheses for experimental validation. By using standardized and widely accepted datasets, the integration of these databases enhances research reproducibility and transparency, allowing scientists to compare and replicate findings across different studies. Additionally, it promotes collaborative efforts and accelerates discoveries by providing a shared foundation of knowledge and resources.

3.6 Successful applications of proteomics and databases in NAFLD research

Advancements in proteomics and database technologies have significantly contributed to the understanding and managing NAFLD. A study analyzing the plasma proteome of 48 patients with or without cirrhosis or NAFLD identified six statistically significantly changing proteins (ALDOB, APOM, LGALS3BP, PIGR, VTN, and AFM). Two of these proteins, AFM and LGALS3BP, have previously been associated with liver disease. AFM is strongly associated with components of metabolic syndrome, NAFL), and alcoholic liver disease (ALD). LGALS3BP has been identified as a candidate biomarker for hepatitis C-related fibrosis and cirrhosis [54]. A global clinical and proteomic data correlation map strongly associated DPP4, ANPEP, TGFBI, PIGR, and APOE with NAFLD and cirrhosis. DPP4, ANPEP, and TGFBI are potential drug targets for liver disease due to their correlation with liver enzymes indicative of hepatic injury in the plasma proteome [54].

The application of annotated databases combined with proteomics can reveal specific protein signatures throughout the progression of NAFLD, aiding in early diagnostic strategies. Serum proteome profiling, leveraging the Plasma Proteome database [55], identified specific protein signatures related to immune system regulation and inflammation (e.g., RBP4), coagulation (i.e., fibrinogen β chain and fibrinogen γ chain), and the structure and function of cellular and extracellular matrices (i.e., Lumican). These signatures also include carrier proteins in the blood (e.g., apolipoprotein C1), enabling the differentiation between various liver disease conditions and improving early diagnosis and prognosis.

In the work conducted by Xing et al., a mass spectrometry (M.S.)-based discovery-verification-validation proteomics workflow in combination with machine learning models was used to identify serum proteomic biomarkers including HABP2, CD163, AFP, and PIVKA-II, distinguishing early-stage HCC from liver cirrhosis and healthy liver [56]. These results indicate that proteomic technologies, supported by the human Plasma Proteome database, hold great potential for liquid biopsy applications, enhancing early detection and management of liver disease, including NAFLD.

Liver tissue proteomics, using the National Center for Biotechnology Information (NCBI) [57] annotated database, revealed significant alterations in mitochondrial proteins, providing critical insights into hepatic disease pathogenesis [58]. For example, chronic ethanol exposure in an animal model led to the differential expression of 43 mitochondrial proteins, with 13 increasing and 30 decreasing, highlighting the extensive impact of ethanol on the mitochondrial proteome [59]. This study emphasized the utility of proteomics and annotated databases in uncovering the intricate responses of mitochondria to stress and identifying specific metabolic pathways involved in liver pathology.

Another helpful tool for understanding the complete set of proteins (proteome) expressed in the human liver is the Human Liver Proteome Project (HLPP) database [60]. The Human Liver Proteome Project, aims to map and understand the complete set of proteins expressed in the human liver, focusing on proteome mapping, functional annotation, and clinical relevance. The HLPP database is a valuable resource for researchers, providing detailed proteomic data and analytical tools to advance the understanding and treatment of liver diseases, including NAFLD [61].

Proteomics is advancing research on NAFLD and other liver conditions by facilitating a comprehensive understanding of protein expression and function. Together, these resources enable a deeper understanding of the molecular mechanisms underlying liver diseases, support the development of targeted therapies, and enhance the potential for personalized treatment strategies. Ultimately, they aim to reduce the significant health and economic burden of NAFLD and related liver conditions.

3.7 Extracellular vesicles in NAFLD: Diagnosis and treatment potential

Recent advancement in cellular and molecular biomarker discovery using proteomics have utilized the role of extracellular vesicles (EVs) in cell-cell communications to understand their potential and roles in the pathophysiology of many diseases such as cancer, neurological disorders, cardiovascular diseases, infectious and chronic metabolic disorders, including NAFLD and chronic liver disease [62–69] (**Figure 2**). Extracellular vesicles, especially exosomes, are nanovesicles secreted by most types of cells, characterized by a cargo of proteins, metabolites, nucleic acids, and miRNAs, They play a vital role in intercellular communication in both healthy and pathogenic cells [70–74]. The pathophysiology of NAFLD, particularly insulin resistance, along with chemotaxis, adhesion, and infiltration of circulating immune cells with the subsequent establishment of a proinflammatory phenotype, are crucial for developing NASH [75]. Exploring extracellular vesicle functions and cargo content can provide new information on the diagnosis and prognosis of NAFLD through circulating exosomes between cells, tissues, and organs, including membrane-bound vesicles containing proteins, lipids, and nucleic acids that may alter the phenotype and function of target cells [76–78].

For in-depth proteome analysis, the samples must be partitioned or investigated at sub-proteomic levels using enrichment of EVs/exosomes, affinity purification of targets, or organelle fractionation. Recent developments in EVs-omics have offered

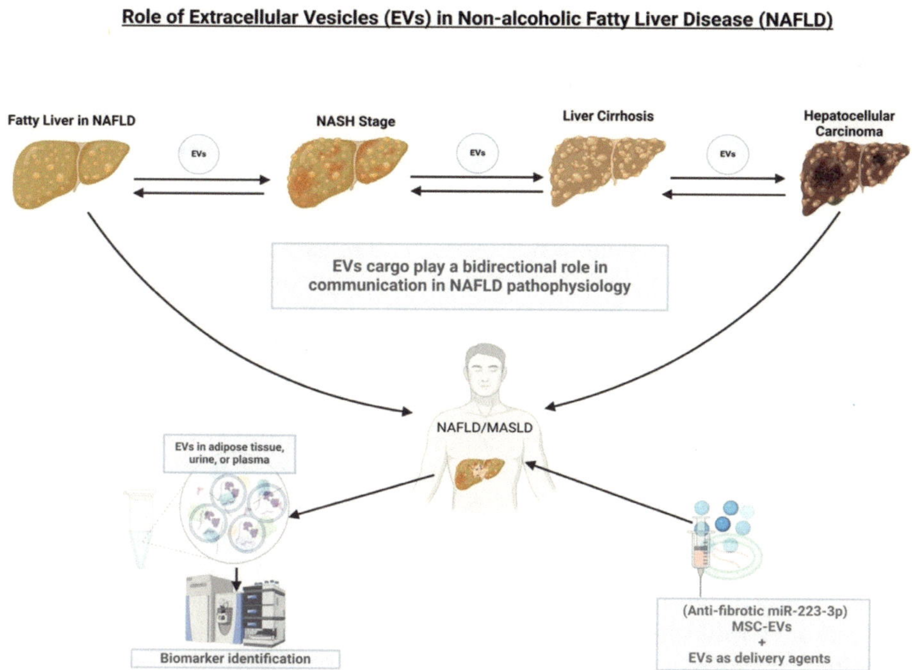

Figure 2.
A schematic for the role of extracellular vesicles in NAFLD. Created in BioRender. Manusov J. *BioRender.com/s18s770*.

great results, and new methods and approaches are continuously being developed. EV-omics success has led to multiple candidate biomarker studies for various diseases. These enrichment approaches have identified thousands of new biomarkers using ultracentrifugation, affinity, antibody-based, and size exclusion (SEC). Although many biomarkers still need to be validated and explored, these approaches offer significant improvements for discovering new analytes. Ultracentrifugation has become the standard method due to ease, low cost, and throughput.

The relevance of EVs in disease progression, coupled with the improved methods of identification and quantification in various biological fluids such as urine, breast milk, semen, saliva, and blood, has presented a critical area of focus for biomarkers in NAFLD [66, 79, 80]. Extracellular vesicles from adipose tissue can pathogenically promote insulin resistance that leads to the progression stages of NAFLD/ Metabolic Associated Fatty Liver Disease MASLD [81].

In vitro studies have shown that adipose tissue-derived EVs inhibit insulin-mediated Akt (A.K. transforming) phosphorylation in hepatocytes, suggesting cell-cell communication between adipose cells and hepatocytes [82]. EVs are also reported to be key players in organ-to-organ communication during liver lipid overload, facilitating crosstalk between the liver and vascular endothelium, leading to cardiovascular complications [81, 83, 84]. The chemotaxis, adhesion, and infiltration of circulating immune cells with the subsequent establishment of a proinflammatory phenotype, are crucial features in NASH, linking immature myeloid cells to the release of EVs in mouse models of NAFLD [85]. EVs are also reported to be key players in organ-to-organ communication during liver lipid overload, facilitating crosstalk between the liver and vascular endothelium, leading to other cardiovascular complications [81, 86]. The formation of liver fibrosis is closely associated with the progression of various liver diseases, including NAFLD. During the development of liver fibrosis, exosomes produced by various cells interact with each other to jointly regulate the changes in cytokines and cell populations and function as the fibrosis regulators in the occurrence and development of liver fibrosis [73]. Hepatocyte-derived exosomes rich in mtDNA are reported to activate Toll-like receptor 9 (TLR9) in Kupffer cells (K.C.s) by triggering the secretion of proinflammatory cytokines, such as Interleukin 1b (IL-1b) and Tumor Necrosis Factor TNF-α, thereby aggravating the progression of NAFLD to NASH [73, 87]. Cultured lipotoxic hepatocytes release EVs containing over 500 differentially regulated miRNAs with a marked upregulation of miR-1. Circulating miRNAs, such as miR-135a-3p in EVs, may serve as potential noninvasive biomarkers for diagnosing NAFLD [88]. This miRNA has been shown to be more sensitive and specific biological marker for NAFLD compared to ALT [88].

Due to their hepatocellular uptake, EVs can serve as potential therapeutic targets by directly carrying liver-alleviating cargo or indirectly as liver-specific delivery agents [69, 89, 90]. EVs derived from adipose tissue mesenchymal stem cells may alleviate specific metabolic abnormalities in NAFLD/MASLD; it was previously demonstrated that these EVs carry and deliver anti-fibrotic miR-223-3p, in their cargoes, which leads to the suppression of E2F1 that contribute to hepatic steatosis thereby providing an opportunity for potential therapy in NAFD [91]. Recently, human milk-derived EVs were also found to alleviate hepatic steatosis and insulin resistance in mice with high-fat diet-induced NAFLD, suggesting the ability of E.V. content to inhibit lipogenesis and increase lipolysis. After treatment with EVs that were isolated from human breast milk, lipid accumulation was also inhibited in hepatocyte [92].

4. The current and future use of genotype-by-environment interactions and gene protein identification

Our group has collected extensive data on liver health in Mexican Americans through two family studies (The Mexican American Family Study [93, 94] and the Rio Grande Valley Family Study [6]). These studies focus on families of Mexican ancestry living in south Texas. Data collected include biometric phenotypic and anthropometric data (blood pressure, height, weight, Body Mass Index, hip-waist ratio, abdominal circumference, instrument data, diet (carbohydrates, total calories, total protein, total fat), physical exercise and energy expenditure, sleep, alcohol and tobacco use, socioeconomic (Duncan Socioeconomic Index), cultural and ethnic background and preference, education levels, social determinants of health data, current and past occupations, marital status, total household income, liver health markers, chronic illnesses, and blood samples.

To search for potential genetically mediating environments of NAFLD risk, we examined two environmental measures. We used the Beck Depression Inventory-II (BDI-II) to assess the degree of depressive symptoms over the past 2 weeks [95, 96]. The BDI-II is a reliable screening tool for assessing the severity of depression. The BDI-II assesses the severity of depression and is an acceptable screening instrument for depression when administered either in Spanish or English [83, 84, 96]. We also examined the Acculturation Rating Scale for Mexican Americans-II (ARSMA-II) which is designed to quantify the acculturation construct and is the basis of many available acculturation scales. The scale comprises two subscales (orientation and marginalization) that can be analyzed individually. Since we are interested in the role of acculturation stress and G × E effects on NAFLD, we analyzed the Marginalization/Separation measure of the ARSMA-II [81].

We measured hepatic fibrosis in the Rio Grande Valley Family Study as the Liver Stiffness Measurement LSM Youden Index (kPa), steatosis (controlled attenuation parameter dB/m CAP), and the FAST (FibroScan-AST) (the most predictive model for risk of fibrosis that combines LSM, CAP, and AST). CAP identifies steatosis with an AUROC of 0.87 (95% confidence interval [CI] 0.82–0.92) for $S \geq S1$, 0.77 (95% CI 0.71–0.82) for $S \geq S2$, and 0.70 (95% CI 0.64–0.75) for S=S3. Youden cutoff values for $S \geq S1$, $S \geq S2$, and $S \geq S3$ were 302 dB/m, 331 dB/m, and 337 dB/m, respectively. LSM identified patients with fibrosis with AUROCs of 0.77 (95% CI 0.72–0.82) for $F \geq F2$, 0.80 (95% CI 0.75–0.84) for $F \geq F3$, and 0.89 (95% CI 0.84–0.93) for F=F4. Youden cutoff values for $F \geq F2$, $F \geq F3$, and F=F4 were 8.2 kPa, 9.7 kPa, and 13.6 kPa, respectively (Echosens, Paris, France) [85–88]. Exclusion criteria included pregnancy, implant, or a cardiac pacemaker. Participants presented fasting for at least 3 hours prior to the exam. The participants lay supine, face-up on the exam table, and fully abducted their right arm. The Fibroscan automatically chooses the correct probe size (M/XL). Ultrasound conduction gel was applied to the abdomen at the 8th–10th intercostal rib space at the mid-axillary line. Measurements were performed by scanning the right liver lobe through the intercostal space. CAP is an average estimate of ultrasound attenuation at 3–5 MHz (dB/m). Liver Stiffness Measurements (LSM) are an average stiffness measurement at a shear wave frequency of 50 Hz (kilopascals). The median value of successful measurements with at least 10 validated measurements and a success rate of at least 30% were selected to represent the LSM [86, 97–99].

Our studies have examined the complex interplay of genetic and environmental interactions that shape the risk for liver disease [3, 6] using variance component models and likelihood-based statistical inference in the phenotypic expression of NAFLD.

Trait	Heritability	Standard Error	p-Value
HbA1C	0.52	0.11	2.5×10^{-06}
Marginalization	0.30	0.08	3.8×10^{-05}
AHC HRSN	0.40	0.13	6.6×10^{-04}
AST	0.25	0.14	2.0×10^{-02}
ALT	0.41	0.13	6.9×10^{-03}
AST/ALT	0.27	0.10	1.9×10^{-03}
BDI-II	0.36	0.10	1.5×10^{-05}
BMI	0.55	0.11	8.0×10^{-07}
CAP	0.34	0.10	3.6×10^{-04}
FAST	0.35	0.13	2.3×10^{-03}
kPa	0.33	0.13	4.3×10^{-03}

Table 1.
Significant heritabilities with p-values [3, 6, 100, 101].

We demonstrated that genes underlying NAFLD progression interact with depression as assessed by the BDI-II, the social determinants of health (AHC HRSN), and acculturation stress (marginalization measured by the ARSMA-II). **Table 1** reviews heritabilities for examined traits [5].

We found consistent evidence of G × E interactions when studying depression, marginalization, and SDOH. Genotype-by-environment interactions were significant for HbA1c, AST/ALT ratio, BDI-II, and CAP, indicating that genetic factors interact with marginalization to influence these traits. Acculturation stress, depression, and the social determinants of health exacerbate the genetic response to NAFLD. These findings underscore the importance of considering G × E interactions in understanding disease susceptibility and may inform targeted interventions for at-risk populations.

Using a novel model to account for genotype-by-environment interactions for dichotomous and continuous environments (G × Sex and G × SDoH interaction influencing depression), we demonstrated that there is G × SDoH interaction for males and that depression is influenced by different sets of genes in males and females. Our results have significant implications for medical research and potential clinical applications [100].

4.1 Transcripts, shared associations, and the future

Recent findings support the molecular basis of how environmental stress modifies gene function. Not only does stress (mental illnesses, poverty, acculturation/marginalization, and adverse effects of the social determinants of health) change our lives, but our genetic makeup reacts at a cellular level, differentially predisposing individuals to chronic illness. Ongoing multiomics research identifies specific genes, mutations, and proteins involved in G × E interaction. We recently have used an integrative approach to evaluate determinants of gene expression measurements of the RGV family study. Each gene expression phenotype was quantitatively decomposed into two complementary components: genetic information (endophenotypes) and environmental response (envophenotype). This variance decomposition approach can be applied to any genetic study, but it is more efficient when there is a substantial genetic relationship with the sample. By separating genetic and environmental effects, we can identify components of environmental risk that may be directly malleable to environmental interventions. Similarly, uniquely genetic components of risk may identify novel pharmacological targets for drug-based interventions.

5. Conclusion

This chapter underscores the complex relationship between genetic predisposition and environmental factors in the development of NAFLD. By exploring genotype-by-environment interactions focused on psychosocial stress—such as social determinants of health, depression, and acculturation—we provide evidence of how stress can exacerbate or mitigate the genetic risk of NAFLD. The chapter reviews how advanced genetic and proteomic techniques are utilized to understand interactions that occur at a molecular level, providing a comprehensive view of the complex interplay between genes and environment in NAFLD pathogenesis. Findings from recent studies, particularly those focusing on the Mexican American population, reveal significant genotype-by-environment interactions influencing NAFLD-related phenotypes. These data highlight the importance of how genetic and environmental factors influence disease susceptibility and progression, especially how acculturation stress, depression, and social determinants of health interact with genetic factors to influence traits such as HbA1c levels, AST/ALT ratio, and steatosis (CAP), which are key indicators of liver health and NAFLD progression. The chapter also emphasizes the potential of integrating multi-omics approaches, including proteomics and transcriptomics, to further understand and address chronic liver disease. These advanced techniques allow for the identification of specific proteins and genetic variants involved in NAFLD, providing information for more targeted and personalized interventions, particularly in high-risk populations. By elucidating the molecular mechanisms underlying gene-environment interactions in NAFLD, this research sets the stage for developing more effective prevention strategies and tailored treatments.

In conclusion, this comprehensive exploration of gene-environment interactions in NAFLD among Mexican Americans not only advances our understanding of the disease's complex etiology but also highlights the potential for personalized medicine approaches in managing this increasingly prevalent condition. The findings presented here underscore the need for holistic approaches to NAFLD prevention and treatment that consider both genetic risk factors and environmental influences, ultimately aiming to improve health outcomes in vulnerable populations.

Funding

The research discussed leveraged state-of-the-art instrumentation and capabilities established as part of the Valley Baptist Legacy Foundation-supported Project THRIVE awarded to SWB. The research was supported by a grant from the Knapp Community Care Foundation to SWB, and the National Institutes of Health U54 HG013247 to S.W.B., and R01 MD912564.

Author details

Eron G. Manusov[1,2*], Vincent P. Diego[1,2], Marcio Almeida[1,2], Jacob A. Galan[1,2], Auwal A. Bala[1,2], Marco A. Arriaga[1], Natasha S. Garcia-Rodriguez[1], Renee Hernandez[1], Satish Kumar[1,2], John Blangero[1,2] and Sarah Williams-Blangero[1,2]

1 Department of Human Genetics, University of Texas Rio Grande Valley, Brownsville, TX, USA

2 South Texas Diabetes and Obesity Institute, School of Medicine, University of Texas Rio Grande Valley, Brownsville, TX, USA

*Address all correspondence to: eron.manusov@utrgv.edu

References

[1] Petrescu M, Vlaicu SI, Ciumărnean L, Milaciu MV, Mărginean C, Florea M, et al. Chronic inflammation-A link between nonalcoholic fatty liver disease (NAFLD) and dysfunctional adipose tissue. Medicina (Kaunas). 6 May 2022;**58**(5):641. DOI: 10.3390/medicina58050641

[2] Pafili K, Roden M. Nonalcoholic fatty liver disease (NAFLD) from pathogenesis to treatment concepts in humans. Molecular Metabolism. 2021;**50**:101122

[3] Manusov EG Diego VP, Abrego E, Herklotz K, Almeida M, Mao X, et al. Gene-by-environment interaction in non-alcoholic fatty liver disease and depression: The role of hepatic transaminases. Medical Research Archives. Sep 2023;**11**(9):10.18103/mra.v11i9.4408. DOI: 10.18103/mra.v11i9.4408. Epub 2023 Sep 28

[4] Loomba R et al. Heritability of hepatic fibrosis and steatosis based on a prospective twin study. Gastroenterology. 2015;**149**(7):1784-1793

[5] Manusov EG et al. Genotype-by-environment interactions in nonalcoholic fatty liver disease and chronic illness among Mexican Americans: The role of acculturation stress. Genes (Basel). 2024;**15**(8)

[6] Manusov EG et al. Non-alcoholic fatty liver disease and depression: Evidence for genotype × environment interaction in Mexican Americans. Frontiers in Psychiatry. 2022;**13**:936052

[7] Abdellaoui A et al. 15 years of GWAS discovery: Realizing the promise. American Journal of Human Genetics. 2023;**110**(2):179-194

[8] Spencer CC et al. Designing genome-wide association studies: Sample size, power, imputation, and the choice of genotyping chip. PLoS Genetics. 2009;**5**(5):e1000477

[9] Fujita H et al. Variations with modest effects have an important role in the genetic background of type 2 diabetes and diabetes-related traits. Journal of Human Genetics. 2012;**57**(12):776-779

[10] Namjou B et al. GWAS and enrichment analyses of non-alcoholic fatty liver disease identify new trait-associated genes and pathways across eMERGE network. BMC Medicine. 2019;**17**(1):135

[11] Thapar A et al. The contribution of gene-environment interaction to psychopathology. Development and Psychopathology. 2007;**19**(4):989-1004

[12] Ambrosini G et al. Insights gained from a comprehensive all-against-all transcription factor binding motif benchmarking study. Genome Biology. 2020;**21**(1):114

[13] Stewart AJ, Hannenhalli S, Plotkin JB. Why transcription factor binding sites are ten nucleotides long. Genetics. 2012;**192**(3):973-985

[14] Rothenberg EV. Transcription factors specifically control change. Genes & Development. 2022;**36**(21-24):1097-1099

[15] Han D Li Z, Luo L, Jiang H. Targeting hypoxia and HIF1α in triple-negative breast Cancer: New insights from gene expression profiling and implications for therapy. Biology (Basel). 31 Jul 2024;**13**(8):577. DOI: 10.3390/biology13080577

[16] Hong J, Medzikovic L, Sun W, Wong B, Ruffenach G, Rhodes CJ, et al. Integrative multiomics in the lung reveals a protective role of Asporin in pulmonary arterial hypertension. Circulation. 15 Oct 2024;**150**(16):1268-1287. DOI: 10.1161/CIRCULATIONAHA.124.069864

[17] Tan MCB et al. Transcriptome-wide association study and Mendelian randomization in pancreatic cancer identifies susceptibility genes and causal relationships with type 2 diabetes and venous thromboembolism. eBioMedicine. 2024;**106**:105233

[18] Harrison PW, Wright AE, Mank JE. The evolution of gene expression and the transcriptome-phenotype relationship. Seminars in Cell & Developmental Biology. 2012;**23**(2):222-229

[19] Tonyan ZN, Nasykhova YA, Danilova MM, Barbitoff YA, Changalidi AI, Mikhailova AA, et al. Overview of transcriptomic research on type 2 diabetes: Challenges and perspectives. Genes (Basel). 30 Jun 2022;**13**(7):1176. DOI: 10.3390/genes13071176

[20] Darci-Maher N et al. Cross-tissue omics analysis discovers ten adipose genes encoding secreted proteins in obesity-related non-alcoholic fatty liver disease. eBioMedicine. 2023;**92**:104620

[21] Xu Z et al. Exploration of the core gene signatures and mechanisms between NAFLD and sarcopenia through transcriptomic level. Frontiers in Endocrinology (Lausanne). 2023;**14**:1140804

[22] Lonardo A, Arab JP, Arrese M. Perspectives on precision medicine approaches to NAFLD diagnosis and management. Advances in Therapy. 2021;**38**(5):2130-2158

[23] Pirola CJ, Sookoian S. Personalized medicine in nonalcoholic fatty liver disease. Clinical and Molecular Hepatology. 2022;**28**(4):935-938

[24] Sookoian S, Pirola CJ. Precision medicine in nonalcoholic fatty liver disease: New therapeutic insights from genetics and systems biology. Clinical and Molecular Hepatology. 2020;**26**(4):461-475

[25] Pang K et al. Role of protein phosphorylation in cell signaling, disease, and the intervention therapy. MedComm. 2020;**3**(4):e175

[26] Raggiaschi R, Gotta S, Terstappen GC. Phosphoproteome analysis. Bioscience Reports. 2005;**25**(1-2):33-44

[27] Nakayasu ES et al. Tutorial: Best practices and considerations for mass-spectrometry-based protein biomarker discovery and validation. Nature Protocols. 2021;**16**(8):3737-3760

[28] Birhanu AG. Mass spectrometry-based proteomics as an emerging tool in clinical laboratories. Clinical Proteomics. 2023;**20**(1):32

[29] Hunter JM, Paramithiotis E. Protein biomarker quantification by mass spectrometry. Expert Opinion on Medical Diagnostics. 2010;**4**(1):11-20

[30] Ou YN et al. Identification of novel drug targets for Alzheimer's disease by integrating genetics and proteomes from brain and blood. Molecular Psychiatry. 2021;**26**(10):6065-6073

[31] Aguilan JT, Kulej K, Sidoli S. Guide for protein fold change and p-value calculation for non-experts in proteomics. Molecular Omics. 2020;**16**(6):573-582

[32] Hasin Y, Seldin M, Lusis A. Multi-omics approaches to disease. Genome Biology. 2017;**18**(1):83

[33] Karczewski KJ, Snyder MP. Integrative omics for health and disease. Nature Reviews. Genetics. 2018;**19**(5):299-310

[34] Hennrich ML et al. Cell-specific proteome analyses of human bone marrow reveal molecular features of age-dependent functional decline. Nature Communications. 2018;**9**(1):4004

[35] Bekker-Jensen DB et al. An optimized shotgun strategy for the rapid generation of comprehensive human proteomes. Cell Systems. 2017;**4**(6):587-599.e4

[36] Kumar S et al. Utility of lymphoblastoid cell lines for induced pluripotent stem cell generation. Stem Cells International. 2016;**2016**:2349261

[37] Kumar S et al. Efficient generation of functional hepatocytes from human induced pluripotent stem cells for disease modeling and disease gene discovery. Methods in Molecular Biology. 2022;**2549**:85-101

[38] Anzai K et al. Foetal hepatic progenitor cells assume a cholangiocytic cell phenotype during two-dimensional pre-culture. Scientific Reports. 2016;**6**:28283

[39] Uto H et al. Clinical proteomics for liver disease: A promising approach for discovery of novel biomarkers. Proteome Science. 2010;**8**:70

[40] Gray J et al. A proteomic strategy to identify novel serum biomarkers for liver cirrhosis and hepatocellular cancer in individuals with fatty liver disease. BMC Cancer. 2009;**9**:271

[41] Consortium, T.U. UniProt: The universal protein knowledgebase in 2023. Nucleic Acids Research. 2022;**51**(D1):D523-D531

[42] Boutet E et al. UniProtKB/Swiss-Prot. Methods in Molecular Biology. 2007;**406**:89-112

[43] Berman HM et al. The Protein Data Bank. Nucleic Acids Research. 2000;**28**(1):235-242

[44] Kumar S, Blangero J, Curran JE. Induced pluripotent stem cells in disease Modeling and gene identification. Methods in Molecular Biology. 2018;**1706**:17-38

[45] Kumar S et al. Highly efficient induced pluripotent stem cell reprogramming of cryopreserved lymphoblastoid cell lines. Journal of Biological Methods. 2020;**7**(1):e124

[46] Paysan-Lafosse T et al. Inter Pro in 2022. Nucleic Acids Research. 2023;**51**(D1):D418-D427

[47] Guilliams M et al. Spatial proteogenomics reveals distinct and evolutionarily conserved hepatic macrophage niches. Cell. 2022;**185**(2):379-396 e38

[48] Lian Q et al. HCCDB: A database of hepatocellular carcinoma expression atlas. Genomics, Proteomics & Bioinformatics. 2018;**16**(4):269-275

[49] Aleksander SA, Balhoff J, Carbon S, Cherry JM, Drabkin HJ, Ebert D, et al. The gene ontology knowledgebase in 2023. Genetics. 4 May 2023;**224**(1):iyad031. DOI: 10.1093/genetics/iyad031

[50] Finn RD et al. Pfam: The protein families database. Nucleic Acids Research. 2014.42 (Database issue): D222-D230

[51] Kanehisa M et al. KEGG for taxonomy-based analysis of pathways and genomes. Nucleic Acids Research. 2023;**51**(D1):D587-d592

[52] Wu CH et al. The protein information resource. Nucleic Acids Research. 2003;**31**(1):345-347

[53] Zinkin NT et al. Serum proteomics and biomarkers in hepatocellular carcinoma and chronic liver disease. Clinical Cancer Research. 2008;**14**(2):470-477

[54] Niu L et al. Plasma proteome profiling discovers novel proteins associated with non-alcoholic fatty liver disease. Molecular Systems Biology. 2019;**15**(3):e8793

[55] Nanjappa V et al. Plasma proteome database as a resource for proteomics research: 2014 update. Nucleic Acids Research. 2014;**42**(Database issue):D959-D965

[56] Xing X et al. Proteomics-driven noninvasive screening of circulating serum protein panels for the early diagnosis of hepatocellular carcinoma. Nature Communications. 2023;**14**(1):8392

[57] Sayers EW et al. Database resources of the national center for biotechnology information. Nucleic Acids Research. 2022;**50**(D1):D20-d26

[58] Venkatraman A et al. Modification of the mitochondrial proteome in response to the stress of ethanol-dependent hepatotoxicity. The Journal of Biological Chemistry. 2004;**279**(21):22092-22101

[59] Bailey SM et al. S-adenosyl-methionine prevents chronic alcohol-induced mitochondrial dysfunction in the rat liver. American Journal of Physiology. Gastrointestinal and Liver Physiology. 2006;**291**(5):G857-G867

[60] Beretta L. The human liver proteome project. Molecular & Cellular Proteomics. 2007;**6**(11):2043

[61] Niu L et al. Dynamic human liver proteome atlas reveals functional insights into disease pathways. Molecular Systems Biology. 2022;**18**(5):e10947

[62] Xiang SY et al. Function of macrophage-derived exosomes in chronic liver disease: From pathogenesis to treatment. World Journal of Hepatology. 2023;**15**(11):1196-1209

[63] Prieto D et al. S100-A9 protein in exosomes from chronic lymphocytic leukemia cells promotes NF-kappaB activity during disease progression. Blood. 2017;**130**(6):777-788

[64] Wang C et al. Role of exosomes in chronic liver disease development and their potential clinical applications. Journal of Immunology Research. 2022;**2022**:1695802

[65] Yuan M et al. The mechanism of exosomes function in neurological diseases: A progressive review. Current Pharmaceutical Design. 2018;**24**(24):2855-2861

[66] Sun B et al. Applications of stem cell-derived exosomes in tissue engineering and neurological diseases. Reviews in the Neurosciences. 2018;**29**(5):531-546

[67] Liu S, Zhang B, Sun Q. Research progress on the mechanism of exosomes in bacterial infectious diseases. Zhonghua Wei Zhong Bing Ji Jiu Yi Xue. 2023;**35**(12):1327-1330

[68] Fleming A et al. The carrying pigeons of the cell: Exosomes and their role in infectious diseases caused

by human pathogens. Pathogens and Disease. 2014;**71**(2):109-120

[69] Hernandez A, Arab JP, Reyes D, Lapitz A, Moshage H, Bañales JM, et al. Extracellular vesicles in NAFLD/ALD: From pathobiology to therapy. Cells. 27 Mar 2020;**9**(4):817. DOI: 10.3390/cells9040817

[70] Niazi V et al. Communication between stromal and hematopoietic stem cell by exosomes in normal and malignant bone marrow niche. Biomedicine & Pharmacotherapy. 2020;**132**:110854

[71] Poe AJ, Knowlton AA. Exosomes and cardiovascular cell-cell communication. Essays in Biochemistry. 2018;**62**(2):193-204

[72] Nicolini A, Ferrari P, Biava PM. Exosomes and cell communication: From tumour-derived exosomes and their role in tumour progression to the use of exosomal cargo for cancer treatment. Cancers (Basel). 16 Feb 2021;**13**(4):822. DOI: 10.3390/cancers13040822

[73] Mahajan A, Gunewardena S, Morris A, Clauss M, Dhillon NK. Analysis of MicroRNA cargo in circulating extracellular vesicles from HIV-infected individuals with pulmonary hypertension. Cells. 21 May 2024;**13**(11):886. DOI: 10.3390/cells13110886. PMID: 38891019; PMCID: PMC11172129

[74] Xiong JL et al. Pituitary-derived small extracellular vesicles promote liver repair by its cargo miR-143-3p. Scientific Reports. 2024;**14**(1):16635

[75] Parthasarathy G, Revelo X, Malhi H. Pathogenesis of nonalcoholic steatohepatitis: An overview. Hepatology Commununications. 2020;**4**(4):478-492

[76] Mladenovic D et al. Adipose-derived extracellular vesicles - a novel cross-talk mechanism in insulin resistance, non-alcoholic fatty liver disease, and polycystic ovary syndrome. Endocrine. 2024;**85**(1):18-34

[77] van Niel G, D'Angelo G, Raposo G. Shedding light on the cell biology of extracellular vesicles. Nature Reviews. Molecular Cell Biology. 2018;**19**(4):213-228

[78] Urban SK et al. Extracellular vesicles in liver diseases: Diagnostic, prognostic, and therapeutic application. Seminars in Liver Disease. 2019;**39**(1):70-77

[79] Newman LA, Sorich MJ, Rowland A. Role of extracellular vesicles in the pathophysiology, diagnosis and tracking of non-alcoholic fatty liver disease. Journal of Clinical Medicine. 29 Jun 2020;**9**(7):2032. DOI: 10.3390/jcm9072032

[80] Wu D, Zhu H, Wang H. Extracellular vesicles in non-alcoholic fatty liver disease and alcoholic liver disease. Frontiers in Physiology. 2021;**12**:707429

[81] Jimenez DE et al. Using the revised acculturation rating scale for Mexican Americans (ARSMA-II) with older adults. Hispanic Health Care International. 2010;**8**(1):14-22

[82] Jiang F et al. Hepatocyte-derived extracellular vesicles promote endothelial inflammation and atherogenesis via microRNA-1. Journal of Hepatology. 2020;**72**(1):156-166

[83] Wiebe JS, Penley JA. A psychometric comparison of the Beck depression inventory-II in English and Spanish. Psychological Assessment. 2005;**17**(4):481-485

[84] Wang YP, Gorenstein C. Psychometric properties of the

beck depression inventory-II: A comprehensive review. Brazilian Journal of Psychiatry. 2013;**35**(4):416-431

[85] Eilenberg M et al. Accuracy of non-invasive liver stiffness measurement and steatosis quantification in patients with severe and morbid obesity. Hepatobiliary Surgery and Nutrition. 2021;**10**(5):610-622

[86] Newsome PN et al. FibroScan-AST (FAST) score for the non-invasive identification of patients with non-alcoholic steatohepatitis with significant activity and fibrosis: A prospective derivation and global validation study. The Lancet Gastroenterology & Hepatology. 2020;**5**(4):362-373

[87] Oeda S et al. Diagnostic accuracy of FibroScan-AST score to identify non-alcoholic steatohepatitis with significant activity and fibrosis in Japanese patients with non-alcoholic fatty liver disease: Comparison between M and XL probes. Hepatology Research. 2020;**50**(7):831-839

[88] Eddowes PJ et al. Accuracy of FibroScan controlled attenuation parameter and liver stiffness measurement in assessing steatosis and fibrosis in patients with nonalcoholic fatty liver disease. Gastroenterology. 2019;**156**(6):1717-1730

[89] Maas SLN, Breakefield XO, Weaver AM. Extracellular vesicles: Unique intercellular delivery vehicles. Trends in Cell Biology. 2017;**27**(3):172-188

[90] Han C et al. Extracellular vesicles in cardiovascular disease: Biological functions and therapeutic implications. Pharmacology & Therapeutics. 2022;**233**:108025

[91] Niu Q et al. Adipose-derived mesenchymal stem cell-secreted extracellular vesicles alleviate non-alcoholic fatty liver disease via delivering miR-223-3p. Adipocytes. 2022;**11**(1):572-587

[92] Jiang X et al. Human milk-derived extracellular vesicles alleviate high fat diet-induced non-alcoholic fatty liver disease in mice. Molecular Biology Reports. 2023;**50**(3):2257-2268

[93] Mitchell BD et al. Diabetes and hypertension in Mexican American families: Relation to cardiovascular risk. American Journal of Epidemiology. 1999;**149**(11):1047-1056

[94] MacCluer JW et al. Genetics of atherosclerosis risk factors in Mexican Americans. Nutrition Reviews. 1999;**57**(5 Pt 2):S59-S65

[95] Beck AT et al. An inventory for measuring depression. Archives of General Psychiatry. 1961;**4**:561-571

[96] Penley JA, Wiebe JS, Nwosu A. Psychometric properties of the Spanish Beck depression inventory-II in a medical sample. Psychological Assessment. 2003;**15**(4):569-577

[97] Cassinotto C et al. Liver stiffness in nonalcoholic fatty liver disease: A comparison of supersonic shear imaging, FibroScan, and ARFI with liver biopsy. Hepatology. 2016;**63**(6):1817-1827

[98] Mikolasevic I et al. Transient elastography (FibroScan((R))) with controlled attenuation parameter in the assessment of liver steatosis and fibrosis in patients with nonalcoholic fatty liver disease - where do we stand? World Journal of Gastroenterology. 2016;**22**(32):7236-7251

[99] Xu Y et al. Comparison of FibroTouch and FibroScan for staging fibrosis in chronic liver

disease: Single-center prospective study. Digestive and Liver Disease. 2019;**51**(9):1323-1329

[100] Diego VP, Manusov EG, Almeida M, Laston S, Ortiz D, Blangero J, et al. Statistical genetic approaches to investigate genotype-by-environment interaction: Review and novel extension of models. Genes (Basel). 25 Apr 2024;**15**(5):547. DOI: 10.3390/genes15050547

[101] Manusov EG, Diego VP, Almeida M, Ortiz D, Curran JE, Galan J, et al. Genotype-by-environment interactions in nonalcoholic fatty liver disease and chronic illness among Mexican Americans: The role of acculturation stress. Genes. 2024:15

Chapter 9

Non-alcoholic-Related Fatty Liver Disease (NAFLD) as a Risk Factor for Atherosclerotic Cardiovascular Disease: The Hidden Link – ASCVD Risk Factors from NAFLD

Paulin Bilonda Kabeya

Abstract

Non-alcoholic fatty liver disease (NAFLD) is a significant independent risk factor for atherosclerotic cardiovascular diseases (ASCVDs). The incidence of ASCVD has increased along with the prevalence of NAFLD. ASCVD events are common and a leading cause of mortality in patients with NAFLD. Numerous observational, cohort, and genetic studies have confirmed an association between NAFLD and ASCVD. Most studies have indicated that NAFLD markedly increases the risk of atherosclerosis and ASCVD. Furthermore, the underlying pro-atherosclerotic mechanisms of NAFLD have been elucidated, with shared pathophysiological factors including insulin resistance, systemic inflammation, and dyslipidemia from NAFLD exacerbating atherosclerosis. Recently, NAFLD has emerged as a risk factor for ASCVD, garnering interest as a potential therapeutic target. This review seeks to elucidate mechanistic insights, present recent clinically significant research, and investigate emerging therapies, including novel anti-diabetic and lipid-lowering agents, that may ameliorate NAFLD and mitigate ASCVD risk.

Keywords: nonalcoholic fatty liver disease, atherosclerotic cardiovascular disease, systemic inflammation, dyslipidemia, lipid-lowering agents, anti-diabetic agents, insulin resistance

1. Introduction

Non-alcohol-related fatty liver disease (NAFLD) is a significant public health issue, with studies linking it to atherosclerotic cardiovascular disease (ASCVD).

Recent scientific studies have revealed the connections between ASCVD and NAFLD.

Non-alcoholic fatty liver disease (NAFLD) is a significant public health issue, and studies have linked NAFLD to atherosclerotic cardiovascular disease (ASCVD).

IntechOpen

NAFLD affects the athérosclérose, one of the etiologies of cardiovascular disorders and metabolic syndrome failure.

The pathophysiological mechanisms of NAFLD and athérosclérеuse cardiovascular illnesses are influenced by cardiology and hepatology.

The correlation between NAFLD and ASCVD is well documented, with shared molecular processes and signaling pathways. Diagnostic studies are needed to study NAFLD and ASCVD, and lifestyle adjustments, pharmacological treatments, and novel therapies are required to treat NAFLD and ASCVD.

Population-based public health approaches to NASH and cardiovascular disease are also discussed.

Understanding the strong association between NAFLD and ASCVD can help health practitioners assess the risk, perform early screening, and implement treatment strategies for patients at risk of ASCVD due to NAFLD.

In contemporary decades, non-alcoholic fatty liver disease (NAFLD) has surfaced as a dysmetabolic syndrome of considerable global relevance, with a pronounced escalation in its incidence particularly observed in the Asian continent [1, 2].

The characterization of NAFLD, irrespective of geographical milieu, pertains to the pathological accumulation of excess lipids within hepatic tissues that cannot be attributed to excessive alcohol intake [2–4].

This chapter lays out NAFLD in two clear categories: non-alcoholic fatty liver disease and non-alcoholic steatohepatitis (NASH), with the latter presenting a spectrum of conditions from fibrosis to cirrhosis and even hepatocellular carcinoma [4].

Right now, our view of NAFLD has moved from recognizing it as a liver marker of metabolic syndrome (MetS) to realizing how it aids the atherogenic mechanism, which ultimately leads to atherosclerotic cardiovascular disease (ASCVD), involving coronary artery disease (CAD), ischemic stroke (IS), and numerous significant cardiovascular events [2–5].

The inquiry into whether NAFLD is independently associated with ASCVD remains an arena of ongoing academic discourse. Yet, a rising assortment of epidemiological, genetic, and observational findings has affirmed the theory that NAFLD could either directly or indirectly aggravate the progression of atherosclerosis and its associated clinical presentations, thereby proposing that NAFLD signifies a newly emerging independent risk factor and a potential target for ASCVD therapy.

Recently, the American Heart Association published a scientific statement that stresses the clinical significance of NAFLD management and prevention as a strategic tactic to diminish the risk of ASCVD [5].

This extensive narrative review clarifies the nuanced relationship between NAFLD and ASCVD by stressing the key pathophysiological mechanisms tying NAFLD to atherosclerosis, alongside assessing the promise of new therapeutic strategies for NAFLD that might concurrently lessen ASCVD risk.

2. Epidemiological role linking NAFLD and ASCVD

A recent study employing a Markov model has projected an escalation in the incidence of non-alcoholic fatty liver disease (NAFLD) from 18% to 29% across eight nations (China, France, Germany, Italy, Japan, Spain, the United Kingdom, and the United States) by the year 2030 [6]. The global prevalence of NAFLD is estimated to be approximately 25%, with a slightly heightened occurrence in Asia (around 29%), particularly in Indonesia (51%) and a cumulative prevalence approaching

30% in China [1]. An expanding corpus of research has documented the prevalence of NAFLD among populations afflicted by cardiovascular disease (CVD). A cohort study based on a specific Finnish population, which included 988 subjects observed from 1991 to 2009, revealed that 10.4% and 11.1% of individuals with severe fatty liver disease experienced fatal and non-fatal coronary heart disease, respectively [7].

A cohort analysis with 22,048 patients carried out in Germany revealed that 12.8% of individuals diagnosed with NAFLD/NASH were found to have coronary heart disease, and 2.9% were diagnosed with myocardial infarction within a decade, rates that notably surpassed those of individuals not having NAFLD/NASH.

A population-based cohort study executed in Minnesota, United States, with an average follow-up period of 7.6 years, indicated that ischemic heart disease (IHD) constituted 25% of mortality among patients with NAFLD, nearly twice the mortality rate associated with liver disease [8]; furthermore, a more extensive national investigation involving 55 million patients revealed that the incidence of myocardial infarction (MI) in individuals with non-alcoholic steatohepatitis (NASH) was 10.2% [9].

A meta-analysis encompassing 2,054,554 participants derived from 392 studies conducted in China illustrated a significantly elevated risk of cardiovascular disease (odds ratio [OR] 3.2, 95% confidence interval [CI] 2.27–4.50; $P < 0.50$; $P < 0.001$) among patients diagnosed with NAFLD [10].

Furthermore, an extensive meta-analysis encompassing 16 observational studies, both prospective and retrospective, with a collective 34,043 subjects and an average follow-up time of 6.9 years indicated that individuals diagnosed with NAFLD had a 64% elevated risk of encountering deadly and non-deadly cardiovascular occurrences [11]. In summary, the collective epidemiological findings derived from multiple populations underscore a clear prevalence and severity of cardiovascular incidents in those suffering from NAFLD, thereby indicating that NAFLD could potentially act as a harbinger of future risk for atherosclerotic cardiovascular disease (ASCVD).

3. Genetic determinants of non-alcoholic fatty liver disease (NAFLD) and atherosclerotic cardiovascular disease (ASCVD)

Prevalent genetic polymorphisms may modulate the pathogenesis of atherosclerosis among individuals afflicted with NAFLD, particularly those variants that have been extensively characterized, including PNPLA3, TM6SF2, and GCKR. Alterations in the PNPLA3 gene are recognized for their propensity to elevate the likelihood of hepatic lipid accumulation and inflammatory responses.

A research investigation conducted within the Chinese Han demographic suggested that the PNPLA3 I148M and TM6SF2 E167K polymorphisms might confer a protective influence against coronary heart disease (CHD) by attenuating serum triglyceride and low-density lipoprotein (LDL) levels [12]. Polymorphisms within the GCKR gene did not correlate with an augmented risk of coronary artery disease (CAD) in NAFLD patients of North Han Chinese descent, as demonstrated through a case-control study [13]. Carriers of the alleles associated with GCKR exhibited no significant alterations in fasting plasma glucose or serum triglyceride concentrations [13]. Likewise, within the framework of the IMPROVE study, genetic variants of PNPLA3, TM6SF2, and GCKR did not demonstrate associations with markers of subclinical atherosclerosis [14]. Furthermore, a comprehensive exome-wide association study encompassing over 300,000 participants revealed that the PNPLA3 variants p.ILE148met and TM6SF2 p.Glu167Lys were linked to a reduction in blood triglycerides and LDL-C levels, alongside a diminished risk of coronary heart disease, notwithstanding elevated hepatic lipid content [15].

In a cohort analysis performed in Italy, the PNPLA3 GG genotype was found to be associated with heightened severity of carotid atherosclerosis in young individuals diagnosed with NAFLD [16]; in contrast, investigations in China identified the PNPLA3 CC genotype, rather than the GG genotype, as being correlated with an increased susceptibility to subclinical atherosclerosis [17]. Dongiovanni and his associates illustrated that individuals afflicted with non-alcoholic steatohepatitis (NASH) who possessed the TM6SF2 E167K variant exhibited lowered serum lipid levels (triglycerides and total cholesterol), were more predisposed to hepatic damage, and had a greater likelihood of developing carotid plaques compared to non-carriers [18].

The methodology of Mendelian randomization has also been employed to clarify the causal nexus between NAFLD and atherosclerosis.

In a cohort study involving the Danish populace (n = 94,708; IHD: 10,897), Lauridsen et al. reported that the risk of ischemic heart disease escalated progressively alongside increasing liver lipid content (OR 2.41, 95% CI 1.28–4.51; P = 0.004), with the corresponding odds ratio for ischemic heart disease among subjects with versus without NAFLD being (OR 2.41, 95% CI 1.28–4.51; P = 0.004). The likelihood difference (LD) was calculated to be 1.65 (95% CI 1.34 to 2.04; $P = 3 \times 10^{-6}$) [19].

The principles of Mendelian randomization have been leveraged to enhance understanding of the causal interplay between non-alcoholic fatty liver disease (NAFLD) and atherosclerosis. In a cohort investigation involving the Danish population (n = 94,708; ischemic heart disease: 10,897), Lauridsen et al. disclosed that the probability of ischemic heart disease augmented progressively in conjunction with rising liver lipid accumulation (odds ratio 2.41, 95% confidence interval 1.28–4.51; P = 0.004), with the respective odds ratio for ischemic heart disease among individuals with NAFLD compared to those without being (odds ratio 2.41, 95% confidence interval 1.28–4.51; P = 0.004). The calculated likelihood differential was ascertained to be 1.65 (95% confidence interval 1.34 to 2.04; $P = 3 \times 10^{-6}$) [19].

A progressive accumulation of hepatic lipids was additionally noted in individuals possessing the PNPLA3 I148M MM genotype in contrast to those with genotype II, demonstrating an odds ratio of 2.03 (95% CI 1.52 to 2.70; $P = 3 \times 10^{-7}$; $P = 3 \times 10^{-7}$) for non-alcoholic fatty liver disease (NAFLD).

4. Potential mechanisms of NAFLD

While the specific proatherogenic pathways associated with non-alcoholic fatty liver disease (NAFLD) continue to be the subject of extensive investigation, a multitude of studies have proposed credible insights into the essential mechanisms that govern the intricate interactions between hepatic function and cardiovascular wellness.

A variety of mechanisms, encompassing insulin resistance (IR), dyslipidemia, systemic inflammation, and oxidative stress attributable to NAFLD, have been identified as facilitators of endothelial cell injury, the activation of inflammatory cells, the promotion of foam cell development, and the stimulation of smooth muscle cell proliferation within arterial walls, ultimately contributing to the advancement of atherosclerosis.

The presence of metabolic syndrome alongside diabetes mellitus can worsen the complex interactions between non-alcoholic fatty liver disease and atherosclerosis, due to shared risk factors.

In **Figure 1**, the complex dynamics of NAFLD and atherosclerosis are shown.

4.1 Proatherogenic mechanism of cardiovascular diseases and direct contributors

Insulin resistance is implicated in a multitude of dysmetabolic phenomena, encompassing lipid metabolism, glucose metabolism, oxidative stress activation, and inflammation, thereby engendering a proatherogenic milieu that predisposes individuals to the development of atherosclerosis [20]. Insulin resistance, which is a pivotal characteristic of non-alcoholic fatty liver disease (NAFLD), is marked by diminished insulin sensitivity not only within hepatic tissue but also in skeletal muscle and adipose tissue, thereby fostering the progression of atherosclerosis [20]. Consequently, insulin resistance instigates lipolysis within adipose tissue, resulting in the catabolism of triglycerides stored in adipocytes, which subsequently liberates free fatty acids [20]. These liberated free fatty acids are subsequently translocated to the liver, where they facilitate the synthesis of apolipoprotein B, a structural protein that constitutes a principal component of very low-density lipoproteins (VLDL) [21].

The impairment of insulin signaling attributable to insulin resistance further hinders the degradation of apolipoprotein B, thereby augmenting the production of VLDL in hepatocytes [22]. VLDLs are secreted by hepatic cells into the circulatory

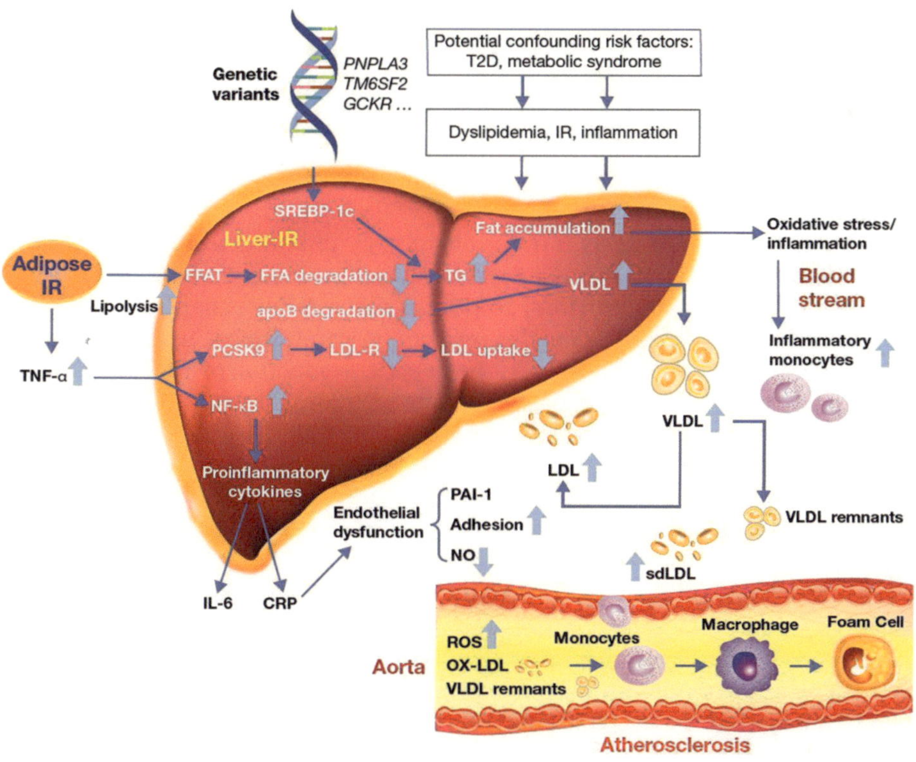

Figure 1.
Proatherogenic mechanisms of NAFLD.

system, with their remnants swiftly permeating the arterial wall, consequently inducing endothelial dysfunction and promoting the recruitment of inflammatory monocytes, which ultimately leads to the accumulation of foam cells [21]. Insulin resistance is a fundamental aspect that underlies various metabolic disorders, including type 2 diabetes (T2D) and metabolic syndrome. Therefore, insulin resistance serves as a common pathophysiological mechanism that interconnects these aforementioned conditions with NAFLD. Insulin resistance can thus be regarded as a critical determinant in atherosclerotic cardiovascular disease (ASCVD), as it is associated with impaired glucose tolerance, visceral adiposity, obesity, metabolic syndrome, and type 2 diabetes, all of which are correlated with an elevated risk of NAFLD.

Atherogenic dyslipidemia is characterized by elevated concentrations of triglycerides, low-density lipoproteins (LDL), and reduced levels of high-density lipoprotein (HDL-C) cholesterol [21]. The liver assumes a pivotal role in the metabolism of lipoproteins, and this metabolic pathway is disrupted in individuals afflicted with NAFLD, leading to the upregulation of sterol-regulatory element-binding protein 1c (SREBP-1c). SREBP-1c is acknowledged for its regulatory roles in de novo lipogenesis as well as in the metabolism of triglyceride-rich lipoproteins [23].

De novo lipogenesis plays a pivotal role in the pathophysiology of non-alcoholic fatty liver disease (NAFLD) by promoting the accumulation of hepatic lipids through enhanced triglyceride synthesis and reduced fatty acid catabolism, consequently exacerbating the atherogenic lipid profile [23]. Beyond the dysregulation of lipoprotein metabolism, low-density lipoproteins (LDL) derived from pro-atherogenic very low-density lipoprotein 1 (VLDL1), a subclass characterized by elevated triglyceride levels, exhibit a propensity to infiltrate the arterial wall, thereby facilitating the development of atherosclerotic plaques in individuals afflicted with NAFLD [21]. Furthermore, the manifestation of inflammation constitutes a critical aspect of NAFLD [24]. The lipid accumulation within hepatic tissue, in conjunction with oxidative stress, has the potential to incite the secretion of inflammatory cytokines.

An augmentation in systemic inflammation has been documented in individuals with NAFLD, as evidenced by elevated levels of tumor necrosis factor (TNF) -α, interleukin (IL) -6, and high-sensitivity C-reactive protein (hs-CRP), among a variety of other biomarkers [24]. These pro-inflammatory cytokines, released into the systemic circulation, exert a direct impact on the advancement of atherosclerosis. TNF-α is integral in facilitating inflammatory responses. Considerable quantities of TNF-α are secreted into the bloodstream by insulin-resistant visceral adipose tissue [25].

This phenomenon, in turn, prompts the hepatic production of TNF-α, which augments the expression of pivotal molecules pertinent to lipid metabolism, inflammatory cytokines, and fibrotic processes within the liver [25]. Elevated concentrations of TNF-α are associated with an increased probability of coronary events. Moreover, in addition to being upregulated by inflammatory mediators, genetic polymorphisms of TNF-α can modulate protein expression, thereby affecting predisposition to cardiovascular disease (CVD). A particular study indicated that the presence of TNF-α polymorphisms at positions 238 and 308 among patients with NAFLD was linked to an elevated risk of developing coronary heart disease (CAD) [26].

Prior investigations have demonstrated that the exposure of hepatocytes to TNF-α leads to the upregulation of proprotein convertase subtilisin/kexin type 9 (PCSK9), a protein that is critical for the regulation of lipid metabolism [27, 28]. PCSK9, secreted by hepatocytes, modifies LDL absorption by facilitating the degradation of LDL receptors. In a specific study, circulating levels of PCSK9 were shown to have a positive correlation with the severity of fatty liver disease [29].

As a result, it is plausible to argue that TNF-α supports the upregulation of PCSK9 expression, which subsequently hinders LDL metabolism, causing a further rise in the elevated LDL cholesterol levels frequently observed in atherosclerotic conditions. With the understanding that medical approaches that focus on reducing PCSK9 can effectively drop cardiovascular mortality figures, and recognizing the data suggesting circulating PCSK9 is a factor in vascular damage, and it is reasonable to think that the irregular secretion of PCSK9 in individuals suffering from NAFLD could be a key factor in the emergence of atherosclerosis [29].

Elevated circulating concentrations of interleukin-6 (IL-6) have been correlated with the incidence of cardiovascular disease, presenting as endothelial impairment, increased arterial rigidity, and the advancement of atherosclerosis [30]. Furthermore, IL-6 serves as the principal hepatic inducer for the biosynthesis of C-reactive protein (CRP). CRP, which is predominantly produced in the liver, is postulated to actively promote the progression of atherosclerosis by enhancing the expression of plasminogen activator inhibitor-1 (PAI-1) and adhesion molecules within endothelial cells, diminishing nitric oxide synthesis, and encouraging low-density lipoprotein (LDL) uptake by macrophages [20, 31]. Elevated circulating levels of PAI-1 have been observed in individuals suffering from non-alcoholic fatty liver disease (NAFLD) [30].

An augmented concentration of PAI-1 exerts a direct influence on atherothrombosis by initiating the coagulation cascade through a reduction in fibrinolytic capacity [32].

Oxidative stress, resulting from the accumulation of hepatic lipids, extended insulin resistance (IR), and hyperglycemia, has been recognized as a contributory factor to the heightened risk of cardiovascular disease (CVD) in patients diagnosed with non-alcoholic fatty liver disease (NAFLD), indicating a shared pathophysiological connection between these two conditions. Oxidative stress arises from a disruption in the balance between the production of reactive oxygen species (ROS) and the impairment of antioxidant defense mechanisms [33].

Within the hepatic milieu, ROS are implicated in the upregulation of proinflammatory cytokines, as well as in the mechanisms of apoptosis and fibrosis, thereby intensifying oxidative stress and perpetuating a detrimental cycle [33].

An elevation in reactive oxygen species (ROS) negatively influences endothelial activity, eventually causing the development and sustained accumulation of oxidized low-density lipoproteins (LDL) in the subendothelial zone [34].

In addition, ROS has the potential to improve the process of converting macrophages into foam cells by means of oxidative modification of LDL, which is a vital contributor to the emergence of atherosclerotic lesions [34], and may lead to lipid degradation, thereby predisposing the tissue to inflammatory responses, which introduces additional atherogenic stimuli into an already oxidative and pro-inflammatory milieu. In aggregate, the pro-inflammatory environment originating from the liver is likely to facilitate plaque formation, alter vascular tone, and compromise endothelial function, potentially contributing to the continuum of atherosclerosis.

4.2 Proatherogenic mechanism of cardiovascular diseases and indirect contributors

Traditional risk factors associated with atherosclerotic cardiovascular disease (ASCVD), including type 2 diabetes mellitus (T2DM) and metabolic syndrome (MetS), concurrently function as determinants of non-alcoholic fatty liver disease (NAFLD) risk, thereby introducing confounding variables in the analysis of atherosclerotic cardiovascular events among individuals diagnosed with NAFLD [35]. Moreover, individuals afflicted with NAFLD exhibit an elevated propensity for the development of diabetes and MetS, both of which are acknowledged as significant risk factors for ASCVD. Empirical investigations have demonstrated a positive association between NAFLD and an augmented risk of ASCVD in patients suffering from type 2 diabetes. A specific meta-analysis contrasting patients with type 2 diabetes, both with and without NAFLD, revealed a synergistic escalation in cardiovascular risk attributable to the concomitant presence of T2D and NAFLD [36]. Likewise, individuals with NAFLD presented an elevated risk of cardiovascular events in comparison with their counterparts without NAFLD, irrespective of the presence of MetS, with the risk being further exacerbated in conjunction with the presence of liver fibrosis [37].

This investigation asserts that in individuals possessing equivalent conventional risk factors for ASCVD, the probability of experiencing atherosclerotic events is markedly heightened in the context of NAFLD, thereby suggesting that NAFLD may confer an additional risk of ASCVD that surpasses the implications of preexisting metabolic disorders.

5. The clinical implications of NAFLD on ASCVD

There is a growing corpus of evidence delineating the relationship between non-alcoholic fatty liver disease (NAFLD), subclinical atherosclerosis, and more overt atherosclerotic manifestations [1–5, 9, 37–40]. Through the assessment of vascular calcification, carotid intima-media thickness (C-IMT), and aortic stiffness, these studies facilitate the evaluation of whether NAFLD constitutes an independent risk factor with the capacity to forecast the onset of atherosclerotic cardiovascular disease (ASCVD) [1–5, 38–40]. A plethora of studies have investigated coronary artery calcification (CAC), which is widely acknowledged as a reliable surrogate marker indicative of atherosclerotic burden in individuals with NAFLD [1–4, 38–40]. Individuals diagnosed with NAFLD appear to have a correlation with the progression of CAC, even when controlling for various confounding variables and metabolic risk factors. A recent meta-analysis encompassing a cohort of 10,060 participants revealed that patients with NAFLD significantly elevated the risk of subclinical atherosclerosis, particularly concerning the progression of CAC (OR 1.50, 95% CI 1.34–1.68; $P = 0.001$) [41], thus implying that NAFLD functions as an independent risk factor in the advancement of CAC.

A prospective community investigation carried out in Kailuan involving Chinese adult participants revealed that non-alcoholic fatty liver disease (NAFLD) was independently associated with an elevation in carotid intima-media thickness (C-IMT) after controlling for traditional cardiovascular risk factors (OR 1.663, 95% CI 1.391–1.989, $P < 0.0001$) [5]. Notably, NAFLD has been recognized as a contributing risk factor for subclinical atherosclerosis across various ethnic groups, as substantiated by a recent meta-analysis encompassing 172,385 individuals across 64 studies [42]. Collectively, this body of research indicates that individuals diagnosed with NAFLD exhibit a more pronounced association with subclinical atherosclerosis, as evidenced by the detection of atherosclerotic plaques, non-calcified plaques, coronary artery calcification (CAC) scores, and C-IMT, in comparison with individuals without NAFLD. The majority of these investigations have determined that this correlation persists independently of established cardiovascular risk factors, which include type 2 diabetes mellitus (T2D), hypertension, and dyslipidemia. An increasing number of studies have elucidated the complexities of the relationship between NAFLD and advanced atherosclerotic phenomena, such as coronary artery disease (CAD), myocardial infarction (MI), and ischemic stroke (IS) [9, 37, 43–46]. Despite the findings of the study conducted by Alexander et al. approaching null results [9], a substantial fraction of these inquiries corroborates the independent influence of NAFLD on atherosclerotic cardiovascular disease (ASCVD) following rigorous adjustments for cardiovascular disease (CVD) risk factors. Consequently, NAFLD is positioned as a pertinent risk factor for cardiovascular events. However, the imperative for long-term, prospective cohort studies with augmented sample sizes remains to elucidate the causal interplay between NAFLD and ASCVD, which could ultimately facilitate the stratification of individual risk profiles and inform therapeutic strategies.

6. Diagnosis

6.1 Diagnosis of non-alcoholic fatty liver disease (NAFLD) is independently *associated with cardiovascular risk*

The identification of non-alcoholic fatty liver disease (NAFLD) is established subsequent to the exclusion of viral, autoimmune, and genetic hepatic disorders (for instance, Wilson's disease, hereditary hemochromatosis, and alpha-1 antitrypsin deficiency), as well as excessive alcohol consumption, defined as ≥30 g per day for males and ≥ 20 g per day for females, in alignment with European clinical practice guidelines concerning the management of NAFLD [47]. The NAFLD fibrosis score (NFS) is computed as delineated by [48]. In essence, the NFS amalgamates variables such as age, body mass index (BMI), the current presence of impaired fasting blood glucose or diabetes, aspartate aminotransferase (AST), alanine aminotransferase (ALT), platelet count, and serum albumin levels to categorize patients based on their likelihood of significant fibrosis. More specifically, individuals with an NFS of less than −1.455 are classified within the F0–2 category, those with an NFS exceeding 0.676 are designated as "F3–4," while patients with an NFS ranging from −1.455 to 0.676 are regarded as "intermediaries." The diagnosis of metabolic syndrome is confirmed when three or more of the following conditions are fulfilled [49]: a fasting blood glucose level of ≥100 mg/dL or the commencement of antidiabetic therapy, a waist circumference exceeding 102 cm in males and 88 cm in females, blood pressure readings of ≥130/85 mmHg or the recent administration of antihypertensive medications, plasma triglyceride concentrations of ≥150 mg/dL, and plasma high-density lipoprotein (HDL) cholesterol levels falling below 40 mg/dL in males and below 50 mg/dL in females.

The non-alcoholic fatty liver disease (NFS) score functions both as a prognostic marker for advanced hepatic fibrosis and as an indicator of cardiovascular risk. Specifically, the NFS has proven effective in discerning patients who are at the highest risk for recurrent cardiovascular events. The evaluation of cardiovascular risk is critical and may be conducted in individuals with cardiovascular disease utilizing the Framingham risk score (FRS), which demonstrates elevated values in patients diagnosed with non-alcoholic fatty liver disease (NAFLD).

The most prominent relationship between cardiovascular risk and NFS is attributed to the fact that this scoring system incorporates a multitude of factors, including age, body mass index (BMI), alanine aminotransferase (ALT), aspartate aminotransferase (AST), platelet count, serum albumin levels, and the presence or absence of diabetes; all these essential elements reflect metabolic processes and underlying inflammatory states. It is imperative to acknowledge that inflammation and fibrosis are acknowledged as defining features of hepatic and cardiovascular pathologies [48], which may ultimately imply the existence of shared systemic mechanisms.

6.2 Cardiovascular risk assessment in patients with non-alcoholic fatty liver disease (NAFLD)

In accordance with the collaborative clinical practice guidelines formulated by EASL-EASD-EASO regarding the management of individuals diagnosed with NAFLD [47], it is imperative that a non-invasive assessment be utilized as a preliminary screening tool to evaluate the severity of the disease. Depending on the outcomes yielded by this assessment, patients will be categorized into distinct groups classified as low, intermediate, and high risk in relation to the likelihood of advanced fibrosis. For those individuals classified within the low-risk group, it is crucial that their specific cardiovascular risk be evaluated employing risk stratification instruments, such as the Framingham risk score (FRS). Target objectives for modifiable risk factors, encompassing, but not limited to, blood pressure, low-density lipoprotein (LDL) cholesterol, body mass index, and glycemic control, should be attained in accordance with established primary prevention protocols [50]. It is vital to recommend that patients identified as being at intermediate or high risk of advanced fibrosis be referred to a hepatology specialist for further specialized assessment. In scenarios where patients present with an advanced stage of fibrosis or cirrhosis, it is prudent that the cardiovascular risk be evaluated by a qualified cardiologist, as suggested by Choudhary and Duseja [51]. All remaining patients will undergo a comprehensive clinical evaluation, stratified according to a cardiovascular risk score and managed in alignment with pertinent prevention guidelines [50].

6.3 Screening for NAFLD in cardiovascular patients

In individuals who have experienced a cardiovascular event (CV) or those demonstrating elevated cardiovascular risk, it is recommended to utilize a systematic methodology for the detection of non-alcoholic fatty liver disease (NAFLD). As an initial screening instrument, the non-alcoholic fatty liver disease (NFS) fibrosis score will be computed. For individuals assessed to be at low risk of advanced fibrosis, it is prudent to advocate for lifestyle modifications. Those categorized at intermediate risk should be referred for liver ultrasound imaging and consultation with a hepatologist possessing expertise in transient elastography.

Should these assessments not reveal fibrosis or suggest a low stage of fibrosis, management should adhere to established protocols pertinent to the low-risk population. In contrast, for individuals with an intermediate NFS score who present with advanced stage fibrosis or cirrhosis upon subsequent evaluations, as well as for those designated with a high-risk NFS score, it is imperative to seek consultation with a hepatologist. It is important to acknowledge that the NFS was initially developed to estimate fibrosis within the framework of NAFLD.

Nevertheless, we propose the NFS as a cost-effective and non-invasive "screening tool" for the detection of NAFLD in patients who have experienced a cardiovascular event or who possess elevated cardiovascular risk. All patients should be managed in accordance with the current guidelines established by the European Society of Cardiology [52].

6.4 How is NAFLD/NASH diagnosed?

Non-alcoholic fatty liver disease (NAFLD) encompasses two distinct clinico-pathological categories: simple steatosis, which typically manifests a benign and non-progressive clinical trajectory, and non-alcoholic steatohepatitis (NASH), which possesses the potential to advance to cirrhosis and hepatocellular carcinoma. The diagnostic criteria for NAFLD are predicated upon three fundamental components: the absence of alcohol consumption, the detection of steatosis through imaging techniques or histopathological assessment, and the comprehensive exclusion of alternative hepatic disorders. The determination of NAFLD is contingent upon the identification of the following three critical criteria: the non-consumption of alcoholic beverages, the recognition of steatosis via imaging methodologies or histological examination, and the meticulous exclusion of other hepatic pathologies [53–55].

The identification of NASH is reliant upon the detection of steatohepatitis through liver biopsy. In light of the present absence of surrogate biomarkers for the diagnosis of NAFLD, it is imperative to exclude other hepatic diseases, including alcoholic liver disease, viral hepatitis, autoimmune liver conditions, and metabolic or hereditary liver disorders. Nevertheless, due to the exceedingly high prevalence of NAFLD, it is frequently complicated by concomitant hepatic conditions such as viral hepatitis, among others, and NAFLD exacerbates hepatic injury while diminishing the efficacy of therapeutic strategies. Epidemiological studies have indicated that alcoholic liver disease may manifest when daily alcohol intake surpasses 20 g for females and 30 g for males. Consequently, NAFLD is diagnosed when alcohol consumption remains below these specified thresholds for each sex. NAFLD is not only correlated with hepatic morbidity and mortality; it is also associated with considerable extrahepatic complications, including cardiovascular disease (CVD) [54].

6.5 The diagnosis of non-alcoholic fatty liver disease (NAFLD) is independently associated with cardiovascular risk

Cardiovascular disease (CVD) is prevalent and ranks among the foremost causes of mortality globally, impacting both the general population and individuals diagnosed with NAFLD [56, 57].

NAFLD exhibits an independent association with various markers of subclinical atherosclerosis, which encompass coronary artery calcification, diminished flow-mediated vasodilation, heightened arterial stiffness, inflammation, and thickening of the carotid artery intima-media, alongside left ventricular hypertrophy and diastolic dysfunction [58, 59].

6.6 The influence of non-alcoholic fatty liver disease and metabolic syndrome on the progression of coronary artery calcification

The coronary artery calcification score (CAC), which is measured through multi-detector computed tomography (MDCT), acts as a metric for the comprehensive accumulation of coronary plaques, with an elevated CAC score indicating future coronary events in an independent and progressive manner [60]. Recent investigations have demonstrated that the advancement of CAC scores is significantly associated with an augmented probability of subsequent cardiovascular disease (CVD) occurrences and overall mortality [61, 62]. Given that atherosclerosis represents a dynamic process, enhancements in the CAC score yield a more precise depiction of atherosclerosis progression relative to the baseline CAC score, thereby aiding in the evaluation of medical interventions' efficacy and the estimation of prospective cardiovascular event risks [61–63]. A recent meta-analysis has established a significant positive correlation between non-alcoholic fatty liver disease (NAFLD) and CAC, thereby sustaining the assertion that NAFLD serves as an independent predictor of CVD [64].

Prior studies have suggested an elevated risk of CAC among individuals diagnosed with NAFLD [61–66].

Although the pathophysiological mechanisms through which non-alcoholic fatty liver disease (NAFLD) exerts an influence on the progression of coronary artery calcification (CAC) are not exhaustively delineated in this chapter, numerous plausible mechanisms have been articulated [67–73]. Endothelial dysfunction within the systemic circulation, acknowledged as the preliminary phase in the onset of coronary atherosclerosis, has been documented in instances of NAFLD [67, 68].

Furthermore, a multitude of studies have demonstrated a positive correlation between hepatic fat content and prothrombotic factors, which encompass factors VII, IX, XI, and XII, in addition to the plasminogen activator inhibitor-1 [69, 70]. Consequently, this procoagulant imbalance linked to NAFLD may signify a causal relationship between NAFLD and cardiovascular diseases.

Elevated oxidative stress may additionally elucidate the heightened cardiovascular risk associated with NAFLD. Plasma homocysteine, identified as a cardiovascular risk factor, induces detrimental effects on the cardiovascular endothelium and smooth muscle cells, with elevated plasma homocysteine levels having been consistently documented in individuals with NAFLD [71, 72].

Lastly, given that the liver contains the highest concentration of macrophages and immune cells, the cytokines generated by the compromised liver have been regarded as one of the primary pathogenic mechanisms responsible for systemic inflammation, which subsequently contributes to cardiovascular disease [73]. While the pathophysiological mechanisms are not thoroughly examined in this paragraph, the aforementioned mechanisms may offer insights into the relationship between NAFLD and the progression of CAC.

The progression of coronary artery calcification (CAC) can be defined as (1) the occurrence of an incident CAC, denoting an Agatston score of zero but revealing detectable CAC upon subsequent evaluations in a cohort that exhibited no CAC at the initial assessment [74, 75] or (2) an increase of ≥2.5 units between the reference value and the final square root of the CAC scores in subjects with detectable CAC at baseline [61–79].

The CAC score can be computed utilizing an automated software application in conjunction with the Agatston scoring methodology [76], and participants classified according to cut-off values established by Greenland et al. [77] (none, 0; mild, 1 to 100; moderate, 101 to 300; severe, >300).

7. Management: NAFLD as a potential target for ASCVD

7.1 Evidence-based guidelines and expert recommendations

Patients diagnosed with non-alcoholic fatty liver disease (NAFLD) display a markedly increased risk of cardiovascular morbidity and mortality; therefore, it is imperative to rigorously address cardiovascular disease (CVD) risk factors concomitantly with the management of hepatic conditions themselves [46]. Within the framework of China, it is recognized that individuals afflicted with NAFLD undergo comprehensive assessments and continuous monitoring regarding the risks and complications associated with atherosclerotic cardiovascular disease (ASCVD) [2]. Lifestyle changes, which comprise adjustments in nutritional intake, weight loss, and waist circumference reduction, are endorsed as both preventive and therapeutic interventions for NAFLD by lessening cardiovascular risk factors [2–4]. The provision of pharmacotherapeutic interventions should be ensured for patients with NAFLD who have not succeeded in managing their metabolic risk factors. The agents that inhibit the renin-angiotensin pathway are recognized for their capacity to enhance insulin resistance (IR), lower blood pressure, and provide protection for individuals affected by NAFLD; additionally, omega-3 polyunsaturated fatty acids are essential for liver fat retention and the management of triglyceride-enriched lipoproteins, which significantly influence the progression of atherosclerosis in patients with NAFLD; moreover, omega-3 polyunsaturated fatty acids affect the accumulation of lipids in the liver and the breakdown of triglyceride-rich lipoproteins, which are pivotal in the discourse surrounding NAFLD. Moreover, GLP-1 receptor agonists have indicated their skill in lowering heart-related mortality and positively affecting NAFLD, whereas statins could be utilized to cut LDL-C levels and lessen heart disease risk, all while ensuring a safe liver profile, except for those experiencing liver failure and decompensated cirrhosis [2–4]. Individuals with NAFLD might find that Metformin and Pioglitazone serve as valuable supplementary drugs for reducing cardiovascular risks. The preceding choice proves effective in managing insulin resistance without adverse effects on the liver, whereas the subsequent consideration is crucial for patients with NAFLD and type 2 diabetes who might display higher vulnerability to cardiovascular issues.

7.2 Stratification of the risk of ASCVD according to the severity of NAFLD

Non-alcoholic fatty liver disease (NAFLD) frequently coexists with various other metabolic disorders. The existence of these accompanying medical conditions may have a multiplicative outcome, thus promoting the swift progression of atherosclerosis. Observations imply that individuals managing both NAFLD and metabolic syndrome (MetS) likely face an increased risk of aggravating atherosclerosis [2, 35].

The presence of elevated fatty liver disease markers or pronounced NAFLD severity is notably tied to a higher risk of cardiovascular outcomes, including heart attacks and ischemic strokes. As a further point, an important association has been noted between the aggravated severity of NAFLD and a marked escalation in type 2 diabetes mellitus (T2D) cases [35, 36]. The implementation of standardized diagnostic modalities for the identification of NAFLD, as well as an accurate evaluation of its severity [2, 4], can facilitate the assessment of ASCVD risk, thereby underscoring the potential advantages of early preventive strategies and therapeutic interventions. Numerous international guidelines advocate for the systematic screening or periodic assessment of patients diagnosed with NAFLD to identify additional metabolic syndromes and cardiovascular risk factors [2, 4]. In alignment with standard clinical practice, the management of ASCVD in patients diagnosed with NAFLD necessitates a comprehensive risk stratification approach to effectively guide the medical management of the condition.

7.3 Lifestyle modification

Lifestyle modifications, including weight reduction, dietary regulation, and enhanced physical activity, constitute the cornerstone of NAFLD management [2–4]. The goal is to improve insulin sensitivity and decrease visceral fat, thus minimizing the likelihood of extrahepatic complications like ASCVD. A body weight reduction of at least 3–5% has shown to improve fatty liver; a decrease of 7% or greater is necessary for lowering serum transaminases and moderating NASH; and losing a minimum of 10% is needed to reverse liver scarring. Pharmacological agents aimed at weight reduction may be suitable and effective in achieving sustained weight loss, particularly among obese patients; however, the adverse effects of such medications necessitate vigilant monitoring, with long-term usage being discouraged [2]. Maintaining a schedule of steady moderate cardiovascular workouts and/or resistance exercises has been proven to significantly decrease liver fat [2, 4]. Taking part in habitual physical activity positively affects typical risk components associated with both NAFLD and ASCVD, encompassing insulin resistance (IR), heightened triglyceride levels, obesity, and lower amounts of high-density lipoprotein cholesterol [80]. With respect to dietary recommendations, guidelines advocate for a caloric intake reduction of 500–1000 kcal to facilitate a weight loss of 0.5 to 1.0 kg per week [2–4]. To lower the chances of worsening liver fibrosis or suffering from acute liver injury, it is smart to limit alcohol intake; however, having alcohol in moderation could potentially have good impacts on NAFLD.

7.4 Therapeutic approaches to reducing ASCVD risk in patients with NAFLD

7.4.1 Hypolipidemic agents

Statins represent a class of pharmacological agents that markedly diminish cholesterol concentrations and have been empirically validated to mitigate the risk of atherosclerotic cardiovascular disease (ASCVD). Given the elevated incidence of atherosclerotic complications in patients afflicted with non-alcoholic fatty liver disease (NAFLD) and non-alcoholic steatohepatitis (NASH), it has been hypothesized that these individuals could experience considerable therapeutic gains from statin intervention. The perspectives offered in the Chinese protocols about the prevention and treatment of non-alcoholic fatty liver disease, when combined with findings from the European Association for the Study of the Liver, indicate that statins are viewed as safe for those facing NAFLD and NASH, promoting a decrease in low-density lipoprotein cholesterol (LDL-C) and diminishing heart-related problems.

It remains essential to note that, as things are today, there have not been any randomized controlled trials that thoroughly assess how statins affect NASH and liver fibrosis. However, two post-hoc analyses derived from robust prospective randomized clinical trials elucidated the impact of statins on NASH; specifically, the IDEAL and GREACE studies demonstrated that statin therapy led to significant enhancements in both NAFLD and cardiovascular outcomes in patients presenting with elevated transaminase levels [81, 82]. Consequently, one may deduce that statins could provide protective effects in both cardiovascular and hepatic domains, notwithstanding a slight risk associated with increased liver transaminases [2–5].

Xuezhikang (XZK), an extract derived from red yeast rice, is predominantly utilized in traditional Chinese medicine and is regarded as a natural hypolipidemic agent for the management of ASCVD, additionally imparting beneficial effects on hepatic health [83, 84]. Within a multicenter assessment, individuals afflicted with dyslipidemia who had XZK treatment experienced a 27% lessening in LDL-C when contrasted with those on a placebo; furthermore, notable reductions in other atherogenic lipoproteins were recorded in this demographic [84]. A thorough examination that followed the Chinese Secondary Prevention of Coronary Heart Disease Study, which was a detailed randomized controlled trial focused on assessing how well XZK could lower cardiovascular incidents in comparison with a placebo, was carried out involving 820 individuals experiencing mild to moderate liver irregularities, indicated by serum alanine aminotransferase values not exceeding three times the normal upper limit. Over a follow-up period of 4.5 years, XZK was found to enhance both lipid and hepatic profiles in individuals with abnormal liver tests; intriguingly, the risk reduction associated with XZK for major coronary events was markedly greater in patients with abnormal liver tests (n = 401) than in those with normal liver tests (n = 1781) (76.3% versus 40.1%, P = 0.009) [83].

The findings presented herein robustly support the clinical advantages and the sustained safety profile of XZK within contexts characterized by hepatic irregularities.

PCSK9 is a protein that has been connected to the intricate relationship between non-alcoholic fatty liver disease (NAFLD) and atherosclerosis, with PCSK9 inhibitors coming forth as a new category of lipid-lowering therapies that successfully cut down LDL-C levels and foster the reduction of cardiovascular incidents. A short while back, PCSK9 inhibitors have been highlighted as encouraging therapeutic interventions that could alleviate NAFLD through the suppression of lipid storage in liver tissue [85]. In a recent retrospective investigation, a cohort of 29 patients receiving PCSK9 inhibitors was scrutinized to ascertain whether this hypolipidemic pharmacological agent could enhance hepatic fatty infiltration. The individuals involved in the study received PCSK9 inhibitor therapy for roughly 23.7 months, which resulted in a statistically relevant uptick in serum alanine aminotransferase and aspartate aminotransferase. In a cohort of 11 persons diagnosed with fatty liver disease, eight noted complete resolution post-treatment with PCSK9 inhibitors. In a distinct analysis, the utilization of berberine, a natural hypolipidemic phytochemical acknowledged for its capacity to reduce PCSK9 levels, was demonstrated to be efficacious in decreasing hepatic fat levels and enhancing the lipid profile [86]. To establish the cardiovascular and liver benefits of PCSK9 inhibitors regarding NAFLD/NASH, extensive and comprehensive randomized controlled trials are crucial.

7.4.2 Novel agents for glucose regulation

GLP-1 receptor agonists (RAs) demonstrate hypoglycemic properties that can substantially diminish body mass while concurrently providing cardiovascular advantages. Research findings imply that GLP-1 receptor agonists may assist in achieving a modest enhancement in the handling of non-alcoholic fatty liver disease (NAFLD) and lessen the probability of encountering significant cardiovascular complications. In the phase IIb LEAN investigation, a sample of 52 obese individuals with a diagnosis of non-alcoholic steatohepatitis (NASH) receiving liraglutide at a regular dosage of 1.8 mg demonstrated considerably elevated rates of NASH resolution throughout a timeframe of 48 weeks in contrast to the control group [87]. Furthermore, it has been noted that liraglutide could be tied to a reduction in carotid intima-media thickness (C-IMT) among those with a diagnosis of type 2 diabetes mellitus (T2DM) and NAFLD [88]. Research indicates that semaglutide, a GLP-1 RA, is effective in addressing NAFLD/NASH by lowering inflammatory cytokine levels in liver tissues and alleviating atherosclerotic changes in mouse models at risk for atherosclerosis. Recent findings regarding the application of semaglutide indicated that a majority of patients were inclined to experience resolution of NASH without exacerbation of fibrosis in a dose-dependent fashion when contrasted with placebo [89]. While the exact therapeutic pathways through which GLP-1 RAs display their influence on NAFLD still lack complete clarity, studies have suggested that these compounds improve key factors associated with NAFLD through an incretin action and directly influence lipid handling in liver cells, all the while reducing inflammation in the liver, thus aiding in the reversal of NAFLD advancement and lowering the chances of atherosclerotic cardiovascular disease (ASCVD) [5, 87, 90]. Further investigations are essential to yield significant mechanistic insights into the capacity of GLP-1 RAs to confer cardiovascular benefits through the resolution of NAFLD or NASH. Sodium-glucose cotransporter-2 (SGLT-2) antagonists achieve their purpose by restricting glucose intake in the kidneys, resulting in decreased blood sugar levels and remarkable weight loss. The SGLT-2 inhibitors elicit a multitude of advantageous effects that mitigate the onset of cardiomyopathy [91–93]. A comprehensive review of randomized trials by Wei and colleagues indicated that SGLT-2 inhibitors resulted in elevated liver enzymes, reduced hepatic fat, and decreased body weight, thereby leading to an improvement in liver fibrosis for individuals with NAFLD and T2DM. An additional modern meta-analysis that included 1498 individuals with NAFLD substantiated these findings, showcasing that SGLT-2 inhibitors contributed to better body mass index (BMI), glucose and lipid metabolism, liver functionality, and liver fibrosis. A preclinical investigation involving mice with atherosclerosis highlighted that treatment with empagliflozin, an SGLT-2 blocker, over 5 weeks significantly curtailed NAFLD progression by boosting autophagy, mitigating endoplasmic reticulum stress, and decreasing liver cell death in susceptible subjects. These studies augment the mechanistic evidence regarding the beneficial impact of SGLT-2 inhibitors on NAFLD and ASCVD.

7.4.3 Innovations in pharmacological management of NAFLD

Contemporary investigations reveal that a considerable array of pharmacological compounds is currently in various stages of development, aimed at targeting specific pathways related to non-alcoholic fatty liver disease (NAFLD). While the predominant emphasis of these compounds is on enhancing histological characteristics of hepatic tissue, it is imperative that cardiovascular parameters are not disregarded, as they warrant greater scholarly scrutiny; this is particularly pertinent given that cardiovascular mortality represents a substantial fraction of extrahepatic mortality linked to NAFLD.

8. Conclusion

This chapter briefly discusses how non-alcoholic steatosis affects atherosclerocardiovascular disease.

Health practitioners can assess risk, perform early screening, and implement treatment strategies for patients at risk of ASCVD due to non-alcoholic steatosis by understanding the strong association between these two diseases.

Author details

Paulin Bilonda Kabeya[1,2]

1 China Medical University, China

2 Sino-Congolese Hospital, Democratic Republic of the Congo, Kinshasa, China

*Address all correspondence to: paulin.bill@gmail.com

References

[1] Sinn DH, Kang D, Chang Y, et al. Non-alcoholic fatty liver disease and progression of coronary artery calcium score: A retrospective cohort study. Gut. 2017;**66**:323-329. DOI: 10.1136/gutjnl-2016-311854

[2] Cho YK, Kang YM, Yoo JH, et al. The impact of non-alcoholic fatty liver disease and metabolic syndrome on the progression of coronary artery calcification. Scientific Reports. 2018;**8**:12004. DOI: 10.1038/s41598-018-30465-y

[3] Gummesson A, Stromberg U, Schmidt C, et al. Non-alcoholic fatty liver disease is a strong predictor of coronary artery calcification in metabolically healthy subjects: A cross-sectional, population-based study in middle-aged subjects. PLoS ONE. 2018;**13**:e0202666. DOI: 10.1371/journal.pone.0202666

[4] Lee SB, Park GM, Lee JY, et al. Association between non-alcoholic fatty liver disease and subclinical coronary atherosclerosis: An observational cohort study. Journal of Hepatology. 2018;**68**:1018-1024. DOI: 10.1016/j.jhep.2017.12.012

[5] Zheng J, Zhou Y, Zhang K, et al. Association between nonalcoholic fatty liver disease and subclinical atherosclerosis: A cross-sectional study on population over 40 years old. BMC Cardiovascular Disorders. 2018;**18**:147. DOI: 10.1186/s12872-018-0877-2

[6] Estes C, Anstee QM, Arias-Loste MT, et al. Modeling NAFLD disease burden in China, France, Germany, Italy, Japan, Spain, United Kingdom, and United States for the period 2016-2030. Journal of Hepatology. 2018;**69**:896-904. DOI: 10.1016/j.jhep.2018.05.036

[7] Pisto P, Santaniemi M, Bloigu R, et al. Fatty liver predicts the risk for cardiovascular events in middle-aged population: A population-based cohort study. BMJ Open. 2014;**4**:e004973. DOI: 10.1136/bmjopen-2014-004973

[8] Adams LA, Lymp JF, St Sauver J, et al. The natural history of nonalcoholic fatty liver disease: A population-based cohort study. Gastroenterology. 2005;**129**:113-121. DOI: 10.1053/j.gastro.2005.04.014

[9] Alexander M, Loomis AK, van der Lei J, et al. Non-alcoholic fatty liver disease and risk of incident acute myocardial infarction and stroke: Findings from matched cohort study of 18 million European adults. BMJ. 2019;**367**:l5367. DOI: 10.1136/bmj.l5367

[10] Zhou F, Zhou J, Wang W, et al. Unexpected rapid increase in the burden of NAFLD in China from 2008 to 2018: A systematic review and meta-analysis. Hepatology. 2019;**70**:1119-1133. DOI: 10.1002/hep.30702

[11] Targher G, Byrne CD, Lonardo A, et al. Non-alcoholic fatty liver disease and risk of incident cardiovascular disease: A meta-analysis. Journal of Hepatology. 2016;**65**:589-600. DOI: 10.1016/j.jhep.2016.05.013

[12] Wu JT, Liu SS, Xie XJ, et al. Independent and joint correlation of PNPLA3 I148M and TM6SF2 E167K variants with the risk of coronary heart disease in patients with non-alcoholic fatty liver disease. Lipids in Health and Disease. 2020;**19**:29. DOI: 10.1186/s12944-020-01207-9

[13] Gao H, Liu S, Zhao Z, et al. Association of GCKR gene polymorphisms with the risk of

nonalcoholic fatty liver disease and coronary artery disease in a Chinese Northern Han Population. Journal of Clinical and Translational Hepatology. 2019;**7**:297-303. DOI: 10.14218/JCTH.2019.00030.21

[14] Castaldo L, Laguzzi F, Strawbridge RJ, et al. Genetic variants associated with non-alcoholic fatty liver disease do not associate with measures of sub-clinical atherosclerosis: Results from the IMPROVE study. Genes (Basel). 2020;**11**:1243. DOI: 10.3390/genes11111243

[15] Liu DJ, Peloso GM, Yu H, et al. Exome-wide association study of plasma lipids in >300,000 individuals. Nature Genetics. 2017;**49**:1758-1766. DOI: 10.1038/ng.3977

[16] Petta S, Valenti L, Marchesini G, et al. PNPLA3 GG genotype and carotid atherosclerosis in patients with non-alcoholic fatty liver disease. PLoS ONE. 2013;**8**:e74089. DOI: 10.1371/journal.pone.0074089

[17] Xia MF, Ling Y, Bian H, et al. I148M variant of PNPLA3 increases the susceptibility to nonalcoholic fatty liver disease caused by obesity and metabolic disorders. Alimentary Pharmacology & Therapeutics. 2016;**43**:631-642. DOI: 10.1111/apt.13521

[18] Dongiovanni P, Petta S, Maglio C, et al. Transmembrane 6 superfamily member 2 gene variant disentangles nonalcoholic steatohepatitis from cardiovascular disease. Hepatology. 2015;**61**:506-514. DOI: 10.1002/hep.27490

[19] Lauridsen BK, Stender S, Kristensen TS, et al. Liver fat content, non-alcoholic fatty liver disease, and ischaemic heart disease: Mendelian randomization and meta-analysis of 279 013 individuals. European Heart Journal. 2018;**39**:385-393. DOI: 10.1093/eurheartj/ehx662

[20] Gaggini M, Morelli M, Buzzigoli E, et al. Non-alcoholic fatty liver disease (NAFLD) and its connection with insulin resistance, dyslipidemia, atherosclerosis and coronary heart disease. Nutrients. 2013;**5**:1544-1560. DOI: 10.3390/nu5051544

[21] Deprince A, Haas JT, Staels B. Dysregulated lipid metabolism links NAFLD to cardiovascular disease. Molecular Metabolism. 2020;**42**:101092. DOI: 10.1016/j.molmet.2020.101092

[22] Haas ME, Attie AD, Biddinger SB. The regulation of ApoB metabolism by insulin. Trends in Endocrinology and Metabolism. 2013;**24**:391-397. DOI: 10.1016/j.tem.2013.04.001

[23] Xu X, Lu L, Dong Q, et al. Research advances in the relationship between nonalcoholic fatty liver disease and atherosclerosis. Lipids in Health and Disease. 2015;**14**:158. DOI: 10.1186/s12944-015-0141-z

[24] Haukeland JW, Damas JK, Konopski Z, et al. Systemic inflammation in nonalcoholic fatty liver disease is characterized by elevated levels of CCL2. Journal of Hepatology. 2006;**44**:1167-1174. DOI: 10.1016/j.jhep.2006.02.011

[25] Stojsavljevic S, Gomercic Palcic M, Virovic Jukic L, et al. Adipokines and proinflammatory cytokines, the key mediators in the pathogenesis of nonalcoholic fatty liver disease. World Journal of Gastroenterology. 2014;**20**:18070-18091. DOI: 10.3748/wjg.v20.i48.18070

[26] Cheng Y, An B, Jiang M, et al. Association of tumor necrosis factor-alpha polymorphisms and risk of coronary artery disease in patients

with non-alcoholic fatty liver disease. Hepatitis Monthly. 2015;**15**:e26818. DOI: 10.5812/hepatmon.26818

[27] Ruscica M, Ricci C, Macchi C, et al. Suppressor of cytokine signaling-3 (SOCS-3) induces proprotein convertase subtilisin kexin type 9 (PCSK9) expression in hepatic HepG2 cell line. The Journal of Biological Chemistry. 2016;**291**:3508-3519. DOI: 10.1074/jbc.M115.664706

[28] Shafiq M, Walmann T, Nutalapati V, et al. Effects of proprotein convertase subtilisin/kexin type-9 inhibitors on fatty liver. World Journal of Hepatology. 2020;**12**:1258-1266. DOI: 10.4254/wjh.v12.i12.1258

[29] Ruscica M, Ferri N, Macchi C, et al. Liver fat accumulation is associated with circulating PCSK9. Annals of Medicine. 2016;**48**:384-391. DOI: 10.1080/07853890.2016.1188328

[30] Simon TG, Trejo MEP, McClelland R, et al. Circulating Interleukin-6 is a biomarker for coronary atherosclerosis in nonalcoholic fatty liver disease: Results from the Multi-Ethnic Study of Atherosclerosis. International Journal of Cardiology. 2018;**259**:198-204. DOI: 10.1016/j.ijcard.2018.01.046

[31] Badimon L, Pena E, Arderiu G, et al. C-reactive protein in atherothrombosis and angiogenesis. Frontiers in Immunology. 2018;**9**:430. DOI: 10.3389/fimmu.2018.00430

[32] Alessi MC, Bastelica D, Mavri A, et al. Plasma PAI-1 levels are more strongly related to liver steatosis than to adipose tissue accumulation. Arteriosclerosis, Thrombosis, and Vascular Biology. 2003;**23**:1262-1268. DOI: 10.1161/01.ATV.0000077401.36885.BB

[33] Ferro D, Baratta F, Pastori D, et al. New insights into the pathogenesis of non-alcoholic fatty liver disease: Gut-derived lipopolysaccharides and oxidative stress. Nutrients. 2020;**12**. DOI: 10.3390/nu12092762

[34] Polimeni L, Del Ben M, Baratta F, et al. Oxidative stress: New insights on the association of non-alcoholic fatty liver disease and atherosclerosis. World Journal of Hepatology. 2015;**7**:1325-1336. DOI: 10.4254/wjh.v7.i10.1325

[35] Lee HH, Cho Y, Choi YJ, et al. Non-alcoholic steatohepatitis and progression of carotid atherosclerosis in patients with type 2 diabetes: A Korean cohort study. Cardiovascular Diabetology. 2020;**19**:81. DOI: 10.1186/s12933-020-01064-x. 23

[36] Zhou YY, Zhou XD, Wu SJ, et al. Synergistic increase in cardiovascular risk in diabetes mellitus with nonalcoholic fatty liver disease: A meta-analysis. European Journal of Gastroenterology & Hepatology. 2018;**30**:631-636. DOI: 10.1097/MEG.0000000000001075

[37] Baratta F, Pastori D, Angelico F, et al. Nonalcoholic fatty liver disease and fibrosis associated with increased risk of cardiovascular events in a prospective study. Clinical Gastroenterology and Hepatology. 2020;**18**:2324-2331.e2324. DOI: 10.1016/j.cgh.2019.12.026

[38] Hsu PF, Wang YW, Lin CC, et al. The association of the steatosis severity in fatty liver disease with coronary plaque pattern in general population. Liver International. 2021;**41**:81-90. DOI: 10.1111/liv.14637

[39] Koo BK, Allison MA, Criqui MH, et al. The association between liver fat and systemic calcified atherosclerosis. Journal of Vascular Surgery. 2020;**71**:204-211 e204. DOI: 10.1016/j.jvs.2019.03.044

[40] Tang K, Lin J, Ji X, et al. Non-alcoholic fatty liver disease with reduced

myocardial FDG uptake is associated with coronary atherosclerosis. Journal of Nuclear Cardiology. 2021;**28**:610-620. DOI: 10.1007/s12350-019-01736-6

[41] Koulaouzidis G, Charisopoulou D, Kukla M, et al. Association of non-alcoholic fatty liver disease with coronary artery calcification progression: A systematic review and meta-analysis. Przeglad Gastroenterologiczny. 2021;**16**:196-206. DOI: 10.5114/pg.2021.109063

[42] Wong MYZ, Yap JJL, Sultana R, et al. Association between non-alcoholic fatty liver disease and subclinical atherosclerosis in Western and Asian cohorts: An updated meta-analysis. Open Heart. 2021;**8**. DOI: 10.1136/openhrt-2021-001850

[43] Kim JH, Moon JS, Byun SJ, et al. Fatty liver index and development of cardiovascular disease in Koreans without pre-existing myocardial infarction and ischemic stroke: A large population-based study. Cardiovascular Diabetology. 2020;**19**:51. DOI: 10.1186/s12933-020-01025-4

[44] Sinn DH, Kang D, Chang Y, et al. Non-alcoholic fatty liver disease and the incidence of myocardial infarction: A cohort study. Journal of Gastroenterology and Hepatology. 2020;**35**:833-839. DOI: 10.1111/jgh.14856

[45] Xu J, Dai L, Zhang Y, et al. Severity of nonalcoholic fatty liver disease and risk of future ischemic stroke events. Stroke. 2021;**52**:103-110. DOI: 10.1161/STROKEAHA.120.030433

[46] Zou B, Yeo YH, Cheung R, et al. Fatty liver index and development of cardiovascular disease: Findings from the UK Biobank. Digestive Diseases and Sciences. 2021;**66**:2092-2100. DOI: 10.1007/s10620-021-06954-y

[47] European Association for the Study of the Liver (EASL), European Association for the Study of Diabetes (EASD), European Association for the Study of Obesity (EASO). EASL-EASD-EASO clinical practice guidelines for the management of non-alcoholic fatty liver disease. Journal of Hepatology. 2016;**64**:1388-1402

[48] Angulo P, Hui JM, Marchesini G, Bugianesi E, George J, Farrell GC, et al. The NAFLD fibrosis score: A noninvasive system that identifies liver fibrosis in patients with NAFLD. Hepatology. 2007;**45**:846-854

[49] Grundy SM, Cleeman JI, Daniels SR, Donato KA, Eckel RH, Franklin BA, et al. Diagnosis and management of the metabolic syndrome: An American Heart Association/National Heart, Lung, and Blood Institute scientific statement: Executive summary. Critical Pathways in Cardiology. 2005;**4**:198-203

[50] Piepoli MF, Hoes AW, Agewall S, Albus C, Brotons C, Catapano AL, et al. 2016 European Guidelines on cardiovascular disease prevention in clinical practice: The Sixth Joint Task Force of the European Society of Cardiology and Other Societies on Cardiovascular Disease Prevention in Clinical Practice (constituted by representatives of 10 societies and by invited experts) Developed with the special contribution of the European Association for Cardiovascular Prevention & Rehabilitation (EACPR). European Heart Journal. 2016;**37**:2315-2381

[51] Choudhary NS, Duseja A. Screening of cardiovascular disease in nonalcoholic fatty liver disease: Whom and how? Journal of Clinical and Experimental Hepatology. 2019;**9**:506-514

[52] Knuuti J, Wijns W, Saraste A, Capodanno D, Barbato E,

Funck-Brentano C, et al. 2019 ESC guidelinesforthediagnosisandmanagement of chronic coronary syndromes. European Heart Journal. 2020;**41**:407-477

[53] Ludwig J, Viggiano TR, McGill DB, Oh BJ. Nonalcoholic steatohepatitis: Mayo Clinic experiences with a hitherto unnamed disease. Mayo Clinic Proceedings. 1980;**55**:434-438

[54] Sanyal AJ, American Gastroenterogical Association. AGA technical review on nonalcoholic fatty liver disease. Gastroenterology. 2002;**123**:1705-1725

[55] Chalasani N, Younossi Z, Lavine JE, et al. The diagnosis and management of non-alcoholic fatty liver disease: Practice guideline by the American Association for the Study of Liver Diseases, American College of Gastroenterology, and the American Gastroenterological Association. Hepatology. 2012;**55**:2005-2023

[56] Roth GA, Johnson C, Abajobir A, Abd-Allah F, Abera SF, Abyu G, et al. Global, regional, and national burden of cardiovascular diseases for 10 causes, 1990 to 2015. Journal of the American College of Cardiology. 2017;**70**:1-25

[57] Ong JP, Pitts A, Younossi ZM. Increased overall mortality and liver-related mortality in non-alcoholic fatty liver disease. Journal of Hepatology. 2008;**49**:608-612

[58] Oni ET, Agatston AS, Blaha MJ, Fialkow J, Cury R, Sposito A, et al. A systematic review: Burden and severity of subclinical cardiovascular disease among those with nonalcoholic fatty liver; should we care? Atherosclerosis. 2013;**230**:258-267

[59] Mantovani A, Pernigo M, Bergamini C, Bonapace S, Lipari P, Pichiri I, et al. Nonalcoholic fatty liver disease is independently associated with early left ventricular diastolic dysfunction in patients with type 2 diabetes. PLoS ONE. 2015;**10**:e0135329

[60] Silverman MG et al. Impact of coronary artery calcium on coronary heart disease events in individuals at the extremes of traditional risk factor burden: The Multi-Ethnic Study of Atherosclerosis. European Heart Journal. 2014;**35**:2232-2241

[61] Budof MJ et al. Progression of coronary artery calcium predicts all-cause mortality. JACC: Cardiovascular Imaging. 2010;**3**:1229-1236

[62] Budof MJ et al. Progression of coronary calcium and incident coronary heart disease events: MESA (Multi-Ethnic Study of Atherosclerosis). Journal of the American College of Cardiology. 2013;**61**:1231-1239

[63] Raggi P, Cooil B, Ratti C, Callister TQ, Budof M. Progression of coronary artery calcium and occurrence of myocardial infarction in patients with and without diabetes mellitus. Hypertension. 2005;**46**:238-243

[64] Jaruvongvanich V, Wirunsawanya K, Sanguankeo A, Upala S. Nonalcoholic fatty liver disease is associated with coronary artery calcifcation: A systematic review and meta-analysis. Digestive and Liver Disease. 2016;**48**:1410-1417

[65] Al Rifai M et al. The association of nonalcoholic fatty liver disease, obesity, and metabolic syndrome, with systemic inflammation and subclinical atherosclerosis: The Multi-Ethnic Study of Atherosclerosis (MESA). Atherosclerosis. 2015;**239**:629-633

[66] Sung KC et al. Arterial stiffness, fatty liver and the presence of coronary

artery calcium in a large population cohort. Cardiovascular Diabetology. 2013;**12**:162

[67] Villanova N et al. Endothelial dysfunction and cardiovascular risk profile in nonalcoholic fatty liver disease. Hepatology. 2005;**42**:473-480

[68] Vanhoutte PM. Endothelial dysfunction: The first step toward coronary arteriosclerosis. Circulation Journal. 2009;**73**:595-601

[69] Kotronen A et al. Increased coagulation factor VIII, IX, XI and XII activities in non-alcoholic fatty liver disease. Liver International. 2011;**31**:176-183

[70] Verrijken A et al. Prothrombotic factors in histologically proven nonalcoholic fatty liver disease and nonalcoholic steatohepatitis. Hepatology. 2014;**59**:121-129

[71] Ganguly P, Alam SF. Role of homocysteine in the development of cardiovascular disease. Nutrition Journal. 2015;**14**:6

[72] de Carvalho SC et al. Plasmatic higher levels of homocysteine in non-alcoholic fatty liver disease (NAFLD). Nutrition Journal. 2013;**12**:37

[73] Francque SM, van der Graaf D, Kwanten WJ. Non-alcoholic fatty liver disease and cardiovascular risk: Pathophysiological mechanisms and implications. Journal of Hepatology. 2016;**65**:425-443

[74] DeFilippis AP et al. The association of Framingham and Reynolds risk scores with incidence and progression of coronary artery calcification in MESA (Multi-Ethnic Study of Atherosclerosis). Journal of the American College of Cardiology. 2011;**58**:2076-2083

[75] Carson AP et al. Hemoglobin a1c and the progression of coronary artery calcification among adults without diabetes. Diabetes Care. 2015;**38**:66-71

[76] Agatston AS et al. Quantifcation of coronary artery calcium using ultrafast computed tomography. Journal of the American College of Cardiology. 1990;**15**:827-832

[77] Greenland P, LaBree L, Azen SP, Doherty TM, Detrano RC. Coronary artery calcium score combined with Framingham score for risk prediction in asymptomatic individuals. JAMA. 2004;**291**:210-215

[78] Kronmal RA et al. Risk factors for the progression of coronary artery calcification in asymptomatic subjects: Results from the Multi-Ethnic Study of Atherosclerosis (MESA). Circulation. 2007;**115**:2722-2730

[79] Hokanson JE et al. Evaluating changes in coronary artery calcium: An analytic method that accounts for interscan variability. AJR. American Journal of Roentgenology. 2004;**182**:1327-1332

[80] Kwak MS, Kim D. Non-alcoholic fatty liver disease and lifestyle modifications, focusing on physical activity. The Korean Journal of Internal Medicine. 2018;**33**:64-74. DOI: 10.3904/kjim.2017.343

[81] Tikkanen MJ, Fayyad R, Faergeman O, et al. Effect of intensive lipid lowering with atorvastatin on cardiovascular outcomes in coronary heart disease patients with mild-to-moderate baseline elevations in alanine aminotransferase levels. International Journal of Cardiology. 2013;**168**:3846-3852. DOI: 10.1016/j.ijcard.2013.06.024

[82] Athyros VG, Tziomalos K, Gossios TD, et al. Safety and efficacy

of long-term statin treatment for cardiovascular events in patients with coronary heart disease and abnormal liver tests in the Greek Atorvastatin and Coronary Heart Disease Evaluation (GREACE) Study: A posthoc analysis. Lancet. 2010;**376**:1916-1922. DOI: 10.1016/S0140-6736(10)61272-X

[83] Li JJ, Lu ZL, Kou WR, et al. Impact of long-term xuezhikang therapy on cardiovascular events in high-risk patients with nonspecific, preexisting abnormal liver tests: A post-hoc analysis from Chinese Coronary Secondary Prevention Study (CCSPS). International Journal of Cardiology. 2012;**154**:362-365. DOI: 10.1016/j.ijcard.2011.11.005

[84] Moriarty PM, Roth EM, Karns A, et al. Effects of xuezhikang in patients with dyslipidemia: A multicenter, randomized, placebo-controlled study. Journal of Clinical Lipidology. 2014;**8**:568-575. DOI: 10.1016/j.jacl.2014.09.002

[85] Theocharidou E, Papademetriou M, Reklou A, et al. The role of PCSK9 in the pathogenesis of non-alcoholic fatty liver disease and the effect of PCSK9 inhibitors. Current Pharmaceutical Design. 2018;**24**:3654-3657. DOI: 10.2174/1381612824666181010123127

[86] Yan HM, Xia MF, Wang Y, et al. Efficacy of berberine in patients with non-alcoholic fatty liver disease. PLoS ONE. 2015;**10**:e0134172. DOI: 10.1371/journal.pone.0134172

[87] Armstrong MJ, Gaunt P, Aithal GP, et al. Liraglutide safety and efficacy in patients with non-alcoholic steatohepatitis (LEAN): A multicentre, double-blind, randomised, placebocontrolled phase 2 study. Lancet. 2016;**387**:679-690. DOI: 10.1016/S0140-6736(15)00803-X

[88] Rizvi AA, Patti AM, Giglio RV, et al. Liraglutide improves carotid intima-media thickness in patients with type 2 diabetes and non-alcoholic fatty liver disease: An 8-month prospective pilot study. Expert Opinion on Biological Therapy. 2015;**15**:1391-1397. DOI: 10.1517/14712598.2015.1067299

[89] Newsome PN, Buchholtz K, Cusi K, et al. A placebo-controlled trial of subcutaneous semaglutide in nonalcoholic steatohepatitis. The New England Journal of Medicine. 2021;**384**:1113-1124. DOI: 10.1056/NEJMoa2028395

[90] Rakipovski G, Rolin B, Nohr J, et al. The GLP-1 analogs liraglutide and semaglutide reduce atherosclerosis in ApoE(-/-) and LDLr(-/-) mice by a mechanism that includes inflammatory pathways. JACC: Basic to Translational Science. 2018;**3**:844-857. DOI: 10.1016/j.jacbts.2018.09.004

[91] Wei Q, Xu X, Guo L, et al. Effect of SGLT2 inhibitors on type 2 diabetes mellitus with non alcoholic fatty liver disease: A meta-analysis of randomized controlled trials. Frontiers in Endocrinology (Lausanne). 2021;**12**:635556. DOI: 10.3389/fendo.2021.635556

[92] Nasiri-Ansari N, Nikolopoulou C, Papoutsi K, et al. Empagliflozin attenuates non-alcoholic fatty liver disease (NAFLD) in high fat diet fed ApoE(-/-) mice by activating autophagy and reducing ER stress and apoptosis. International Journal of Molecular Sciences. 2021;**22**:818. DOI: 10.3390/ijms22020818

[93] Mo M, Huang Z, Liang Y, et al. The safety and efficacy evaluation of sodium-glucose cotransporter 2 inhibitors for patients with non-alcoholic fatty liver disease: An updated metaanalysis. Digestive and Liver Disease. 2021. DOI: 10.1016/j.dld.2021.08.017. Online ahead of print